Documenting
Physical Therapy:
The Reviewer Perspective

Documenting Physical Therapy: The Reviewer Perspective

Angela M. Baeten, PT

Reimbursement Consultant Director, MJ Care, Inc., Racine, Wisconsin

Michael L. Moran, ScD, PT

Associate Professor, Department of Physical Therapy, College Misericordia, Dallas, Pennsylvania

Lynn M. Phillippi, MS, PT

Former Vice President of Career Development, MJ Care, Inc., Racine, Wisconsin

With Foreword by

Mark A. Brimer PhD, PT

Orthopedic Institute, Administrator, Holmes Regional Medical Center, Inc, Melbourne, Florida

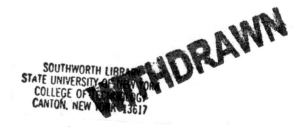
BUTTERWORTH
HEINEMANN

Boston   Oxford   Auckland   Johannesburg   Melbourne   New Delhi

Copyright © 1999 by Butterworth–Heinemann

 A member of the Reed Elsevier group

Every effort has been made to ensure that the drug dosage schedules within this text are accurate and conform to standards accepted at time of publication. However, as treatment recommendations vary in the light of continuing research and clinical experience, the reader is advised to verify drug dosage schedules herein with information found on product information sheets. This is especially true in cases of new or infrequently used drugs.

Butterworth–Heinemann supports the efforts of American Forests and the Global ReLeaf program in its campaign for the betterment of trees, forests, and our environment.

Recognizing the importance of preserving what has been written, Butterworth–Heinemann prints its books on acid-free paper whenever possible.

Library of Congress Cataloging-in-Publication Data
Baeten, Angela M. (Angela Marie), 1964–
     Documenting physical therapy : the reviewer perspective / Angela M.
   Baeten, Michael L. Moran, Lynn M. Phillippi ; with foreword by Mark
   A. Brimer
          p.   cm.
     Includes index.
      ISBN 0-7506-9950-7 (paperback : alk. paper)
      1. Physical therapy—Practice.   2. Medical records.   I. Moran,
   Michael L.   II. Phillippi, Lynn M.   III. Title.
   RM713.B34   1999
   615.8'2'068—dc21   99-23379
                                                                        CIP

British Library Cataloguing-in-Publication Data
A catalogue record for this book is available from the British Library.

The publisher offers special discounts on bulk orders of this book.

For information, please contact:
Manager of Special Sales
Butterworth–Heinemann
225 Wildwood Avenue
Woburn, MA 01801-2041
Tel: 781-904-2500
Fax: 781-904-2620

For information on all B–H medical publications available, contact our World Wide Web home page at: http://www.bh.com

10 9 8 7 6 5 4 3 2 1

Printed in the United States of America

Dedication

This book is dedicated to the memory of
Lynn Marie Phillippi (1947–1997)
and in honor of her family and friends.

Contents

Foreword

As health professionals, physical therapists have long been known for their commitment to quality and dedication to attaining rehabilitation outcomes. In recent years, however, health care reform has significantly affected the profession of physical therapy and placed increased emphasis on costs and outcomes associated with service provision. This change, which is expected to continue well into the next decade, will require therapists to devote more attention to documenting the need for care and outlining functional results that can be anticipated if services are to be eligible for reimbursement. As professionals, therapists are beginning to realize that documentation of services provided is becoming almost as important as the care delivered to the patient.

Documentation has long been recognized as the cornerstone of the profession of physical therapy. A properly developed clinical record is one of the most effective mechanisms for accurately portraying treatments delivered and the response to treatment, and for identifying the need for skilled care. The book *Documenting Physical Therapy: The Reviewer Perspective* gives us an excellent opportunity to see how important attention to detail is in documenting the delivery of rehabilitative services. Documentation for purposes of ensuring quality, continuity of care, response to treatment, identifying barriers to recovery, and recording attainment of functional outcomes are some of the critical areas of current and future professional focus. This book provides a clinical framework for identifying what constitutes quality, response to treatment, and the attainment of functional outcomes, and then translates this framework into strategies for improved documentation.

Documenting Physical Therapy: The Reviewer Perspective is an important text for therapists in all health care settings regardless of years of professional experience. The book examines "our" profession from the "reviewer's perspective" and provides guidelines as to how we can make patient documentation more clearly delineate the objectives and goals of treatment. The text examines how the results of the care provided to a patient should be recorded in the medical record and how they are typically reviewed for quality and effectiveness. Students and established professionals will find examples of how to use "key words and phrases" to outline a course of treatment and reduce the likelihood of reimbursement denial.

Documenting Physical Therapy: The Reviewer Perspective is a valuable addition to our professional literature. As health care reform continues to evolve, we can expect to be called on to provide "treatment rationales" to qualify the value of services provided. We can increasingly expect reviewers to examine whether physical therapy services are reasonable, or whether they could more appropriately be provided by nonskilled personnel. This text provides numerous examples of how to make documentation work as an advocate for the profession by educating third-party payers concerning the long-term benefits of physical therapy. Case studies are included that allow the reader to develop an ability to analyze and interpret physical therapy documentation in home health, the hospital setting, industry, outpatient and pediatric facilities, skilled nursing care, and the subacute environment. Most importantly, as health care becomes more dynamic, this text will become an invaluable reference for updating documentation skills and abilities as professional job opportunities and employment settings change.

Mark A. Brimer, PhD, PT

Preface

Documentation is the foundation of physical therapy practice and serves multiple purposes. As the health care dollar continues to shrink, the physical therapist's ability to obtain payment for services is contingent on functional documentation that describes the need for skilled care. With this in mind, understanding the essential elements of physical therapy documentation from the reviewer's perspective can be helpful.

In the early 1990s co-author Lynn Phillippi began to expand her knowledge of reimbursement. Although it started by advocating for denied physical therapy services involving the elderly, Lynn realized firsthand the need for educating third-party payers and physical therapists regarding coverage issues and documentation. Recognizing these needs, Lynn began to share her knowledge with others through lectures and writing. She also became a peer physical therapist reviewer.

We are fortunate to have learned many documentation tips from Lynn through the years. Both having worked with Lynn in varying capacities, we share her enthusiasm for improving documentation. We started this book with Lynn during a time when she was experiencing health challenges. Although Lynn did not see the finished manuscript, it is a privilege to share her vision and advocate for improving documentation from a reviewer's perspective.

All practicing physical therapists and physical therapist assistants, as well as those with an understanding of basic documentation principles, will benefit from this text. It is our intention to provide the reader with the skills to analyze documentation from a reviewer's perspective. This will improve functional writing and help provide a clear picture of the patient to the reviewer. This text is not intended to portray all documentation as being deficient or to address all payers and coverage issues. It is intended to show that how and what therapists document can affect reimbursement, and to advocate professional involvement in policy development and coverage issues at both the state chapter and national association level.

In this book, the essential elements of documentation from a reviewer's perspective for a variety of patient types and settings are presented. Chapter 1 begins by providing insight into the purposes, definitions, and essential elements of documentation. This is followed by explanations of the need for medical review, who reviewers are, and the purposes of peer review in Chapter 2. Actual patient data are used for examples and provide insight into the challenges reviewers face when determining the need for skilled care.

Chapter 3 provides insight into how to improve documentation skills, a proactive approach to appeal processing, and documentation tips, with emphasis on descriptive writing. In addition, the use of functional phrases and the appearance of documentation are explored. These tips will help to prepare the reader for analyzing documentation in the case studies provided in Chapter 4.

In the case studies, data commonly seen by reviewers are presented. Readers are encouraged to review all case studies, but may choose a patient type or setting that meets their clinical needs. It is through documentation analysis that the challenges faced by reviewers are experienced.

In Chapter 4, readers are asked to analyze documentation by identifying the essential elements, and then to provide a coverage determination. An interpretation of the data by the authors is provided for the reader. The authors recognize the type of review performed may vary for the settings and patient types provided. However, the authors chose a consistent approach to documentation review, because they feel that quality documentation must exist in all settings and for all patient types.

The book concludes by providing strategies for incorporating essential elements into documentation formats used in the clinical setting. Improving documentation skills requires a commitment to learning. The results of such efforts may be to decrease denials and improve functional documentation efficiency. Although technology may advance, the need to describe accurately why the skills of a physical therapist are needed will not change.

Physical therapy documentation from the reviewer's perspective emphasizes that if documentation is functional and accurately presented, the skilled nature of the service will be evident. It is critical that a clear picture of the patient be presented to the reviewer for determining medical necessity. Documentation skills evolve over time and require an ongoing commitment to excellence. They must not be lost because of the changes that occur in health care. Physical therapists must continue to improve and maintain high standards of documentation quality. The efficacy of our profession may depend on that.

Angela M. Baeten, PT
Michael L. Moran, ScD, PT

Acknowledgments

The authors extend special thanks to their families (David, Amber, and Ashley Baeten and Jeanne, Katie, and Mike Moran) for their love and support throughout this project.

The authors acknowledge MJ Care, Inc. for their commitment to this project and for providing the technical support to see it to completion. Especially we recognize Mary Cavicchi, Curt Klade, and Michele Thorman.

The authors are grateful for the contributions of many others (family, friends, and peers) who provided sample reports, research, consultation, and technical assistance.

Chapter 1
Reviewer Expectations

Introduction

Documentation is the foundation for communication between third-party payers and the providers of physical therapy services. Health care reform has heightened rehabilitation professionals' awareness of the need to communicate effectively regarding treatment interventions and the necessity for skilled service. Documentation not only is needed for reimbursement, but is a reflection of treatment. Physical therapists are now confronted with providing documentation of reasonable and predictable functional outcomes in a concise, cost-effective manner to avoid claim denials.

In order to effectively analyze documentation from a reviewer's perspective, it is important to first establish a baseline of knowledge. This chapter will review the purposes of documentation, define documentation, and review essential elements for documentation. By focusing on these areas, the physical therapist will develop the skills necessary to identify insufficient documentation and assist in the education of peers to ensure quality documentation of skilled physical therapy services.

Purposes of Documentation

Documentation is one of the most challenging areas for physical therapy professionals because it serves multiple purposes: ensuring quality care, continuity of care, marketing, legal aspects, research, educational, and reimbursement. Because of these multiple purposes, ensuring quality documentation can be time consuming and is not necessarily a favorite task. The proper climate must be present and attention to documentation issues needs to be ongoing at both the staff and supervisory levels.[1] All professionals need to realize the role of documentation as a communication tool. Although the focus of this book is from a reviewer's perspective, it is important to first explore the purposes of documentation.

Documentation of physical therapy services provided to the patient and the patient's response to intervention are important for communicating with the interdisciplinary team to ensure quality care. Scott[2] reinforces that from a clinical and legal perspective, documentation of patient care is as important as the rendition of care itself. It is the patient who benefits from effective communication among interdisciplinary team members. Documentation in the medical record defines problems, identifies barriers to recovery, outlines the approach of care, and defines goals for efficient delivery of skilled care.

Quality of care is also analyzed through the review of the medical record to assess the standards of practice. This process is valuable both internally and externally. Internally, protocols and procedures can be reviewed to ensure therapist compliance, assess department efficiency, and monitor the effectiveness of the care provided. Externally, documentation allows functional outcomes and the approach of care to be assessed and studied. Analysis of functional outcome data is a key component in the business aspect of contract negotiations with potential referral sources. It also serves as a basis for research, as the record can be used for retrospective studies that measure outcomes to determine the cost-effectiveness of patient care.[3]

Continuity of care is another important purpose of documentation. Documentation reflects the history of patient care. Through quality documentation, the physical therapist can determine the previous response to treatment, and continue or modify care as established in a previous treatment setting, in an efficient and cost-effective manner.

Documentation can also be a marketing tool. For example, in the area of industrial rehabilitation Saunders[4] noted that, "When done correctly, documentation can be one of the more powerful marketing tools the therapist has available." The unique nature of each patient, the referral source, and the cost of programming play a role in selecting an industrial rehabilitation setting for skilled treatment. However, the importance of documentation should not be minimized, in terms of marketing, in any practice setting. The professional appearance and clinical content of documentation are a reflection on the therapist and the marketed service. The quality of the care and functional outcomes achieved can be overlooked by potential referral sources because of the poor appearance of documentation.

The legal aspect of documentation must be considered by physical therapy providers. In the event of a lawsuit or malpractice issue, the documentation of care provides the objective evidence of care rendered to the patient.[2] This issue in itself requires much depth and will not be explored in this book. However, the authors encourage all therapists to independently seek information on this topic, as it is extremely important to understand the legal aspects of documenting in the medical record. One suggested reference is *Legal Aspects of Documenting Patient Care* by Ronald W. Scott.[2]

There are other, and unfortunately often less formally stated, purposes of documentation that are of value to the profession of physical therapy. For instance, documentation provides useful information for research and education.[2] Although these are implied within the other purposes listed in this section, it is important to remember the importance of research and education separately. Accurate data pave the way for analyzing the effectiveness of physical therapy treatment strategies.

Last, the focus of this book and the final purpose of documentation to explore is reimbursement. Documentation in the medical record provides the basis for coverage decisions. Through a medical record review or prior authorization process, the third-party payer ensures that the physical therapy services provided meet standards of practice and are reasonable and medically necessary. The cost-effectiveness of the skilled services provided within the guidelines of the payer are also reviewed. Ultimately, to receive coverage, the burden of proof rests with the provider of service.

Payments received from a third-party payer for physical therapy services are linked to clinical decision making through documentation. Payment is often denied when the treatment records submitted to the payer do not clearly provide the rationale to support the care that was provided.[3] Providers of physical therapy services often overlook the essential elements necessary for quality documentation.

To ensure reimbursement for physical therapy services, it is necessary to achieve and maintain a high standard of documentation. The effectiveness of the services delivered is measured in terms of how well the patient can function in his or her environment and is documented in the description of the patient's functional abilities. This is first accomplished by understanding the definition of documentation.

Definition of Documentation

The definition of documentation is clear in the policy, *Guidelines for Physical Therapy Documentation*, provided by the American Physical Therapy Association (APTA). The APTA's 1997 policy defines documentation as "Any entry into the client record, such as: consultation report, initial examination report, progress note, flowsheet/checklist that identifies the care/service provided, reexamination, or summation of care."[5]

Within the policy, guidance is given regarding general documentation guidelines. For instance, making entries in ink, obtaining informed consent, and the manner of referral are some of the items outlined. The guidelines also specify the need for an evaluation at the onset of physical therapy care and the elements to include in an initial examination and evaluation/consultation, continuum of care note(s), and summation of care report. In this book the authors will not separate examination and evaluation. The language used will be *initial evaluation* or *evaluation*. The continuum of care note(s) will include *daily/weekly notes* and *progress report(s)* and the summation of care

report will be referred to as a *discharge report*. To read the APTA's *Guidelines for Physical Therapy Documentation*, refer to Appendix 1. A copy of the latest policy can be obtained by contacting the APTA at 1-800-999-2782.

Defining documentation, in any patient care setting, through the development of a documentation policy is a necessity. The documentation format developed and used will vary depending on the players. For instance, the format will vary in presentation for an industrial health setting involved in providing skilled physical therapy for the work hardening or work conditioning patient versus physical therapy provided to an acute care hospital inpatient.

The industrial health setting may involve multiple players, including the patient (employee), the employer, and the third-party payer. The duration of service may be longer than for an acute hospital inpatient, and legal aspects may also surface. Therefore, the documentation format for the industrial rehabilitation team needs to relay a clear purpose of the program to the patient and record data in a concise nonjudgmental manner, as well as maintain the essential elements for quality documentation and provide for a positive functional outcome. As a result, the documentation format may be lengthy and detailed.

Conversely, the hospital inpatient may be involved in a diagnostic-related group (DRG) In this case, the focus of the physical therapy documentation is primarily on providing quality service delivery and improving functional outcomes in a timely manner. As the needs of the players are different, there is often a shorter treatment duration with less emphasis on the legal aspects of documentation. Therefore, efficiency in delivering care is important, and to be cost-effective the format used is generally more concise.

When a documentation policy and format are developed, functional outcomes must be presented regardless of the players involved, the format used, or the setting. There is much debate about how a functional status measure should be used in payment systems for rehabilitation.[6] This book will not address measurement tools, but rather will emphasize functional writing for any documentation system. Although the need for functional outcomes seems clear for the physical therapist and physical therapist assistant in any practice setting, the ability to document functional outcomes and the need for skilled service is often lacking. As a result, reviewers of documentation are challenged when rendering coverage decisions.

Managed care and the shrinking health care dollar have brought the need for documentation to the forefront. Data without descriptions of how the patient will improve functionally are being scrutinized for medical necessity. The focus of the third-party payer is now on the cost of the functional outcome achieved, and the need for good documentation skills has become even more essential for reimbursement. The challenge is to improve on already defined physical therapy guidelines and interventions and evaluate, on each patient visit, what is being done and why it is being done.

It has become essential to justify the need for skilled physical therapy intervention for the third-party payer. Regardless of the format used, there are four documentation reports to examine:

- Initial evaluation
- Daily/weekly notes
- Progress report(s)
- Discharge report

The authors will also present information on individualized education programs (IEPs).

Each of these reports and the IEP contain essential elements for documentation from a reviewer's perspective. Before describing the essential elements, an overview of each report's role in the medical review process will be explored. The information provided emphasizes elements from a reviewer's perspective and does not focus on any specific state, federal, and/or payer guidelines.

Initial Evaluation

The initial evaluation is the cornerstone for all future documentation. The baseline data obtained are the foundation on which comparative progress will be documented. Allen et al.[7] indicate this by stating, "Documentation is the only tangible evidence of the critical link between the therapist's clinical reasoning and the patient's functional performance outcome." It is through the evaluation process that a physical therapist establishes the primary purpose for intervention and outlines the expectations for progress to the reviewer. These expectations are obtained through analyzing measurable data, developing a plan of care, and establishing functional goals.

An initial evaluation should contain all basic identifying information specific to the patient and the practice setting. The documentation may include information such as the patient's full name (including first, last, and often the middle initial), date of birth, age, gender, medical records number, health insurance claim number, room number, employer, site of service (e.g., facility or school name), billing provider name, billing provider number, and referring physician's name. Accuracy of this information is essential for ensuring reimbursement. For instance, to omit or mistakenly enter a patient's name could result in a billing submission error or a claim denial by certain payers.

The evaluation report then needs to describe data for the essential elements of documentation, including the referral, data accompanying referral, physical therapy intake/history, referral diagnosis, prior therapy history, baseline evaluation data, prior level of function, treatment diagnosis, assessment, problems, and plan of care. For the purposes of this book the initial evaluation format (Table 1.1) outlines the essential elements required for successful documentation from a reviewer's perspective. When clinically relevant and appropriately described, these elements provide the reviewer with the basis for rendering coverage decisions.

Providing documentation for relevant essential elements is important, as the evaluation is routinely requested by third-party

Table 1.1 Essential Elements of an Initial Evaluation

Referral
Reason
Specific treatment requested

Data Accompanying Referral
Diagnosis/onset date
Secondary diagnoses
Medical history
Medications
Comorbidities (complicating or precautionary information)

Physical Therapy Intake/History
Date of birth
Age
Gender
Start of care
Primary complaint

Referral Diagnosis
Mechanism of injury
Prior diagnostic imaging/testing

Prior Therapy History

Baseline Evaluation Data
Cognition
Vision/hearing
Vital signs
Vascular signs
Sensation/proprioception
Edema
Posture
Active range of motion/passive range of motion (AROM/PROM)
Strength
Pain
Coordination
Bed mobility
Balance (sit and stand)
Transfers
Ambulation (level and elevated surfaces)
Orthotic/prosthetic devices
Wheelchair use
Durable medical equipment (DME) (using or required)
Activity tolerance
Wound description, including incision status
Special tests
Architectural/safety considerations
Requirements to return to home, school and/or job

Prior Level of Function
Mobility (home and community)
Employment
School

Treatment Diagnosis

Assessment
Reason for skilled care

Problems

Plan of Care
Specific treatment strategies
Frequency
Duration
Patient instruction/home program
Caregiver training
Short-term goals and achievement dates
Long-term goals and achievement dates
Rehabilitation potential

payers for adjudication of claims. The data provided in the evaluation serve as the basis for all future progress comparisons and are the primary source for determining the reasonableness of skilled care. Payment is strongly related to the data described.

Daily/Weekly Notes

Daily and/or weekly treatment notes are generally brief entries. Depending on the payer, these entries may or may not be seen by a reviewer. However, certain payers may require or request daily entries for proof of services rendered. The format used and the frequency of documentation will vary depending on the practice setting, the patient type, and the payer involved.

Like the initial evaluation, the notes need to contain basic identifying information. The identifying information may only include the patient's full name (including first, last, and often the middle initial), date of birth, medical records number, and room number. The amount of identifying information is often facility- and payer-specific.

In general, there are two approaches to the daily/weekly treatment notes that will be addressed in terms of a reviewer's perspective. They are the SOAP note and the narrative format.

SOAP Note

The SOAP note follows the sequence of data organization corresponding to **s**ubjective, **o**bjective, **a**ssessment and **p**lan. For the reviewer, this structure provides consistency. When treatment is documented appropriately, the reviewer can focus easily on finding objective data, goals, and any changes to the treatment plan.

The SOAP note format, however, tends to limit direct comparisons in the data reported. In this format the reviewer must compare SOAP notes over a period of time to identify functional progress, usually leading to a lot of paper shuffling and inference. The SOAP note also tends to foster repetitive data entry.

Narrative Format

The narrative format as a daily/weekly summary may vary in its structure. When documentation is provided consistently, this format allows the reviewer to focus on finding objective data, goals, and additions/deletions to the treatment plan. This strategy tends to foster progress comparisons directly within the note and decreases the need for a reviewer to search other reports for functional progress comparisons.

The narrative format can become challenging for a reviewer if not organized properly. For instance, if comparisons are not made, the reviewer may draw erroneous conclusions because of the need to search for data in previous notes. There is a tendency for narratives to become lengthy, thus decreasing the ease of the review process. Therapists also may vary in their focus from day to day or week to week when using a narrative approach (Table 1.2).

Table 1.2 An Example of a Narrative Approach That Lacks Focus

For example, an initial evaluation may identify three problem areas: decreased strength, decreased transfers from bed to chair, and decreased ambulation. In week two, the therapist reports lower extremity range of motion measurements and emphasizes the need for moderate assistance to correct balance. In week three, the therapist describes range of motion measurements, transfers from chair to toilet, and gait deficits. This type of "problem jumping" is truly a reviewer nightmare and leaves the question of, "What is the focus of treatment?"

In either format, SOAP or narrative, documentation needs to reflect treatment and functional progress in an organized and consistent manner. Emphasis must be placed on components such as daily/weekly functional progress comparisons in direct relationship to the problems identified, variables or complicating factors affecting treatment, and education/training provided to the patient, family, caregiver, nursing, and/or employer.

Daily and/or weekly treatment notes are often required by payers, although they may or may not be requested in the review process. These notes prove that physical therapy services were delivered on each patient visit and reflect the results of ongoing treatment. They often serve as additional evidence in the event a claim denial is received. To avoid redundancy, this book will place emphasis on progress reports, as they are the documents most often seen by the reviewer. The strategies explored for progress reports also apply to daily/weekly treatment notes.

Progress Report(s)

Documentation of the continuum of care provides the reviewer with comparative data to justify the skilled physical therapy services rendered. The format used may vary. However, measurable and functional progress should be reflected in the essential elements of documentation.

A progress report should contain the same basic identifying information found in the initial evaluation: the patient's full name (including first, last, and often the middle initial), date of birth, age, gender, medical records number, health insurance claim number, room number, employer, site of service (e.g., facility/school name), billing provider name, billing provider number, and the referring physician's name.

Progress reports are commonly completed weekly, biweekly, and/or monthly. The essential elements in a progress report that are required for successful documentation from a reviewer's perspective are outlined in Table 1.3. When clinically relevant and appropriately described, these elements provide the reviewer with the basis for rendering coverage decisions.

The focus of the progress report is on the problems identified in the initial evaluation or any new problems that have developed since the last formal reevaluation. Documentation describing the skilled intervention provided, complicating factors that may have affected the duration of skilled care, and comparative data are needed.

Table 1.3 Essential Elements of a Progress Report

Attendance

Current Baseline Data

Cognition
Vision/hearing
Vital signs
Vascular signs
Sensation/proprioception
Edema
Posture
AROM/PROM
Strength
Pain
Coordination
Bed mobility
Balance (sit and stand)
Transfers
Ambulation (level and elevated surfaces)
Orthotic/prosthetic devices
Wheelchair use
DME (using or required)
Activity tolerance
Wound description, including incision status
Special tests
Architectural/safety considerations

Treatment Diagnosis

Assessment

Reason for skilled care

Problems

Plan of Care

Specific treatment strategies
Frequency
Duration
Patient instruction/home program
Caregiver training
Short-term goals and achievement dates
Long-term goals and achievement dates
Rehabilitation potential

Describing the skilled intervention the patient receives demonstrates the complexity of the treatment. What was done, what was monitored, and what parameters are defined may be a few of the questions to be answered. Reviewers and the interdisciplinary team find it helpful to understand what treatment has been provided and the measurable functional outcome.

Complicating factors are often documented in daily/weekly notes but are frequently forgotten in the progress report. It is important to understand what documents are received by a reviewer for determining a coverage decision. With this in mind, the progress report must describe events since the last report or treatment authorization to assist in justifying skilled care. Factors that affect the treatment duration may include illness, attendance/compliance, exacerbation of a present diagnosis, change in medication, side effects from medications, new diagnosis, recent fall, change in weight bearing restrictions, and/or a new physician's order. By including complicating factors in the progress report, the therapist paints a clear picture of the patient's functional progress and leaves nothing to inference.

Progress reports are strengthened when comparative data are presented. The comparative data are often presented in chart or statement form (Table 1.4). The documentation format used by the therapist is often driven by the third-party payer and how often documentation is requested for coverage decisions. For example, in the outpatient setting, duration may be limited to days or weeks. Therefore, comparative data may be provided in chart form. On the other hand, in a subacute setting a narrative format may be used. In either case and in any practice setting, the reviewer must be able to easily identify progress through comparative documentation.

Along with the functional progress comparisons, a progress report needs to reflect upgraded short-term goals and restorative nursing/home program recommendations. If the short-term goals are not met, does the documentation demonstrate sound clinical judgement in changing the plan of care or does the report identify the complicating factor(s) involved? Is there a clear necessity for skilled care and an expectation that the patient's condition will improve in a reasonable period of time? Indeed, these questions must be answered or provided for

Table 1.4 Examples of Comparative Data Presented in Chart and Statement Form

Comparative data allow the reviewer to identify functional progress or regression without the need to search through multiple reports. Data are often presented in chart or statement form. Example of chart form:

Essential Element	03-29-98	04-29-98
Strength	BLE Poor. Requires maximal assist of 2 to stand in parallel bars.	BLE Fair. Requires moderate assist of 1 to stand with walker.
Bed mobility	Moderate assist of 1 and moderate verbal cuing for upper and lower extremity placement.	Moderate assist of 1 and minimal verbal cuing for upper and lower extremity placement.

Example of statement form:
Balance (sit and stand): Patient performs dynamic standing activity with RUE. Previously required RUE support in standing with walker. (Case 17: Subacute, p. 208)
OR
Currently performs gait training with minimal assist of one, using a cane, for fifty feet. (Previously maximal assist of one for ten feet.)

within the progress report. A clear response assists the reviewer in determining the reasonableness of continued skilled care.

Discharge Report

The discharge report is the last of the four reports to be explored. The written summary helps to ensure continuity of care between providers and describes the success of the physical therapy services provided. Has the functional outcome established for the patient at the time of evaluation been achieved? If not, what barriers to progress were present?

For a discharge report to be successful, like the other reports, it must have basic identifying information and provide a functional summary of progress. The comparative data provided should be from the initiation of service to the time of discharge as well as functional progress that has occurred since the last report. The essential elements of a discharge report that are required from a reviewer's perspective are outlined in Table 1.5.

Table 1.5 Essential Elements of a Discharge Report

Attendance

Current Baseline Data
Cognition
Vision/hearing
Vital signs
Vascular signs
Sensation/proprioception
Edema
Posture
AROM/PROM
Strength
Pain
Coordination
Bed mobility
Balance (sit and stand)
Transfers
Ambulation (level and elevated surfaces)
Orthotic/prosthetic devices
Wheelchair use
DME (using or required)
Activity tolerance
Wound description, including incision status
Special tests
Architectural/safety considerations

Treatment Diagnosis

Assessment
Reason for skilled care

Problems

Plan of Care
Specific treatment strategies
Frequency
Duration
Patient instruction/home program
Caregiver training
Short-term goals and achievement dates
Long-term goals and achievement dates
Discharge prognosis

The discharge report is quite similar to the progress report. Comparative data should be included and the focus on patient instruction/home program and caregiver training evident.

The four reports described-the initial evaluation, daily/weekly notes, progress reports, and the discharge report—are all unique for each practice setting and third-party payer. Yet, despite all the documentation formats and policies that exist in physical therapy, when reviewing documentation there are essential elements for documentation success.

Essential Elements of Documentation

From a reviewer's perspective, there are essential elements for documentation that when adequately presented will help to provide the necessary insight into the need for skilled physical therapy services. In this chapter a description of the essential elements of an initial evaluation, progress report, and discharge report as outlined in Tables 1.1, 1.3, and 1.5 will be provided. In addition, this will be followed by the essential elements of an individualized education program. The elements for all reports will be further explored in examples in Chapter 2 of what reviewers frequently encounter and through case studies in Chapter 4 to allow practical application for a variety of settings and patient types. It is through an understanding of the essential elements from a reviewer's perspective that documentation skills can be developed.

Essential Elements of an Initial Evaluation

Referral

To identify the reason for referral to physical therapy and the specific treatment requested are the first steps in justifying the need for skilled physical therapy intervention. The reviewer needs to identify that as a practical matter the patient is receiving necessary skilled care that is properly supervised within the coverage guidelines of the payer.

Reason. The reviewer will assess the reason for referral to ensure that the physical therapy services are reasonable and could not be performed by nonskilled personnel. The reviewer will also assess that the referral is consistent with the payer's coverage guidelines.

One aspect to describe is the referral source. This may include information regarding self-referral/direct access or from a referral source defined in state regulations. For example, is the referral being initiated by the physician, patient, family, employer, teacher, and/or caregiver?

Another aspect is to briefly define the treatment objective. This is helpful to the reviewer for understanding the need for skilled intervention in relationship to functional deficits. Esposto[8] indicates that a statement of the reason for referral ". . . must be made to assure that it is obvious to the reviewer that the *professional judgement* of the physical therapist is needed." For example:

- Have other treatment interventions been attempted?
- Were other treatments unsuccessful?
- What difficulties are being experienced or have been reported by the referral source?
- What will be accomplished? (Return to home, work and/or integration into the classroom)

Specific Treatment Requested. Documenting the specific treatment requested by the physician helps the reviewer determine that coverage is within the payer's guidelines. Most payers require a physician's order prior to initiation of an evaluation. Often the physician's involvement in establishing and/or approving the plan of care is also necessary prior to treatment intervention.

Knowing the specific treatment requested helps the reviewer to determine the appropriateness of the plan of care established by the therapist and to assess possible overutilization of services. The payers that require physician involvement may deny services billed if the documentation does not reflect that an order specifying the modalities for treatment was received prior to treatment delivery. It is therefore important that therapists understand the payer's guidelines regarding referrals. It is also important to determine the appropriateness of the order received from the physician, as not all evaluations are coverable.

Data Accompanying Referral

In an initial evaluation, data accompanying a referral help the reviewer justify the need for skilled care and understand the complexity of the patient. It defines the diagnosis/onset date, secondary diagnoses, medical history, medications and comorbidities (complicating or precautionary information). Thorough descriptions provide the reviewer with data that may directly affect the patient's participation in rehabilitation. The following explores each of these areas in detail.

Diagnosis/Onset Date. Identifying the patient's diagnosis and onset date is an essential element in the review process. The accuracy of the diagnosis and onset date is also a key element in the billing process. It provides the first insight into the physical therapy frequency and anticipated duration of treatment. The referral diagnosis may be commonly recognized as the medical diagnosis or primary diagnosis, depending on the documentation format used and the third-party payer's terminology. For purposes of this book the term diagnosis will be used.

Accuracy of the diagnosis and onset date is important as the health care industry progresses toward managed care and prospective payment systems. Guccione[9] noted that, "Physical therapy interventions cannot be shown to be effective for any condition unless there is a clear statement of what the condition is." This is especially true in the review process.

On the surface identifying a diagnosis and onset date may seem like an easy task, but depending on the setting this can be quite challenging. Most often the diagnosis is established by the physician and is acute in nature, with an onset date that is easily identified. For example, the initial physician's order may specify the diagnosis and onset, such as with a work-related injury or fracture. In other cases, where there is a functional regression or a developmental delay, the identification of the diagnosis and onset may be difficult. When necessary, the therapist may need to contact the physician to clarify these data. In either case, the therapist must document the diagnosis based on professional standards of practice and expectations of the payer.

The APTA defines diagnosis in the *Guide to Physical Therapist Practice.*[5] The information provided indicates specific guidelines for the diagnostic process in terms of professional standards (Table 1.6). It is important for therapists to identify the diagnosis resulting in the need for skilled services.

An accurate diagnosis and onset date are expected by third-party payers. Distinguishing between acute and chronic diagnoses by identifying the onset date is also needed. In general, to authorize or approve physical therapy intervention, a reviewer will determine if there is an acute diagnosis that has developed, a recent functional regression, an exacerbation of a chronic condition, or a defined developmental delay.

Chronic diagnoses are especially challenging to physical therapists during the evaluation process. Clearly the therapist must present an accurate onset date. Usually onset dates are acute in nature and are within six months of the start of physical therapy services. With that in mind, chronic diagnoses such as low back pain, Parkinson's disease, dementia, multiple sclerosis, multiple cerebrovascular accidents, chronic obstructive pulmonary disease, and arthritic conditions need to be closely assessed and an onset date identified that corresponds to the need for skilled care (i.e., is there a current or recent exacerbation,

Table 1.6 Diagnosis as Defined by the APTA (Reprinted from Guide to Physical Therapist Practice; *Phys Ther*; Alexandria, Virginia, APTA; 1997; 77(11): 1183, with permission of the American Physical Therapy Association.)

A *diagnosis* is a label encompassing a cluster of signs and symptoms, syndromes, or categories. It is the decision reached as a result of the diagnostic process, which includes evaluating the information obtained during the examination; organizing it into clusters, syndromes, or categories; and interpreting it.

The purpose of the diagnosis is to guide the physical therapist in determining the most appropriate intervention strategy for each patient/client. In the event that the diagnostic process does not yield an identifiable cluster, syndrome, or category, intervention may be guided by the alleviation of symptoms and remediation of deficits. Alternatively, the physical therapist may determine that a reexamination is in order and proceed accordingly.

In carrying out the diagnostic process, physical therapists may need to obtain additional information (including diagnostic labels) from other professionals. In addition, as the diagnostic process continues, physical therapists may identify findings that should be shared with other professionals, including referral sources, to ensure optimal care. If the diagnostic process reveals findings that are outside the scope of the physical therapist's knowledge, experience, or expertise, the physical therapist refers the patient/client to an appropriate practitioner.

hospitalization, or fall associated with the need to initiate therapy?). Justification of the onset date may be further described in the medical history.

If the exact date of onset is not known, as for a chronic condition, this should be clarified within the documentation. However, note that the onset date is most often *not* the date of evaluation. Usually the reason for referral is identified prior to the scheduling of physical therapy services. Therefore, the accuracy of the onset date may be questioned by a reviewer if it corresponds to the start of care date, as it may imply treatment for a chronic condition.

An onset date is also necessary for billing purposes. From a reviewer's perspective the physical therapist should identify the exact onset date whenever possible. One common strategy used when an exact date cannot be identified is to provide the month, first day of that month, and the year. Therapists should consult with their payer for education on how to most accurately represent the onset date if such a situation occurs. It is also important from a billing perspective to identify the diagnosis as specifically as possible corresponding with the ICD 9 CM (*International Classification of Diseases, 9th Revision, Clinical Modification*)[10] coding manual.

The ability to accurately identify the referral diagnosis and onset date is an essential element in the review process. Third-party payers may request information based on the diagnosis and onset date provided. For example, chronic conditions may imply the need for a short duration of care to establish or reestablish home programming or restorative nursing recommendations, unless additional documentation of the need for skilled care is provided. It is usually easier to justify skilled therapy intervention when an acute diagnosis that has a direct relationship to therapy, such as an orthopedic injury or acute neurological deficit, is documented.

It is common for payers to identify parameters that are reasonable in relationship to the diagnosis presented. The APTA has also proactively defined an expected range of number of visits per episode of care in the *Guide to Physical Therapy Practice*.[5] Although the parameters and guide begin to provide insight into the patient's deficits and need for skilled intervention, it is the additional measurable and functional data in the documentation that provide the justification for reasonable and necessary care.

Secondary Diagnoses. Secondary diagnoses provide the reviewer with insight into the patient's multiple deficits that may affect the frequency, duration, and/or tolerance of an intensive rehabilitation program. Additional data describing their impact may be defined in the medical history, baseline data, and/or assessment sections of the evaluation.

It is has become increasingly important for therapists to view the entire patient, meaning the multiple diagnoses involved. Secondary diagnoses have grown in importance with the emergence of managed care and with the implementation of prospective payment systems. Despite the system used, providers must pay greater attention to monitoring costs by diagnosis and length of stay, as the admitting diagnosis may no longer be the sole criterion for eligibility. Providers are now shifting from recording a single admitting diagnosis to recording the multiple diagnoses that may require care. This holds true for many, if not all, physical therapy settings.

Medical History. The medical history provides the reviewer with insight into therapeutic interventions associated with the need for physical therapy and the patient's rehabilitation potential. Data relating directly to the reason for referral must be described.

The medical history is obtained through interview and/or medical record review. The cognitively intact patient may subjectively report an accurate medical history. In the pediatric setting, additional medical history is obtained from parents and/or teachers. In a structured setting such as a hospital or skilled nursing facility, prior therapy records or the information provided by other members of the interdisciplinary team in the medical record is used. For the cognitively impaired patient, the caregiver or responsible party may provide the history. The data reported by the physical therapist in the medical history may include items such as the following:

- Past and present medical conditions/complications
- History of hospitalization for the present and/or a related diagnosis
- Surgical history
- Barriers to progress
- Prior/present therapeutic intervention for the present diagnosis
- Caregiver support
- Birth history
- Developmental history
- Functional deficits and their relationship to the diagnoses presented
- Living/working/school environments

Pertinent medical history must be described in the evaluation. However, the therapist may vary the length of the history based on the overall availability of documentation. For instance, in the acute care setting, documentation may not be highly reviewed because of the payment structure of diagnostic-related groups, and details of the medical history are provided by other members of the interdisciplinary team in the medical record. In this situation the history may be briefly stated by the therapist. In contrast, records reviewed for a pediatric patient in an outpatient setting would require additional detail, as the reviewer may not have a detailed account or direct access to the birth and developmental history.

By describing the medical history, the therapist helps the reviewer understand the barriers to progress and challenges that may affect the frequency and duration of skilled care. Also important are the use of medications and the presence of comorbidities. These two areas will be addressed separately because of their importance.

Medications. It is important to document the use of medications that may affect rehabilitation. It is helpful for the reviewer to have an understanding of all interventions provided to the patient when determining the need for skilled care. For example, potential complications of medications that may affect the duration of skilled care or influence functional improvement should be noted.

Comorbidities (Complicating or Precautionary Information). The presence of comorbidities reinforces the need for the skills of a therapist to safely perform activities that will improve function. Documenting complicating and precautionary information is helpful for communication with the interdisciplinary team in terms of patient safety and to the reviewer for determining the need for skilled care.

Examples of data may include seizure status, weight-bearing restrictions, cardiac parameters, oxygen dependency, use of positioning devices, bone metastases, angina, and/or diet restrictions. The presence of such data helps justify why the skills of a therapist are needed for safe performance of therapeutic intervention. If comorbidities are not identified in the examination process, this area should be listed as "none" to demonstrate that it was addressed.

Physical Therapy Intake/History

Additional data are obtained in the admission to physical therapy to help the reviewer assess rehabilitation potential. The data include identifying information such as date of birth, age and gender. The start of care date should also be listed and the patient's primary complaint described.

Date of Birth, Age, and Gender. Patient identifying information is important, not only clinically for assessing rehabilitation potential, but also for reimbursement. It is common for physician offices and third-party payers to file or trigger data retrieval based on date of birth. It is especially important in situations where different patients may have the same name.

Age and gender are also relevant. They help the therapy billing specialist, the therapist, and the reviewer identify the possibility of another payer. It is important to differentiate the primary payer source from a secondary payer. For example, an outpatient who is over sixty-five years of age may innocently report that Medicaid is his or her primary payer. Knowing the patient's age will point out the need to explore Medicare eligibility. In this example the review and/or coverage criteria may be quite different.

Age and gender also help to identify norms such as for fine motor skills (i.e., grip and pinch strength). They also are important for determining age-appropriate skills for the pediatric patient who presents with a developmental delay.

Start of Care. The start of care date reflects the first day of the physical therapy evaluation. It serves as a baseline to determine future attendance and is needed for billing purposes. The reviewer finds this date helpful and will compare it to the onset date of the diagnosis. Although the onset date and the start of care date are usually not the same, a significant delay (i.e.,

months or years) will trigger the need for further information explaining the delay in initiation of skilled care. As examples, were other treatment approaches attempted prior to the order for physical therapy, or were complicating factors present, or is this a chronic problem?

Primary Complaint. Documentation of the patient's primary complaint helps the reviewer to determine the need for skilled care and to identify potential barriers to progress. It also helps the therapist establish reasonable treatment strategies and goals. The primary complaint should be specific and provide an adequate description of the patient's functional deficits. With the need to focus treatment and control costs, it is important that the therapy services provided emphasize the patient's concerns in relationship to function.

Referral Diagnosis

How the referral diagnosis is established, as defined by the mechanism of injury and/or prior diagnostic testing/imaging, is relevant to the review process for most patients. This process justifies the appropriateness of the diagnosis provided by the physician and provides clinical insight into the treatment approach.

Mechanism of Injury. How and where an injury occurs can be relevant information. This is especially true for motor vehicle accidents, work-related injuries, and orthopedic injuries. From a reviewer's perspective this data helps to determine if another payer is the primary source of reimbursement. It is important to identify the primary payer and the secondary payer, as coverage criteria may vary. It can also provide clinical insight into the sudden or gradual onset of the diagnosis and the treatment approach needed.

For pediatric and neurologically impaired patients, the mechanism of injury may provide insight into complicating factors. For example, if a developmental delay exists, what was the cause (e.g., anoxia or prenatal drug dependency), and will it have an effect on the patient's rehabilitation potential? Or in the case of a cerebrovascular accident, was the insult related to hypertension, thrombosis, or a hemorrhage?

Prior Diagnostic Imaging/Testing. Describing relevant data pertaining to the results of prior diagnostic imaging/testing (e.g., MRI, x-ray, CAT scan, EKG, stress test) provides insight into treatment strategies, the duration of care, and patient safety. For instance, x-ray results may prove valuable in determining realistic range of motion goals for orthopedic patients, and results of cardiac stress tests may help determine safe aerobic capacities for cardiopulmonarily challenged patients.

Prior Therapy History

It is helpful for the reviewer to know the patient's prior therapy history for the present diagnosis or any related condition. The frequency, duration, and functional outcomes of prior therapy intervention help to establish the patient's rehabilitation potential.

Prior therapy history should always be addressed in an evaluation. It is important for the therapist to obtain this information to ensure reimbursement and an efficient approach to care. As shorter length of stays are the trend in health care today, the potential for patients to "provider hop" will increase. Also, therapists need to ensure that the most effective treatment approach is being used. If the patient received skilled care in another setting, what treatment strategies were successful or unsuccessful? What was the impact of therapy intervention on previously established goals for the same or similar diagnoses? Data should be specific regarding functional activities such as transfers, ambulation, and bed mobility in order to be beneficial for the reviewer. If prior therapy was not received, this area should be listed as "none" to demonstrate that it was evaluated.

Baseline Evaluation Data

Establishing objective data and functional deficits is the foundation for subsequent physical therapy reports. The following will address areas that may be pertinent to a patient's rehabilitation from a reviewer's perspective. The information provided will serve as a basis for writing measurable and functional documentation for progress and discharge reports. Baseline data are needed to justify skilled intervention and establish medical necessity for skilled physical therapy service.

Cognition.   Providing data on a patient's cognition provides insight into the patient's ability to participate in and benefit from an intensive rehabilitation program. From a reviewer's perspective, cognition may be a complicating factor, a barrier to functional progress, or irrelevant to the case. The impact of cognition on safety and functional deficits should be noted.

When presented appropriately, cognition may be a complicating factor that justifies the need for the skills of a physical therapist. The presence of diagnoses such as dementia, Alzheimer's disease, or psychiatric disorders tend to foster the philosophy of short treatment durations. However, documentation that supports the patient's ability to participate and benefit from rehabilitation is needed to extend coverage.

The therapist also needs to describe the patient's ability to respond to commands and determine the potential for carryover of functional progress gained. If the patient is unable to follow simple commands and presents with poor memory, then cognition is likely to be a barrier to progress. If progress is hindered, a reviewer will expect documentation emphasizing training of caregivers and adaptive equipment options to ensure patient safety. The duration of care must be reasonable and necessary based on the expected improvement in the patient's condition.

Cognition, in certain settings and for certain diagnoses, does not need to be addressed. This may be true of most outpatient settings when the diagnosis is unrelated to a cognitive impairment and the potential effects of aging are not a factor. However, if a diagnosis or medication is present that may affect cognition, then data must be provided. For example, dehydration in the elderly or a history of multiple cerebrovascular accidents may require baseline data to ensure that confusion has

resolved or is not a factor that will affect participation in the therapy program.

Vision/Hearing.   Data describing vision/hearing deficits may help the reviewer in determining another need for skilled therapy. If deficits exist, their presence may be a complicating factor that influences the duration of skilled care. This is especially true for neurologically involved patients and when balance is a defined problem. Vision/hearing deficits, particularly with the elderly and/or pediatric patient, may directly affect function and safety and need to be described.

Vital Signs.   Monitoring vital signs to allow safe participation in physical therapy demonstrates a need for the skills of a physical therapist in order to achieve functional goals. Data such as number of respirations, pulse rate, percentage of oxygen saturation, and blood pressure may be relevant, depending on the patient's diagnoses and clinical presentation. The interpretation of the data gathered demonstrates skilled care. It is reasonable for a reviewer to expect data when edema or cardiopulmonary diagnoses are present. Baseline data at rest, during, and after activities allow for future progress comparisons.

Vascular Signs.   Baseline data describing vascular signs are needed for patients with impaired circulation and edema. Data describing skin color, tissue temperature, capillary refill time, and the functional impact deficits have on the patient's performance in rehabilitation are important to a reviewer in determining the need for skilled care. Girth measurements may also be needed. Describing the deficits helps the reviewer to have a clear picture of the present and potential challenges that may exist (e.g., skin integrity, positioning needs). Data may also justify the need for the skills of a therapist to safely administer treatment modalities such as whirlpool or the use of intermittent pressure devices.

Sensation/Proprioception.   Deficits in sensation and proprioception may be complicating factors that have a direct affect on rehabilitation potential. Data describing the deficits and their impact on treatment and function are needed. For a reviewer to adequately assess a patient's functional limitations, data in areas such as sharp/dull discrimination, light touch, pressure, movement/position sense, and two-point discrimination may be needed. The relationship of any limitations in these areas to the performance of functional activities should be described. These activities may include self-care, bed mobility, transfers, and ambulation.

Deficits may also help to justify the need for a physical therapist's supervision in order to safely perform treatment modalities such as whirlpool or electrical stimulation. They may also justify the need for additional patient training to prevent skin breakdown when a positional, orthotic, or prosthetic device is used.

Edema.   Baseline data describing edema and any resulting functional limitations are helpful for future progress comparisons. They also have a role in assisting the reviewer in determining the effectiveness of the treatment modalities provided.

The objective data regarding edema need to be measurable. Data such as the location of edema, circumference measurements, and whether the edema is pitting or nonpitting are needed for future comparisons. The relationship of the edema to functional deficits is essential. Does the edema limit range of motion, transfers, ambulation, and/or safety? Adequate documentation demonstrates the need for skilled care.

Posture.   A description of postural deficits and how they influence function help the reviewer determine the need for skilled care. To adequately address posture, it is reasonable to expect data in sitting and standing. Deficits have the potential to affect aerobic capacity, joint integrity, and mobility.

Data may describe structural abnormalities, righting reactions, and their effect on function. Functional activities may include lifting, reaching, crawling, ability to safely maneuver a wheelchair or scooter, and ambulation. Data should be detailed. What is the direction of the spinal curve? Does physical assistance or verbal cuing improve posture, and if so, how much help is needed?

AROM/PROM.   An adequate description of range of motion is important to a reviewer for determining future progress and the present functional limitations. Data must describe the body part measured, with opposite limb measurements for comparison, and must differentiate active and passive range of motion. It is helpful to the reviewer if measurements are described in terms of norms such as "left shoulder flexion is 70°/180°." Providing this detail allows the reviewer to easily understand the degree of loss.

Along with the objective data, the therapist should provide the functional loss experienced by the patient. Is the patient able to perform job duties, self-care skills, home management, or school activities? Also, what are the complicating factors that require the skills of a therapist versus a home program to increase range of motion (e.g., pain, muscle tone, adhesions)?

Strength.   Baseline data pertaining to muscle strength are important to the reviewer. As with range of motion, the data help in making future progress comparisons and determining the patient's present functional limitations. Data must describe the body part tested and opposite limb grades for comparison. It is helpful to the reviewer if the manual muscle test results are described in terms of a norm such as "shoulder flexor strength is 3/5." Providing this detail lets the reviewer easily understand the strength deficit.

The relationship of the strength deficits to functional limitations is needed to determine if skilled care is reasonable and necessary. For example, can the patient ambulate, climb stairs, and/or perform work duties? Is an assistive device needed?

Data describing complicating factors that require the skills of a therapist in order to improve the functional strength deficit are also needed. Is pain present? Are there changes in muscle tone? If so, they need to be described (e.g., cogwheeling rigidity, muscle spasms).

Pain.   When describing pain, it is helpful to identify the pain rating scale being used, the location of pain, when pain occurs, and how it limits function. These data are important to the reviewer in determining future improvements and the need for skilled care.

Depending on the practice setting, the scale used for measuring pain may include the use of a questionnaire and/or graph, or perhaps patient reporting on a zero to ten scale. It is also helpful to the reviewer to define the pain rating in terms of a norm (e.g., 6/10, with 10 being the most painful).

Details of when pain is exacerbated, such as with movement or at rest, and how it limits the patient's function are needed. Is pain affecting job performance, sleeping patterns, activities of daily living or play? Providing baseline data regarding pain displays the need for rehabilitation.

Coordination.   It is helpful to the reviewer in determining the need for skilled care to have an understanding of the impact impaired coordination may have on functional progress. Establishing this relationship, if applicable, at the time of evaluation is important.

Coordination may be described in terms of gross or fine motor skills. What is of interest to the reviewer is how deficits affect the patient's safety and functioning at home, school, and/or in the community. Describing positions or activities that improve coordination is helpful.

Bed Mobility.   The patient's ability to perform bed mobility activities such as transitioning to and from sitting and supine, rolling, and bridging are important for skin integrity and self-care. The patient's ability to perform these activities can be described measurably in terms of physical assistance and verbal cues for instruction in safe technique. Reviewers find it helpful to know what factors limit bed mobility, as it provides the justification for skilled intervention. For example, does pain, strength deficits, or trunk/pelvic immobility affect safe performance?

Balance (Sit and Stand).   Data pertaining to balance are important to a reviewer, as they directly affect patient safety. Baseline data must be descriptive. Data may include the direction of loss, amount of assistance to correct, trunk righting skills, ability to shift weight, presence of pain, postural limitations, and/or strength deficits.

Balance needs to be addressed in sitting and standing, when applicable, and relate to function, as deficits may affect activities of daily living, safety, transfers, and/or ambulation. DeWane[11] reinforces this: "It is return of function and therapy that require the skills of a therapist that are critical to third-party payers." To provide for future comparisons, data need to be described in the evaluation. Standardized tests may be used as measurement tools, but a description of balance in relation to function is needed.

Transfers.   Transfers are a common functional activity. Evaluation data indicating the amount of physical assistance, verbal cuing, use of an assistive device, posture, and the type of transfer performed are needed. Types of transfers may include toilet, wheelchair to and from bed/mat, car/bus, and transitioning skills such as on/off the floor. A description of safety factors such as appropriate hand placement with sit to/from standing and the ability to apply wheelchair brakes also enhance the need for skilled teaching and training.

Ambulation (Level and Elevated Surfaces).   Ambulation is another common functional activity. Data may pertain to level or elevated surfaces. For community integration, data pertaining to negotiation of curbs, stairs, and ramps are relevant, as carry-over into daily activities is an important functional outcome.

Baseline data that are essential for future comparison include a description of the gait deficits, amount of physical assistance required, amount of verbal cuing, type of assistive device, orthotic/prosthetic device use, weight-bearing restrictions, distance, and safety. An additional description of the factors limiting standing/ambulation also must be written. As examples, are changes in strength, range of motion, posture, muscle tone, activity tolerance, or pain contributing factors?

Including descriptive data enables the reviewer to determine the complex nature of the functional limitations that require the skills of a physical therapist. In general, nonskilled personnel can provide assistance, verbal cues, apply an orthotic/prosthetic device, and increase ambulation distance, unless additional data are provided. The data should describe the need for the skills of a therapist to analyze and improve gait deficits. For example, data such as decreased heel strike, inability to weight shift, and/or a narrow base of support demonstrate skilled need, especially when the relationship to limited standing/ambulation is described.

Orthotic/Prosthetic Devices.   The need for skilled care is enhanced when baseline data are provided regarding orthotic or prosthetic devices. Depending on the circumstances, patient/caregiver education and instruction may be required. Teaching and training are evidence of skilled care. More importantly, the skills of a therapist are required *during gait training* to ensure proper fit of the device, skin integrity, and gait quality.

A description of the therapist's evaluation findings and the therapist's role in coordinating care with vendors, orthotists, and prosthetists is helpful to the reviewer in understanding the complexity of the patient's needs for improving ambulation. However, it is important to remember that duplication of service is to be avoided when another health professional is providing service(s) of a similar nature. The roles of each professional should be documented. It is a reasonable expectation of the reviewer to ensure that payment is for *physical therapy treatment time* based on the patient's established plan of care.

Wheelchair Use.   Baseline data regarding use of a wheelchair must be documented. Relevant data include the type of wheelchair, specialized adaptations/seating systems, ability to propel, amount of physical or verbal assistance, and safety. Evaluation of wheelchair needs may be performed by another professional. Depending on the payer, the reviewer will determine if the skills of a physical therapist are reasonable and necessary. Often the

therapist's expertise is needed to control muscle tone, improve trunk mobility, address range of motion and strength deficits, and/or provide training for safe use. Once again, it is important to avoid duplication of service.

DME (Using or Required).   The use of durable medical equipment helps the reviewer determine the functional limitations of the patient. The presence of and/or the need for equipment should be described. If the skills of a therapist are needed for safe implementation or instruction in use, this would also justify the need for skilled care.

Activity Tolerance.   The patient's ability to tolerate functional activity is important for participation in rehabilitation and integration/reintegration into the community. Endurance-building alone is scrutinized by reviewers, as it may be performed by nonskilled personnel. However, monitoring of vital signs, improvement in the distance for ambulation, and ability to tolerate functional activities at home and in the community are important. Establishing a baseline for future comparison will be important for discharge planning.

Wound Description, Including Incision Status.   Baseline data pertaining to wounds gives the reviewer an objective measure of the effectiveness of the treatment strategies provided. Payers often utilize reverse staging of wounds as evidence of healing.[12] Data pertaining to the wound's location, size (i.e., length, width, depth), drainage, odor, and tissue description are also needed. If treatment is initiated at the time of evaluation, details pertaining to the treatment modalities used and/or results of debridement should be documented.

For the surgical patient, the status of an incision is relevant information for the reviewer. Complications may affect the treatment approach and/or result in soft tissue restrictions that may hinder functional progress.

Special Tests.   Baseline data indicating the results of special tests help provide additional information regarding the patient's deficits. If applicable, the test results and their effect on rehabilitation must be described. This is important, as the relevance of many special tests may not be understood by the reviewer.

Architectural/Safety Considerations.   Depending on the practice setting and patient type, architectural barriers and safety considerations need to be documented in the evaluation. A reviewer finds it helpful to know how the patient is negotiating and functioning at work, home, school, or in the community. This provides insight into the patient's functional limitations and need for skilled intervention.

Requirements to Return to Home, School, and/or Job.   Providing the reviewer with documented insight into requirements for return to home, school, or job helps in determining the extent of the patient's functional limitations. Are there lifting or reaching requirements for job performance? Can these requirements be varied? Can the caregiver provide the necessary assistance for safe return to home or school? By defining these requirements, the reviewer is able to assess the reasonableness of the goals established in the evaluation.

Prior Level of Function

The most important essential element in an initial evaluation is identifying the prior level of function, or for the pediatric patient, an age-appropriate skill. The prior level of function should be clearly and functionally stated. When combined with the analysis of baseline data, the prior level of function allows the therapist to identify the patient's problems, develop an appropriate plan of care, and establish reasonable functional goals.

The data may be obtained from the patient, family, responsible party, medical record, and/or other interdisciplinary team members such as nursing, social services, admission coordinators, or physicians. If the prior level of function is unavailable or unclear at the time of evaluation, then a statement indicating the need to pursue this data should be provided. Depending on the rehabilitation setting, the prior level of function may be specific to mobility, employment, and/or school activities.

Mobility (Home and Community). The prior level of function is important to the reviewer in determining the need for skilled care and assessing the reasonableness of the established goals. The data must be specific to the diagnoses and reason for referral. For instance, what functional activities were performed by the patient prior to the need for skilled care?

The baseline data provided must be measurable and specific to a functional activity. For example, was the patient ambulatory? If so, did the patient use a device? Was assistance required? Was the patient able to ambulate safely in the community? Were gait deficits present prior to this referral? Answers to these types of questions provides the reviewer with insight into whether the established plan of care and goals are realistic.

Employment. The effect of functional deficits on the ability to perform job responsibilities is important to the reviewer. Data pertaining to the place of employment, previous and present work status, and details specific to functional abilities are needed. For example, how much could the patient lift before the reported injury?

School. For the pediatric patient, prior level of function takes a different approach, as often skill level has yet to be achieved. Comparing a child's development to that of age-matched peers can give the proper perspective for contrasting typical and atypical motor development. The patient's present level of educational performance is also important. It should be defined in terms of a functional activity and related to areas of mobility, self-help, and play skills.

Treatment Diagnosis

The treatment diagnosis identifies the diagnosis for which physical therapy services are rendered. This concept may be described by some therapists as the rehabilitation diagnosis, rehabilitation condition, or treatment condition.

The treatment diagnosis is beneficial to identify a functional regression or when the medical diagnosis that resulted in the regression is not specifically related to physical therapy. For example, a patient may be hospitalized for dehydration that results in a decrease in functional gait skills and the need for use of a walker. The identified referral diagnosis of dehydration is given by the physician and is established by the acute onset date. Although dehydration is the medical reason that is directly related to the functional regression, the treatment diagnosis for physical therapy may actually be a gait disturbance or a functional strength deficit. For circumstances such as this, both the referral and treatment diagnosis should be provided to the payer. Often the billing mechanism will allow for the listing of multiple diagnoses.

Assessment

The assessment is the therapist's clinical impressions of the patient's progress and summarizes the expected outcome from skilled intervention. From a reviewer's perspective, this is defined by focusing on the reason for skilled care.

Reason for Skilled Care. The reason for skilled care justifies the need for physical therapy intervention, provides the rationale for the treatment plan, and describes the expectations for functional progress. This provides the reviewer with information on medical necessity. The therapist's insight into the evaluation findings and expectations for progress helps to justify the need for treatment and define the potential barriers that may hinder functional progress.

Problems

Providing a problem list helps to focus physical therapy treatment. Following analysis of the baseline data, the problems identified as the highest priority should be emphasized. To adequately focus treatment, a maximum of five problems are recommended. It is from the problem list that the plan of care is developed.

Plan of Care

The plan of care provides the final elements for the reviewer in rendering a coverage decision. The plan provides the therapist's expertise into what is needed for a successful functional outcome. The plan includes specific treatment strategies, frequency, duration, patient instruction/home program, caregiver training, short-term goals and achievement dates, long-term goals and achievement dates, and the rehabilitation potential.

Specific Treatment Strategies. The treatment strategies are specific procedures and modalities that will be used to address the problems identified and to achieve the stated goals. Most payers expect the physician to agree that the strategies chosen are reasonable and necessary. Certain payers may require physician certification prior to the initiation of treatment; others allow practice without a direct referral. Knowing the guidelines of the payer is important to ensure payment.

The treatment strategies established in the evaluation should be specific and related to a functional outcome. Experimental or treatment modalities that have not been proven to produce a predictable and reproducible result will be questioned by the reviewer. Also, overutilization of similar modalities or a vague representation such as "modalities as needed" should be avoided. From a reviewer's perspective, the strategies will be assessed as what is needed and what is not. This information, along with data provided in other areas, such as the prior therapy history and the assessment, will allow the reviewer to ensure that the modalities described will be the most effective for treatment of the patient's present functional limitations. The modalities used need to relate to the goals and foster carryover into functional activities or home programming.

Frequency. Establishing how often the patient will receive skilled care in order to achieve the established goals is a necessary element of documentation. The frequency should be nonvariable and stated in terms of times per week or, depending on the payer, a number of visits within a defined time frame, for example, six visits before a certain date.

The reviewer will determine if the data presented warrants the established frequency of treatment. The reviewer will analyze the diagnoses, onset date, history, baseline data, and the assessment in this process. In general, a new diagnosis and/or acute diagnosis will result in a higher frequency. However, a complete review of the data and justification for skilled care needs to be considered.

Some payers may provide guidelines or expectations to assist the therapist in establishing a frequency. It is important to be aware of these guidelines; however, ensuring that the patient receives the treatment needed for a positive functional outcome is a necessary practice consideration. As every patient is unique, communication with the payer may be necessary to ensure quality care.

Duration. Documenting the anticipated duration of skilled service provides the reviewer with insight into the reasonableness of the treatment strategies for meeting the established long-term goal. This often is expressed in terms of days or weeks and is described in nonvariable terms.

Establishing a duration based on the evaluation data is not an easy task for therapists. Multiple factors are involved in the decision, including the diagnoses, onset date, history, baseline data, rehabilitation potential, payer expectations/limitations, the therapist's clinical experiences, and standards of practice. It is important to establish the duration knowing that in subsequent documentation an increase or decrease may be warranted. This is acceptable and expected, but once again, the factors that may alter the duration established at the evaluation must be appropriately justified.

Patient Instruction/Home Program. As an emphasis is being placed on shorter durations of skilled physical therapy, it is vital that home programming and/or restorative nursing recommendations be initiated/established at the evaluation. The details of the program and relevance of the exercises to improving function need to be described. Future additions and/or deletions to the program will provide additional justification for skilled care.

Caregiver Training. Teaching and training are skilled elements of rehabilitation. The training may be provided to the patient, family, caregiver, teacher, nurse, and/or employer. Documentation of what exercise or functional activity was taught, who was trained, and when the training occurred are relevant. Training is a component of quality care. Payment for such service may vary depending on the third-party payer.

Short-Term Goals and Achievement Dates. Short-term goals are the stepping stones to achieving the functional outcome/long-term goal. The goals should systematically correspond to the problem list identified. The goals must be measurable, be related to function, and include a time frame for achievement. These three components need to be present for each goal and should not be inferred.

To be measurable, baseline data must be present in the evaluation. The terms of measurability will vary with the functional activity presented. The terms may be assistance levels, percentages, ratios, ratings, grades, degrees, and/or units of length. The measurable component of the goal allows the reviewer to determine future functional progress.

The functional component reflects what the patient is expected to ultimately achieve. This helps the reviewer understand the relationship between the baseline data and treatment strategies described. The function needs to be realistic based on the data provided and the prior level of function.

An achievement date is the last of the three goal components. It is a projected date or time frame that the therapist anticipates for goals to be met. Time frames may vary from days to weeks. They are influenced by the rehabilitation setting/patient type, diagnosis, the payer source, and the documentation format used. It is helpful to establish goals that may be achieved by the next formal report, as this demonstrates to the reviewer that functional progress is being made.

Long-Term Goals and Achievement Dates. The long-term goal is often a statement that summarizes the functional outcome expected, such as return to work, home, or school. Establishing a long-term goal for each short-term goal is not usually expected or necessary for the reviewer. However, just like the short-term goals, the long-term goal needs to contain all three goal components. The goal must be measurable, functional, and time specific. If a time frame is not provided, the reviewer will usually infer the duration to be the achievement date. If the duration of care is limited (e.g., three weeks or less), the long-term goal may be omitted.

Rehabilitation Potential. It is important to identify the patient's rehabilitation potential, as it helps the reviewer determine the need and duration of skilled care. Often this is a one-word response-excellent, good, fair, or poor. Although these responses are not measurable, they are commonly accepted.

Multiple factors affect rehabilitation potential. These factors may include the diagnosis/onset date, history, comorbidities, mechanism of injury, and baseline data. If the patient does not demonstrate good rehabilitation potential, an explanation of the need for skilled care should be provided in the assessment. The therapist must ensure that the progress anticipated and the functional skills to be learned by the patient have a practical application for improving function.

Essential Elements for a Progress Report

Attendance

Patient attendance is important to the reviewer because of the consequences that may have resulted from any absences. Attendance is a factor that may affect the duration of care and the patient's functional outcome.

It is important to describe attendance in relation to the number of visits scheduled and indicate any reasons for absence. Reasons for absence may include illness, cancellation, refusal, and/or unavailability. Identifying these data gives the reviewer insight into potential barriers to progress. The reviewer can compare dates of service, or number of visits, with the billing statement to ensure payment accuracy.

Current Baseline Data

Providing measurable and comparative data with a functional relationship is helpful to the reviewer in determining patient progress and the need for skilled care. The problem list provides a guide to areas of priority. Data must be presented for all pertinent areas since the last formal report and must include complicating factors that affect the patient's ability to achieve the established goals. The following information will address areas that may be pertinent to rehabilitation from a reviewer's perspective.

Cognition. If cognitive deficits exist, comparative data describing any changes in the patient's ability to participate in rehabilitation and/or effects on safety should be documented. Data pertaining to complicating factors, such as medication changes and/or improvements in cognition related to improved nutritional intake, will influence the duration of skilled care. It may also be necessary to provide expectation statements in the assessment area of the report to clarify the effects on goal achievement.

Data regarding changes to the approach of care may also be helpful. The skills of a therapist may be required to determine the type of stimuli helpful to ensure patient safety. For example, a patient who strikes out may display tactile defensiveness to light touch but respond well to elimination of visual or auditory distractions, or respond to gestures versus verbal cues. Documenting the skilled approach to patient care demonstrates that goal achievement requires the expertise of a qualified therapist.

Vision/Hearing. As vision/hearing deficits may affect balance and safety, any changes that influence rehabilitation need to be described. To ensure that the reviewer has a full understanding of events, a summary of any consultations and pertinent findings that affect participation in rehabilitation should be documented. Did the patient obtain a hearing aid, allowing him or her to follow complex commands? Did cataract surgery improve vision and increase safety on elevated surfaces? Comparative data with emphasis on functional improvement are helpful to the reviewer.

Vital Signs. Based on the patient's history and diagnoses, it is important to include vital signs data such as respirations per minute, pulse rate, and blood pressure to ensure safe participation in rehabilitation. Although monitoring vital signs may be routine, comparative data provide the reviewer with another reason for skilled care.

Vascular Signs. It is reasonable for a reviewer to expect comparative baseline data such as girth measurements, skin color, and temperature when edema and/or circulatory deficits exist. This is especially necessary if the treatment strategies provided are for improving circulatory deficits or skin integrity. Data demonstrating improvement may reflect positively on the effectiveness of the modalities provided by the therapist and justify the need for continued skilled care.

Sensation/Proprioception. Comparative data for sensation/proprioception are appropriate if the deficits have an impact on the performance of functional activities. This data provides the reviewer with insight into complicating factors that are influencing patient safety and the duration of care. For example, instructing a patient to check skin integrity of the lower extremity before and after orthotic use is justified in the presence of sensory deficits. Deficits may also reinforce the need for the skills of a therapist to safely administer treatment modalities such as electrical stimulation or hot packs.

Edema. Data regarding edema must include the treatment strategy or strategies performed, comparative data, and the effect on function. Objective, measurable data are required, such as the location of edema, circumference measurements, and whether the edema is pitting or nonpitting. The measurable data should be compared to the last report. It is also helpful to include measurements of the uninvolved extremity, whenever possible, as they help the reviewer understand the extent of the involvement.

Posture. Comparative data regarding postural changes and any effect on functional activities are relevant. The comparative data may include the amount of physical or verbal cuing, improvements in body mechanics, and results of postural analysis measurements. The effects of posture on cardiopulmonary status and mobility need to be described, as well the treatment strategies used to improve posture.

AROM/PROM.   A comparative description of range of motion measurements and the relationship to function are needed. It is helpful to provide data pertaining to the body part measured and active and passive range of motion measurements, and to establish norms through uninvolved limb measurements or established parameters.

The documentation should also describe the skilled techniques utilized to improve range of motion, such as contract/relax, proprioceptive neuromuscular facilitation (PNF), or manual therapy. Any complicating factors, including pain, increased muscle tone, or contractures, are also needed. By documenting the complicating factors and the skilled techniques, the reviewer is provided with insight into why nonskilled personnel are unable to effectively or safely perform range of motion activities.

Strength.   As with range of motion, a comparative description of strength grades and the relationship to function is needed. It is helpful to provide data pertaining to the muscle or group of muscles with the strength deficit and establish norms through uninvolved limb strength grades or established parameters.

The documentation should also describe the skilled techniques utilized to improve strength or facilitate movement, such as progressive resistive exercise, isometric exercises, electrical stimulation, vibration, and/or manual resistance. The quality of muscle performance, such as noting quivering or inconsistent contractions, and any complicating factors, including pain or muscle spasm, are also needed. Documentation of the complicating factors and the skilled techniques provides the reviewer with insight into why the patient is unable to effectively or safely improve strength with just a home exercise program. This may further justify the need for skilled care.

Pain.   A reviewer finds it helpful when the treatment strategies to decrease pain are described, comparative data are provided, and the effect on function is indicated. To develop a full understanding of functional limitations and functional improvements, the following should be documented: the location of pain, comparative pain scale ratings, and when pain occurs. The reviewer needs to determine if the present treatment strategies are effective, and if not, what alternative strategies have been attempted. A thorough description assists the reviewer in establishing a need for continued skilled care.

Coordination.   Comparative data regarding coordination provides the reviewer with another reason for skilled care. The data must describe the functional impact of the deficits. For example, does limited fine motor or gross motor coordination affect safety? Also, what strategies have been used to improve coordination?

Bed Mobility.   Bed mobility is often described in terms of levels of assistance and amounts of verbal cuing for safety. Comparative data help demonstrate functional progress. It is also helpful to describe how any deficits in strength, trunk mobility, range of motion, or presence of pain affect performance.

Balance (Sit and Stand).   The key to providing comparative data for balance is to start with an adequate description in the evaluation or prior reports. Comparative data may include changes in the direction of balance loss, the amount of assistance to correct, improvement in trunk righting skills, improved weight shifting, improved posture, and/or increased strength. The data should be measurable and relate to improved function or safety. Balance deficits demonstrate another functional challenge requiring the skills of a therapist.

Transfers.   A complete description of transfers includes comparative data indicating the type of transfer, level of assistance, amount of verbal cuing, use of an assistive device, and postural changes. Data describing the skilled instruction needed for safe performance enhance the justification for skilled intervention.

Ambulation (Level and Elevated Surfaces).   A reviewer finds it helpful to have a description of gait deficits and comparative statements of progress. Items for consideration include the instruction in safe use of an assistive device or a change in the device, a description of the effect of skilled intervention on gait deficits, the reduction in weight bearing restrictions, how complicating factors affect function, and the number of physical and/or verbal cues. Ambulation distance is usually not important to a reviewer in demonstrating skilled care or functional progress unless a specific functional objective is defined—for example, the patient lives alone and must be able to ambulate an established distance in order to return home and perform activities of daily living.

Depending on the long-term goal, teaching and training for safe community ambulation is expected by the reviewer. Any deficits that occur in carryover to the community, home, school, and/or job may provide another need for continued skilled care.

Orthotic/Prosthetic Devices.   Comparative data regarding skin integrity and analysis of gait quality provide another justification for skilled care. If this is not a problem area, it is still important to document the presence of the device either in this area or in conjunction with ambulation data. Any consultations by other health care professionals, such as an orthotist or prosthetist, should be documented. Also, adjustments to the device and any effects on rehabilitation should be described.

Wheelchair Use.   Instruction in wheelchair propulsion skills and ensuring proper positioning requires the skills of a therapist in the presence of challenges such as postural deficits, neurological involvement, abnormal muscle tone, diminished functional strength, and/or range of motion deficits. A description of these challenges and comparative measurable data allow the reviewer to determine the need for skilled care.

DME (Using or Required). The need for and presence of durable medical equipment helps the reviewer understand the patient's functional limitations. When this is properly documented, the skills of a therapist are evident in determining the medical necessity of the equipment used or to be purchased.

Activity Tolerance. The patient's ability to perform functional activities such as job responsibilities, wheelchair propulsion, and/or ambulation are affected by activity tolerance. Comparative data will reinforce the benefits gained from skilled intervention. However, improvements in activity tolerance need to be reflected in conjunction with other functional activities and are rarely the sole basis for skilled care.

Wound Description, Including Incision Status. It is important to comment on the current status of a surgical incision or wound. This is especially relevant if soft-tissue restrictions exist that affect function or if modalities are being used to promote healing.

For wounds, comparative data are required. The data should be measurable and descriptive. The data may include descriptions of the wound location, size, drainage, odor, and tissue appearance. The parameters used for the modality provided and precautionary information (e.g., sensory deficits) should also be documented as evidence of the need for skilled intervention.

Special Tests. If special tests were documented in the evaluation or a prior report, any follow-up testing results or an anticipated retesting date should be indicated. The relevance of the test data to rehabilitation must be described, as specialized tests may be unfamiliar to a reviewer.

Architectural/Safety Considerations. Defining architectural and safety barriers is needed, as return to work, home, and/or school is an important functional outcome. Data may provide evidence of a home assessment (including the date of the assessment and a summary of findings) and/or a discussion with the patient and/or family regarding safety issues. Identifying barriers and documentation of recommendations or patient/family/employer education is another justification of the need for skilled care.

Treatment Diagnosis

It is important to identify the treatment diagnosis for which physical therapy services are rendered, as it may change during the course of intervention. A change in the focus of treatment may influence the duration of intervention.

Assessment

The assessment is the therapist's clinical impressions of the patient and the summary of the expected outcome from skilled intervention. From a reviewer's perspective, this is defined by focusing on the reason for skilled care.

Reason for Skilled Care. The reason for skilled care justifies the need for physical therapy intervention, provides the rationale for the treatment plan, and describes the expectations for continued functional progress. The therapist's insight into therapeutic expectations help in justifying the effectiveness of treatment and/or defining the potential barriers that may hinder functional progress. An explanation of the complicating factors that are affecting progress or potential barriers to progress may need to be given. This provides the reviewer with insight into the patient's functional progress and/or reason for regression and the need for continued intervention.

Problems

The problem list helps to focus physical therapy treatment and goals. The problems established at the evaluation should be restated. Any additions or deletions to the problem list need to be clarified for the reviewer. This is done by documenting if the problem is resolved or listing a new problem. The date of the change should also be indicated.

Plan of Care

The plan of care helps the reviewer in determining reasonable and necessary physical therapy service. The plan is based on the therapist's expertise as to what is needed for a successful functional outcome. The plan includes specific treatment strategies, frequency, duration, patient instruction/home program, caregiver training, short-term goals and achievement dates, long-term goals and achievement dates, and the rehabilitation potential.

Specific Treatment Strategies. The treatment strategies are specific procedures/modalities that will be used to address the problems listed and to achieve the stated goals. It is common for payers to require physician involvement for any additions and/or deletions to the plan of care. The strategies must correspond with billing. With this in mind, therapists should have an understanding of the payer's guidelines to ensure payment.

The treatment strategies should be specific and related to a functional outcome. Revisions to the plan of care are expected by the reviewer when functional progress is not achieved within a reasonable period of time. Defining a reasonable period of time is a common dilemma for therapists and is not easily answered.

There are many variables involved in determining a reasonable period of time. Patient progress, complicating factors and comorbidities are only a few of the variables used. It is through good documentation and sound clinical judgement that quality care is rendered. The key is to be optimistic but not unrealistic as most payers will not provide coverage for multiple interventions over an extended duration.

The reviewer may also compare the strategies and baseline data to ensure accurate billing has occurred. If it is not documented then it was not done! The reasonableness of the charges may also be assessed.

Frequency.   As defined in the evaluation, establishing how often the patient will receive skilled care in order to achieve the established goals is a necessary element of documentation. The frequency should be nonvariable and stated in terms of times per week or, depending on the payer, a number of visits within a defined time frame, for example, six visits before a certain date. A reviewer can reasonably expect that the frequency of skilled care will decrease as the patient progresses. The documentation should reflect when the frequency change occurred. However, there are certain instances when maintaining a higher frequency will foster goal achievement in a shorter duration and is acceptable because it may prove to be cost-effective for the patient, facility, and/or payer.

Duration.   Documenting the anticipated duration of skilled service provides the reviewer with insight into the reasonableness of the treatment strategies for meeting the established long-term goal. This often is expressed in terms of days or weeks and is described in nonvariable terms. In the event the duration of care is extended, a reviewer would expect justification in the assessment area of the report.

Patient Instruction/Home Program.   The involvement of the patient in a home or restorative nursing program demonstrates carryover of functional progress gained from skilled intervention. This is important to the reviewer, as program revision often requires the skills of a therapist. Documenting details of program revisions provides another reason for skilled care.

Caregiver Training.   Evidence of ongoing training of the patient, family, caregiver, teacher, nurse, and/or employer is important to the reviewer. Documentation of what exercise or functional activity was taught, who was trained, and when the training occurred is needed. Teaching and training with the patient present are considered skilled services by most payers.

Short-Term Goals and Achievement Dates.   It is helpful to indicate when goals are achieved or revised, as short-term goals are the stepping stones to achievement of functional outcomes. The three components for goal writing are needed (i.e., measurable, functional and an achievement date). By documenting new goals, the reviewer is able to assess progress. Therefore, it is important to demonstrate goal progression (Table 1.7).

Long-Term Goals and Achievement Dates.   The long-term goals need to be restated from the evaluation. Any changes to long-term goals should be clarified in the assessment area of the report. The goals need to be measurable and functional. A time frame is recommended. However, in the absence of a time frame, the reviewer will infer that the duration of treatment is the anticipated achievement date.

Rehabilitation Potential.   The patient's rehabilitation potential should be documented. It is customarily a one-word response such as *excellent* or *good*. As with the long-term goal,

Table 1.7 Strategies for Documenting Short-term Goal Progression

The easiest way for the reviewer to identify progress is to see when a goal was achieved, and new goals. The date of the new goal should be provided. For example:

Child will maintain correct alignment in tall kneeling for 3 minutes with verbal cues to improve standing posture in 2 weeks. Goal met.

NEW GOAL (Date): Child will maintain correct alignment in half kneeling for 3 minutes with moderate assistance and verbal cues to improve standing posture in 2 weeks.

As limited space is often an issue, the second strategy suggested is to acknowledge the goal is upgraded and only state the new goal.

Goal met. NEW GOAL (Date) Child will maintain correct alignment in half kneeling for 3 minutes with moderate assistance and verbal cues to improve standing posture in 2 weeks.

any change since the time of the evaluation should be clarified in the assessment area of the report.

Essential Elements of a Discharge Report

The essential elements of a discharge report are similar to those of the progress report. The attendance, treatment diagnosis, and problems are documented as for a progress report. However, although the reports are similar, the current baseline data differ: the comparisons include not only data since the last formal report, but also an overall comparison since the start of care. To avoid redundancy, emphasis will be placed on the assessment and plan of care areas because of their special role in a discharge report.

Assessment

In a discharge report the assessment is the summary of the therapist's clinical impressions of the patient and the outcomes achieved from skilled intervention. From a reviewer's perspective this is defined by focusing on the reason for skilled care.

Reason for Skilled Care.   In a discharge report, complications that were present, an explanation of why goals were not met (if applicable), the need for skilled care, the reason for discharge, and an expectation statement of the therapist's insight regarding successful carryover to home, school, and/or work are helpful items to describe. Data to support the effectiveness of the treatment provided since the last report are also helpful to the reviewer in determining if the care provided was medically necessary and skilled.

Plan of Care

A summary of the plan of care helps the reviewer in determining if the care provided was reasonable and necessary. The plan includes specific treatment strategies, frequency, duration, patient instruction/home program, caregiver training, short-term goals and achievement dates, long-term goals and achievement dates, and the discharge prognosis.

Specific Treatment Strategies. In a discharge report, the obvious plan is that of discharge from physical therapy. However, from a reviewer's perspective this information alone makes it difficult to determine if skilled care was provided. It is recommended that a summary of the treatment strategies used through the time of discharge be provided to help the reviewer determine the reasonableness of the plan of care in relationship to the functional progress reported. Restating the treatment strategies can also help when analyzing documentation and the corresponding services billed.

Frequency. In a discharge report the frequency of further care is not applicable. However, from a reviewer's perspective this makes it difficult to determine if the frequency was reasonable in relationship to the functional progress reported for the period in question. Therefore, it is recommended that a summary of the frequency be provided to help the reviewer determine the reasonableness of care and to help when analyzing documentation and the corresponding services billed.

Duration. At the time of discharge there is no anticipated duration of care. However, it is suggested that a summary of the duration be provided, as it helps the reviewer determine the reasonableness of care in relationship to the functional progress reported. It also helps when analyzing documentation and the corresponding services billed.

Patient Instruction/Home Program. Carryover of the functional benefits from skilled rehabilitation to home, school, and/or job is essential at discharge. A detailed description of the home exercise program or restorative nursing program justifies the skilled care provided. Data should contain a summary of the activities that were or are to be performed, the frequency of performance, and dates the therapist provided training and/or changes to the program.

Caregiver Training. Evidence of ongoing training of the patient, family, caregiver, teacher, nurse, and/or employer through and at the time of discharge is important to the reviewer. Documentation of what exercise or functional activity was taught, who was trained, and when the training occurred is needed. Teaching and training with the patient present are considered skilled services by most payers.

Short-Term Goals and Achievement Dates. The short-term goals from the last report should be restated. The goals should contain all three components and be measurable, functional, and time specific. The status of the goals at discharge is needed (i.e., met or not met). If a goal is not achieved, the reasons the goal was not met, and the functional impact that may have on the patient should be explained in the assessment.

Long-Term Goals and Achievement Dates. The status of the long-term goal at discharge is important to the reviewer in assessing the success of the skilled services provided. If the goal was not achieved, the reason for discharge should be provided in the assessment.

Discharge Prognosis. The discharge prognosis is generally a one-word response such as *excellent*, *good*, *fair*, or *poor*. It provides the reviewer with the therapist's insight into the patient's ability to maintain the functional skills achieved without continued skilled intervention. This helps to assess the reasonableness of skilled care and allows the reviewer to determine whether the benefits of skilled service will be sustained long enough to warrant the efforts invested.[13]

In essence, if the patient follows the recommendations provided by the therapist, what is the potential for a successful outcome beyond the therapy environment? This is an important question that should be considered even at the time of initial evaluation when the plan of care/frequency/duration are established.

Essential Elements of an Individualized Education Program

An IEP is a systematic planning tool used in the educational setting for children with disabilities who demonstrate the need for specialized educational services. Federal law requires that school districts provide children with disabilities with a public education that includes special education and related services.[14] The IEP is developed from the collaborative effort of a diverse group that may include the teacher, parent(s), physical therapist, occupational therapist, speech language pathologist, school psychologist, and/or director of special education. Although IEP formats vary from state to state, several essential elements are commonly found: the present levels of educational performance, an annual goal, short-term objectives, schedule (goal time frames), and specific special education and related services that will contribute to meeting the established goals.

Present Levels of Educational Performance. This area should contain a narrative statement that is written in objective and measurable terms. It needs to include an easily understood description of the child's ability to function in the school environment.

Annual Goal. The annual goal needs to be measurable and focus on a functional outcome in order to justify skilled physical therapy intervention. It is linked to the child's present level of performance and provides a reasonable expectation of what the child may achieve within one year.

Short-Term Objectives. The short-term objectives are the milestones to be achieved in order to reach the annual goal. These objectives need to be stated in measurable and functional terms that are easily observed and understood by teachers and parents. They should relate specifically to the educational setting.

Schedule. The schedule refers to the time frame anticipated for achievement of the short-term objectives. Quarterly reviews are reasonably expected by reviewers.

Specific Special Education and Related Services That Will Contribute to Meeting This Goal. Identification of all contributing services that will be involved in facilitating one or more of the objectives is required. Those who may be involved are teachers, parents, classroom aides, and/or therapists. As educational goal achievement is a team effort, all members providing input into the child's skill development are to be included.

Summary

Documenting physical therapy services from a reviewer's perspective means to accurately describe what is observed, what was performed, and what was achieved. Documentation is not just a game to provide the payer with the information they need in order to determine coverage. It is a reasonable professional expectation to ensure quality care.

This chapter has provided a foundation for beginning the process to effectively analyze documentation from a reviewer's perspective. A baseline of knowledge has been provided that includes an understanding of the multiple purposes of documentation, definitions of documentation through accepted standards of practice, and a review of the essential elements for documentation from a reviewer's perspective.

Based on this knowledge, it is now important to explore the medical review process. Chapter 2 will focus on the reviewer. It will address the need for review, guidelines for review processing, who reviewers are, what essential elements are generally lacking in documentation, and how to improve on data that are lacking.

References

1. Morrissey-Ross M. Documentation: if you haven't written it, you haven't done it. *Nurs Clin North Am* 1988; 23(2): 367.
2. Scott RW. *Legal Aspects of Documenting Patient Care*, Gaithersburg, Maryland: Aspen Publishers, Inc., 1994, 32–34.
3. Lukan M. *Documentation for Physical Therapist Assistants*, Philadelphia, Pennsylvania: F.A. Davis Company, 1997, 8–9.
4. Saunders R. *Industrial Rehabilitation Techniques for Success*, Chaska, Minnesota: The Saunders Group, 1995, 43.
5. American Physical Therapy Association. Guide to Physical Therapist Practice. *Phys Ther* 1997; 77(11): 1183–1636.
6. Wilkerson DL, Batavia AI, DeJong G. Use of functional status measures for payment of Medicare rehabilitation services. *Arch Phys Med Rehabil* 1992; 73:111.
7. Allen C, Foto M, Moon-Sperling T, Wilson D. A medical review approach to Medicare outpatient documentation. *Am J Occup Ther* 1989; 433(12):793.
8. Esposto L. Applying functional outcome assessment to Medicare documentation. In Stewart DL, Abeln SH (eds). *Documenting Functional Outcomes in Physical Therapy.* St. Louis: Mosby—Year Book, Inc., 1993, 142.
9. Guccione AA. Physical therapy diagnosis and the relationship between impairments and function. *Phys Ther* 1991; 71(7): 502/13.
10. *International Classification of Diseases, 9th Revision, Clinical Modification,* fifth edition. Salt Lake City: Medicode Publications, 1997.
11. Dewane JA. Documenting balance and functional outcomes: tips from the clinic. *Top Geriatr Rehabil* 1997; 13(1):24.
12. Thorman M. Documenting wound care for pressure ulcers. *Top Geriatr Rehabil* 1997;13(1):35.
13. Kane RL. Looking for physical therapy outcomes. *Phys Ther* 1994; 74(5):428.
14. Wisconsin Department of Public Instruction. Occupational therapy and physical therapy: a resource and planning guide. Milwaukee: Wisconsin Department of Public Instruction, 1996, 9.

Review Questions

1. Documentation is important for many reasons. List seven purposes of documentation.
2. Who defines documentation policies and formats?
3. Explain why the need for good documentation skills has become essential for reimbursement.
4. Why is an initial evaluation important from a reviewer's perspective?
5. List the two approaches that are commonly used for documenting daily/weekly treatment notes and explain their differences from a reviewer's perspective.
6. List five or more complicating factors that may affect treatment duration.
7. Describe two ways to present comparative documentation. Provide an example of each.
8. Why are the diagnosis and onset date important to a reviewer?
9. Explain why the prior therapy history is important to a reviewer.
10. Should objective data be related to function?
11. What is the most important essential element to document in an initial evaluation?
12. When should patient instruction/home programming begin?
13. List the three goal components.
14. Are terms such as "increased" or "decreased" acceptable to a reviewer? Why or why not?
15. Discharge reports should compare data from evaluation through discharge. What other data should be compared to help the reviewer?

Review Question Answer Sheet

1. The seven purposes of documentation include ensuring quality care, continuity of care, marketing, legal aspects, research, educational, and reimbursement.

2. The definition of documentation is defined by the American Therapy Association in the policy *Guidelines for Physical Therapy Documentation.* This policy provides the starting point for developing documentation formats in any practice setting. Further policy and format development arise defined by the players. The players may include the patient (employee), the employer, and the third-party payer.

3. The need for good documentation skills has become essential for reimbursement because scrutiny by third-party payers into the cost of achieving functional outcomes has increased. Managed care and the shrinking health care dollar have brought the need for documentation of medical necessity to the forefront.

4. The initial evaluation provides baseline data for future progress comparisons. It establishes the reason for intervention and outlines expectations for progress. For these reasons it is routinely requested by third-party payers for adjudication of claims.

5. The two approaches commonly used are the SOAP note and the narrative summary. The SOAP note provides a predictable format. However, it does not foster comparative writing, may be repetitive in nature, and usually requires the reviewer to shuffle through a lot of paper to determine progress. In contrast, the narrative approach may foster progress comparisons and decrease the need for a reviewer to search through a lot of notes. However, if not organized properly the narrative approach may be lengthy and lack focus because of "problem jumping."

6. Complicating factors may include illness, attendance/compliance, exacerbation of a diagnosis, new diagnosis, side effects from medications, change in medication, recent fall, change in weight bearing, and/or a new physician's order.

7. Comparative data are frequently presented in a chart or statement form. Examples are provided in Table 1.4.

8. The diagnosis and onset date are important to a reviewer for identifying the need for skilled rehabilitation and whether the condition requiring treatment is acute or chronic. Both are important for billing purposes.

9. The prior therapy history is important to a reviewer because information regarding frequency, duration, and functional outcomes help to establish the patient's rehabilitation potential.

10. Yes, objective data should be related to function. This will help paint a clear picture of the patient for the reviewer and justify the need for skilled care.

11. Prior level of function. It should be specific and functionally stated.

12. Home programming and/or restorative nursing recommendations and patient education need to be initiated at the initial evaluation.

13. Goals should be measurable, functional, and have an achievement date (time frame).

14. Vague terms such as "increased" or "decreased" are not acceptable to a reviewer. These terms are not measurable and do not demonstrate that functional progress (or a regression) has occurred.

15. It is important to include comparisons not only from the start of care through discharge, but also since the last formal report.

Chapter 2
The Review Process and Documentation Deficiencies

Introduction

In Chapter 1 the purposes, definition, and essential elements for physical therapy documentation from a reviewer's perspective were presented. Emphasis was placed on describing the essential elements necessary to provide accurate and thorough records focusing on functional outcomes. This chapter will address the reviewer and the medical review process as changes in health care systems are driving the increase in scrutiny of rehabilitation services. Consideration will be given to the need for review, general guidelines for review, who reviewers are, and the purposes of physical therapy peer review, regardless of the payer source. The essential elements of documentation will be revisited, with emphasis placed on areas of inadequate documentation commonly found by reviewers. Examples will be provided to help foster the development of functional writing skills.

The Need for Medical Review

The rising cost of health care is the primary driving force that has influenced the need to rethink clinical practice. The increasing anxiety rehabilitation professionals express regarding documentation is symptomatic of the major transformations within the health care delivery system.[1] One major transformation is in the arena of managed care. Payers and the insured (i.e., the patient) are expecting positive functional outcomes, in a reasonable period of time, for a fair price. As rehabilitation professionals, there is a need to adapt to the increased financial restrictions managed care is creating. This can be accomplished by placing emphasis on justifying the need for skilled intervention and the long-term efficacy that can result from treatment interventions.

The need to advocate physical therapy as a viable profession has increased in urgency with health care reform. One method of advocacy is to provide third-party payers with descriptive and accurate documentation. This will help in educating payers about the role of physical therapists, the treatment strategies used, and the effectiveness of the care delivered. This is evident in the 1997 Medicare coverage issue change concerning electrical stimulation for the treatment of wounds. The Health Care Financing Administration (HCFA) initially denied coverage of this modality for wound care. However, a mass effort was initiated to educate this regulator as to the efficiency of this treatment intervention. The action taken resulted in a favorable coverage decision. Taking a proactive role in coverage issues, education of third-party payers, and the development of coverage criteria is essential to ensure that future patients will benefit from skilled physical therapy services.

There are several players involved in the review process. All have unique responsibilities in achieving a positive functional outcome. These players are the providers of physical therapy service, the insured, the third-party payer, and the reviewer. In addition to their individual roles, the need for increased communication between all players is crucial to the survival of quality health care delivery. Any past resistance of an individual player to change needs to be replaced with an attitude of openness to new ideas and methods of compromise.

The provider of physical therapy services has multiple responsibilities that must be considered on a daily basis. These responsibilities include clinical and also legal and ethical practice considerations. The American Physical Therapy Association (APTA) outlines these considerations in the *Guide to Physical Therapist Practice*[2] by defining standards of practice (Appendix 2) and providing codes of ethics (Appendixes 3 and 4) and guides for professional conduct (Appendixes 5 and 6). Within the scope of practice is the obligation to provide clinical documentation that supports the rationale for treatment and reflects the medical necessity and appropriateness of the intervention provided. Within these responsibilities lies the true nature of providing quality rehabilitative service.

The insured has the responsibility to provide insurance information and is responsible for any copayments or deductibles unique to the specific coverage. The insured may not fully recognize these responsibilities. Therefore, it is important for the provider to have policies and procedures to confirm insurance information. Orientation of the insured to their individual insurance policies and their role in advocating services will enhance the billing process.

In addition to following the regulations of an individual contract, the payer has a responsibility to the patient to investigate claims submitted for payment. One method of protecting the patient's interest is for the payer to hire reviewers to perform retrospective or prospective reviews of selected cases. In retrospective review the case is evaluated and reimbursed after the service has been provided. In prospective reimbursement the individual case reimbursement may be based on discounted rates, capitation rates, or specific visits for a certain diagnosis. By performing a review the payer ensures that only medically necessary and reasonable physical therapy services are provided within the scope of the insurance plan's coverage criteria. This is financially beneficial to the patient and to the payer, as costs are controlled.

The final player is the reviewer. The reviewer has a responsibility to the provider of service and the payer to render an opinion regarding the need for or the appropriateness of physical therapy intervention. This opinion is based on the documentation presented and the reviewer's interpretation of the data regarding medical necessity and the payer's guidelines. If the guidelines are not defined or are vague and allow interpretation, the reviewer's personal experience, local, state, or national standards of practice, and/or common sense may be deciding factors. Although the final authority for the coverage or payment decisions may vary depending on the payer, this reinforces the need for quality documentation of physical therapy services.

The need for review of physical therapy services is driven by the multiple players to control costs and provide quality care. To achieve positive functional outcomes all players including the provider of physical therapy service, the patient, the payer and the reviewer must work together. Documentation is the key to justifying the physical therapy services received and/or the need for additional skilled service.

The review process for physical therapy services is evolving, and the establishment of national standards for utilization review is in its infancy. Involvement of physical therapists at the policy level will help shape future trends and coverage. As physical therapists become peer reviewers and/or educate reviewers, consistency of care delivery will improve throughout the profession.

To help understand the reviewer's perspective in determining the need for skilled care, it is necessary to examine criteria that exist for review processing. It is not within the scope of this book to identify the individual guidelines of all payers. Instead, this book discusses general criteria common to most of them. The following section will identify general guidelines for review.

General Guidelines for Review

Despite the lack of national standards/criteria for review of physical therapy services, there are several common criteria used by various payer sources in assessing the appropriateness of rehabilitation services. These criteria (Table 2.1) are summarized best by HCFA in the Medicare Skilled Nursing Facility Manual, Section 214.3, which pertains to skilled physical therapy.[3] These criteria were designed primarily for skilled nursing facilities, but apply to most settings.

Table 2.1 Medicare Part A Skilled Physical Therapy Coverage Guidelines (from Department of Health and Human Services, Health Care Financing Administration. *Medicare Skilled Nursing Facility Manual*, Laurel, Maryland: Government Printing Office, Publication 12, Revision 262, Section 214.3, 1987, 2-17.3–2-17.4.)

A. Skilled Physical Therapy
  1. General.—Skilled physical therapy services must meet all of the following conditions:
  - The services must be directly and specifically related to an active written treatment plan designed by the physician after any needed consultation with a qualified physical therapist;
  - The services must be of a level of complexity and sophistication, or the condition of the patient must be of a nature that requires the judgement, knowledge, and skills of a qualified physical therapist;
  - The services must be provided with the expectation, based on the assessment made by the physician of the patient's restoration potential, that the condition of the patient will improve materially in a reasonable and generally predictable period of time, or the services must be necessary for the establishment of a safe and effective maintenance program;
  - The services must be considered under accepted standards of medical practice to be specific and effective treatment for the patient's condition; and
  - The services must be reasonable and necessary for the treatment of the patient's condition; this includes the requirement that the amount, frequency, and duration of the services must be reasonable.

In addition to Medicare, the APTA provides a written document to promote standardization for peer review training and performance. The document, *Guidelines for Peer Review Training*[4] (Appendix 7), provides a description of peer review, training content, training methods, and recommended resources. It provides principles for performing peer review. The APTA's guidelines recommend that peer reviewers have an understanding of documentation, billing and coding, record review, report writing, claims appeal, legal and ethical issues, and how to market the value of peer review to payers and providers. They also stress the educational role of the peer reviewer in communicating with payers and providers.

The APTA's guidelines provide a foundation for state associations, as standards and guidelines for review vary between payers and geographical locations. By becoming involved at the state level, associations can help educate and facilitate review criteria to foster quality care. The association's involvement may include consultation services to third-party payers, such as peer reviewer services, professional consultation for policy development, or education regarding physical therapy practice as it relates to diagnoses treated, procedures used, documentation expectations, and billing practices.

The verbiage used by third-party payers, as evident in the Medicare and APTA guidelines presented, implies the need for ongoing professional judgment in determining the appropriateness of care to meet coverage criteria. This is a clinical challenge! Physical therapists, in providing quality care, must determine and render services that are medically necessary. The justification of such services is provided through documentation and functional outcomes.

Defining "medically necessary" is not an easy task for the physical therapist or the reviewer and is driven by the payer's interpretation. During the review process, the reviewer is called upon to provide an opinion on the medical necessity of physical therapy services provided or proposed to be provided to an individual patient. The definition of medical necessity is usually determined by the payer based on the language found in the insurance policy covering the patient and varies between payers and policies.

Within the context of the payer's definition of medical necessity, the reviewer makes a determination of compliance for coverage based on the documentation submitted by the physical therapist, the patient, and/or the physician. Reviewers, if knowledgeable in rehabilitation, will use resources provided by the APTA or state associations to define the standard for documentation. Physical therapists are expected to provide documentation that meets this standard for the purposes of review.

The following information, adapted from the Wisconsin Physical Therapy Association (WPTA) in their *Guidelines for WPTA Peer Review*,[5] establishes that medical necessity review could be used to determine the following:

1. *The appropriateness of planned/delivered procedures for the treatment of the identified diagnosis and/or deficits identified in the initial or subsequent evaluations.* Reviewers may use commonly accepted clinical references, their own clinical expertise, other qualified reviewers, and materials submitted by treating therapists in making these determinations. In general, reviewers do not evaluate a therapist's selection of a treatment approach when the therapist has made a choice between one or more appropriate treatment strategies.

2. *If treatment has resulted in progressive improvement as demonstrated by objective comparative clinical findings of physiological and/or anatomical changes in the patient's status that correlate with functional improvements in the area of activities of daily living, mobility, pain and/or safety.* Essentially, is it documented that the services provided have been effective and resulted in carryover into functional activities?

3. *If the active physical therapy intervention at the frequency and duration indicated in the plan of care is required for progressive improvement of the patient's condition.* This could be affected by variability of the patient's condition, patient cognitive ability, patient safety, complexity of the treatment technique required, rate of change, and frequency with which the plan of care needs to be revised. These factors are contrasted with the patient's ability to progress on a supervised or independent home exercise program.

4. *If duplicated services are being delivered by multiple providers.* Duplication of services could be between one or more providers from the same discipline or different disciplines. Generally, when services are duplicated by two providers the patient would be requested to choose between providers.

5. *If the patient had a beneficial response to any previous physical therapy treatment for the same diagnosis.* It is reasonable for a reviewer to expect the treatment approach to be revised if prior intervention was unsuccessful or presented limited carryover into functional activities.

Kane[6] provides insight that medically necessary service is being redefined and with it the need for better data on the appropriateness and the effectiveness of care. According to Kane's criteria, "medically necessary" contains two components. The first is "appropriateness," which refers to doing the right thing and is difficult to measure, as clinical situations have multiple variables. The second component, "effectiveness," addresses outcomes directly. Therefore, positive functional outcomes are the result of doing things well. Kane challenges physical therapists to pursue more studies to specifically establish the role of physical therapy versus other rehabilitation professionals in what is effective care. One problem is that marginal functional gains that require heavy expenditures are being scrutinized. Determining medically necessary services may prove difficult in the future without supportive data regarding outcomes.

The guidelines presented are intended to be an overview to help physical therapy providers in understanding the expectations of various payer sources. As variability exists among payers, such as in the state workers' compensation programs that are unique to each state, expectations need to be carefully analyzed by the provider. Knowledge of more specific guidelines and requirements for individual payer sources is the responsibility of the individual therapist to research through direct communication with the payer sources.

Who Are Reviewers?

Reviewers of physical therapy claims vary depending on the third-party payer. Historically, reviewers have included registered nurses, physicians, peers, and nonmedical personnel. Knowing who is reviewing documentation and their rehabilitation background is helpful to the physical therapist in ensuring that the patient's needs and functional gains are understood.

Reviewers may be individuals who do not have thorough knowledge of physical therapy services. Stewart and Abeln[7] indicates that most reviewers have had a general course on medical terminology, but probably do not understand the relationship between anatomy and the need for continued therapy intervention. Therefore, it is necessary that the therapist be extremely careful to provide documentation that is clear and concise, and that reflects the patient's functional deficits as well as the need for skilled physical therapy intervention. When adequate and objective data are presented, the reviewer is better equipped to make sound coverage decisions based on fact, not broad interpretation.

Within most payer organizations there are typically two to three levels of reviewers. The first level typically are nonmedical personnel with minimal training in medical terminology and even less training in the principles of rehabilitation. At this level technical data are analyzed, such as timely physician certification/recertification, if applicable, that services were performed by qualified therapists and that the modalities performed are covered in the patient's plan.[8] The second level of reviewers consists of medical personnel. They may include registered nurses, licensed practical nurses, and physical therapist peer reviewers to determine the medical necessity of treatment intervention. Reviewers beyond the second level will generally require the involvement of a peer or medical director associated with the insurance plan. Samples of forms reviewers may use are presented in Figures 2.1, 2.2, and 2.3 (see end of chapter) to illustrate different formats and questions commonly asked by various payers.

The review forms used by payers will vary depending on the needs of the insurance plan and the experience of the review team. Forms help to foster consistency in the review process. Although reviewers are commonly nonpeers, there is an increasing need for peer reviewers to ensure the medical necessity and appropriateness of the services delivered.

Who reviewers are may be redefined in the future. Presently, not all payers are aware of or recognize the APTA's guidelines for documentation or for peer reviewers. As physical therapists begin to take a more active role in the development of review criteria to shape appropriate clinical practice, use of the guidelines by payers will increase. It is the responsibility of all reviewers, peer or nonpeer, to be current in as many areas of the field of physical therapy as possible. If a reviewer is not comfortable in reviewing a case, he or she should recommend another peer more qualified to do so. An example of this would be an individual who works primarily in geriatrics (in home health) may have some difficulty reviewing a pediatric case in the school setting, particularly if they have never worked with children. Who reviewers are, their clinical experience, their rehabilitation knowledge, and their understanding of outcomes all influence coverage decisions. Therefore, it is necessary to foster more peer review processing, as it serves multiple purposes.

Purposes of Physical Therapy Peer Review

The purposes of being a peer reviewer for physical therapy are fourfold.

1. It offers an opportunity for physical therapists to network and build trust with third-party payers.

Understanding the multiple challenges faced in both the delivery of care and its reimbursement helps the provider, the payer, and the patient. As a peer reviewer, networking and understanding the payer's challenges will help to educate other physical therapists. The result may be less time spent in denial processing and improved delivery of care.

For example, the payer may realize the importance of a treatment modality. However, without appropriate documentation by the treating therapist, coverage within the plan may be denied or delayed. The peer reviewer can educate the membership, through the state or national association, regarding the payer's guidelines and how to document appropriately. This may facilitate coverage decisions and help all players.

2. It provides an excellent opportunity to offer education regarding the field of physical therapy.

As a peer reviewer, Lynn Phillippi, MS, PT, had many positive experiences inservicing case managers (often registered nurses) on various modalities and treatment techniques, describing gait deficits, muscle and balance difficulties, and relating these to function. Reviewers were overwhelmingly grateful, and the education often resulted in extended coverage for a particular patient, or at a minimum, a closer review of the case.

3. Being involved in peer review displays a commitment to monitoring the profession and ensuring that the highest standards for delivery of care are being followed.

Physical therapists who review claims are often astonished by the documentation submitted. Their expectations of peers are generally higher than those of other reviewers. Providing expertise in the field as a reviewer reveals the weaknesses of practice. Most evident is the need for improved documentation skills to justify medical necessity.

4. Lastly, interaction with third-party payer sources often places therapists in a position to make recommendations and/or review coverage for services, modalities, treatment techniques, and equipment.

Again, as a reviewer, Phillippi participated in the development of several policies affecting coverage for ultrasound and wound healing as well as the treatment of fibromyalgia. These policies are being used by select resources only, but it is a beginning, and every individual can attempt to participate in this process.

The need for peer reviewers is increasing. Establishing rapport with third-party payers is needed to ensure that quality of care is preserved. Therapists should begin at the state chapter level or the reimbursement division of the APTA (1-800-999-2782) for information regarding how to become involved in the review process.

Being a reviewer is an important, although often unpopular, role. As outlined in this chapter, the coverage decisions affect the insured, the provider, and the payer. The process begins with a review of physical therapy documentation. Insufficient documentation of skilled service and functional progress is a real and significant challenge for reviewers. Therefore, the ability to identify essential elements that are lacking in documentation is needed.

Reviewer Findings

Reviewers of documentation frequently find that data are lacking when reviewing physical therapy initial evaluations, progress reports (including daily/weekly notes), and/or discharge reports. As coverage decisions result from what is or is not written in reports, inadequate documentation makes it difficult to determine whether skilled care was reasonable and necessary. The best chance for approval of services occurs when there is documentation of skilled need and functional progress.

In the upcoming section the focus will be on reviewer findings and how to improve physical therapy documentation. The essential elements for initial evaluations, progress reports, discharge reports, and individualized education programs will be described in terms of identifying areas that are often inadequately documented from a reviewer's perspective. Recognizing the areas lacking in documentation provides an appreciation of the challenges faced by reviewers.

Readers should note that the examples of essential elements are from the case studies presented in Chapter 4 and closely represent the verbiage and abbreviations used by the original documenter to best demonstrate what a reviewer encounters. Some of the abbreviations listed may not be common or recommended for use in all settings. A list of abbreviations used is provided in Appendix 8.

Essential Elements Lacking in an Initial Evaluation

Referral

The reason for referral to physical therapy and the specific treatment requested are two areas included in referral data. From a reviewer's perspective it is difficult to justify the need for skilled intervention and whether the care is properly supervised, within the payer's guidelines for coverage, when the data are lacking.

Reason. Reviewers find it difficult to understand the need for skilled therapy intervention when the referral source and the treatment objective are not described. This is especially relevant if data such as the prior level of function, medical history, and/or long-term goal are also undefined. Without referral information the reviewer will speculate what the reason for skilled care is and whether nonskilled personnel or a home program could provide a similar functional result.

Example 1: P.T. was initiated 03-15-96 upon healing of fracture and order from ortho physician. (Case 17: Subacute, p. 203)

In Example 1 the referral source is described as the ortho physician. However, the treatment objective is not described. This unclear description provides a challenge to the reviewer. First, the reviewer may want to know the location of the fracture and the impact on functional activities, as not all healed fractures require skilled physical therapy intervention. Second, it would be helpful to know whether the patient's functional goal may be to walk, reach for objects, and/or return to home, work, or school. The reviewer will need to scrutinize the documentation thoroughly to understand the need for skilled care in this case.

Example 2: Was referred for functional capacity assessment (FCA) and work hardening by Dr. ABC, with the goal of improving work tolerances to return to modified work as a Finish Carpenter. (Case 6: Industrial Health—Work Hardening, p. 118)

It is always helpful to provide a clear statement of the reason for referral as demonstrated in Example 2. Example 2 describes the referral source and the need for skilled intervention in relationship to a functional activity. In this case, Dr. ABC provided

the referral because of the patient's inability to perform job responsibilities as a finish carpenter. The goal of return to work is indicated for the reviewer, and the purpose of skilled intervention is clear.

Specific Treatment Requested. Describing the specific treatment requested by the physician helps the reviewer determine that coverage is within the payer's guidelines and that an appropriate plan of care has been established. This is an easily overlooked area of documentation and is frequently lacking.

Although many states allow direct access to physical therapists, and therefore do not require a written physician order, many therapists experience difficulties with third-party payers reimbursing for services without a physician's order. It is the responsibility of each therapist to know the individual requirements of each payer source. When a physician's order is required, a copy of the order or evidence of the physician's involvement are important to include when submitting the patient claim.

The evidence of physician involvement may be obtained in several ways. Depending on the documentation format used by the provider and the third-party payer's expectations, the physician's signature may be provided in the original physical therapy initial evaluation and subsequent reports. For other formats the physician may sign a separate certification or authorization that specifies the necessary patient data to comply with the third-party payer's guidelines. Often patient identifying data such as the patient's name, date of birth, diagnosis, specific treatment modalities, frequency, duration, and goals are minimal requirements. The frequency for obtaining the physician's signature, if a necessary requirement, will depend on the payer's guidelines.

The reviewer may also examine the referral data to identify the specific treatment requested by the physician. The documentation will be examined for data regarding the treatment modalities or procedures, frequency, and duration of treatment. This helps the reviewer in knowing that the physician is aware of the specific approaches to treatment and that the skilled intervention of a therapist is required. The reviewer will also decide if the treatment strategies are appropriately related to the patient's diagnosis or treatment diagnosis and are not experimental. If not appropriate, data will be expected regarding additions and/or deletions to the plan of care. Depending on the payer, documentation that the physician was involved in approving the plan of care may be necessary prior to treatment to ensure payment. If so, documentation indicating that orders are being pursued or have been received is often beneficial to the review process.

Example 1: PT to see patient 2x/wk for 2 wks for gait and balance training and to resume home exercise program. (Case 1: Home Health, p. 74)

Example 1 demonstrates a specific order from the physician. The reviewer can easily identify the treatment strategies, frequency, and duration deemed necessary by the physician. If billing occurs for more modalities or procedures than indicated, the reviewer may seek additional data to ensure that overutilization has not occurred and that the physician approved the plan of care as medically necessary.

Example 2: PT for evaluation and treatment. (Case 12: Pediatric, p. 164)

The specific treatment requested in Example 2 allows the therapist to determine the specific treatment approach and establish the plan of care. In this example the reviewer will examine the plan of care established by the therapist and determine if it is appropriately related to the diagnosis for which treatment is rendered.

Data Accompanying Referral

From a reviewer's perspective, data accompanying the referral to physical therapy are needed in the billing process and help to establish medical necessity. The reviewer will look for data in the following areas to understand the complexity of the patient: the diagnosis/onset date, secondary diagnoses, medical history, medications, and comorbidities (complicating or precautionary information). Data in these areas are often missing or lacking in detail.

Diagnosis/Onset Date.   The diagnosis and onset date are important not only clinically, but also for reimbursement. The diagnosis and onset are entered by the billing provider when requesting payment from the third-party payer. The appropriateness of the diagnosis for skilled physical therapy service is the beginning point for ensuring that appropriate service is provided. Reviewers often find that the diagnosis and corresponding onset date do not reflect the reason for functional decline or appear inaccurate based on the documentation provided.

Once the specific treatment requested is identified, the diagnosis needs to be differentiated from the secondary diagnoses and the treatment diagnosis. Often the reviewer will investigate a case flagged by the nurse case manager or office personnel simply because the diagnosis appears chronic or inappropriate for therapeutic intervention. Common examples of such a diagnosis may include chronic obstruction pulmonary disease (COPD), congestive heart failure (CHF), and diabetes.

The diagnosis chosen by the therapist is often driven by the onset date, such as a decline in function as the result of an exacerbation, frequent falls, or a recent hospitalization. The onset date is important. If the onset date of the diagnosis is over six months old, implying that the diagnosis is not acute, and no further explanation is provided to substantiate present skilled intervention, this can be a red flag to a reviewer. The onset date needs to reflect the most recent functional decline or probable start of the developmental delay.

Example 1: Diagnosis/onset date: Cerebral Palsy/02-10-93.

Date of birth: 02-10-93. (Case 12: Pediatric, p. 164)

Reviewers will often compare the patient's date of birth and/or start of care date to the onset date of the diagnosis. Inaccuracies may result in the reviewer searching the documentation for

an explanation, or additional evidence may be requested. For instance, in Example 1 it is questionable that the onset date is accurate, as cerebral palsy is generally diagnosed after the patient has demonstrated a developmental delay. It is reasonable to expect that the date of onset for most diagnoses is not the start of care date.

Example 2: COPD exacerbation/04-07-95. (Case 8: Outpatient, p. 138)

In Example 2 a clear diagnosis is provided. As COPD is a chronic pulmonary condition, a reviewer may question the need for skilled care. However, because the documentation indicates an exacerbation, the reviewer will seek further information regarding the treatment diagnosis and functional deficits described in the documentation in order to determine the appropriateness of skilled care.

Secondary Diagnoses.   Reviewers find that secondary diagnoses tend to be omitted. As billing forms customarily allow the coding of multiple diagnoses, secondary diagnoses help the reviewer understand the complicated nature of the patient. Often secondary diagnoses are omitted by the billing provider, but may be found later during the review process in the area of medical history, or are inappropriately listed as indicated in Example 1.

Example 1: Diagnosis/onset date: S/P Multiple CVA's/08-09-92.

Secondary Diagnosis: Recent decline in status. (Case 1: Home Health, p. 74)

In Example 1 the secondary diagnosis is not specific. The statement provided may be misinterpreted by the reviewer as a general decline that may not require the skills of a therapist. As managed care and prospective payment models increase in prominence, accuracy of the diagnosis, the secondary diagnoses, and the treatment diagnosis in documentation and billing submissions will be vital for maximizing reimbursement.

Example 2: Diagnosis/onset date: S/P femoral/popliteal bypass surgery LLE/11-18-95.

Secondary diagnoses: CABG, CAD, ASHD, diabetes, chest pain. (Case 3: Hospital, p. 92)

The reviewer is provided with the patient's complicating diagnoses in Example 2. Although the influence the secondary diagnoses have on participation in rehabilitation needs to be documented elsewhere in the evaluation, the list of diagnoses provided is helpful to the reviewer. Based on this list it would appear that the skills of a therapist are needed for safe progression of functional activities. However, it is suggested that abbreviations not be overutilized, as many reviewers have minimal health care training and may not recognize all the diagnoses provided.

Medical History.   Reviewers find that the medical history is often briefly stated and does not provide insight into the patient's past and present medical conditions, living or work environment, and/or barriers to progress in relationship to the present need for skilled physical therapy. As reviewers often do not have access to the complete medical history, it is helpful when details relevant to rehabilitation are provided.

Example 1: Prior hospitalization unknown. (Case 9: Outpatient—Managed Care, p. 147)

Example 1 provides data that are brief and lack description. The reviewer would find it helpful to know if alternative interventions, other than hospitalization, were prescribed for the diagnosis, which in this case happens to be lumbar degenerative disc disease. Has the patient seen a physician in the past for this diagnosis? Where does this patient live? In a long-term care facility? Is the patient active in the community, work, or at school? Do other medical conditions exist that interfere with function? The reviewer is left with many unanswered questions in Example 1.

A detailed yet brief medical history can provide valuable insight to the reviewer in determining the need for skilled care. Example 2 describes such a history.

Example 2: He is the product of a premature delivery. He was born a twin at 28 weeks gestation with a birth weight of 2 lbs., 1 oz. He spent three months in the neonatal nursery, two of those months on a ventilator. The mother describes that he had a very small bleed while in the nursery, has had no seizures. He did have a patent ductus surgery when he was one week old. He was on an apnea monitor at home from June through October. Other than that, he has been fairly healthy. (Case 12: Pediatric, p. 164)

In Example 2 the reviewer is given a clear and pertinent history for this patient. The past and present medical history are described. This helps in justifying the present need for a physical therapy evaluation.

Medications. Documentation often does not include the patient's use of medications that may affect rehabilitation. It is important for the therapist to document the use of medications and any complicating effects, as reviewers may not understand them.

Example 1: A patient presents with symptoms of chronic edema of the lower extremities and the focus of treatment is to decrease edema. Medications are not mentioned in the documentation. (Case 2: Home Health, p. 83)

In Example 1 it is reasonable to expect that cardiac or pulmonary conditions exist that require the use of medications such as diuretics. In such circumstances an understanding of the medication's effect on edema control is indicated to help determine the need for skilled care.

Example 2: Diagnosis: Lumbar Degenerative disc disease/One month.

Medications: Glucophage™, Metoprolol™, Premarin™, Synthroid™, Diclofenac™ and Imipramine™. (Case 9: Outpatient—Managed Care, p. 147)

Reviewers also find medications described in an evaluation such as in Example 2. However, the list lacks significance to the reviewer. Further detail is needed for the reviewer to understand the effect the medications have on rehabilitation. For instance, Metoprolol™ is for controlling hypertension. Is blood pressure controlled, or is it a complicating factor? Are the skills of a therapist needed to monitor safe exercise parameters? Imipramine™ is an antidepressant. A reviewer may want to know the therapist's assessment of the patient's level of compliance if a home program is initiated. Providing data regarding medications can provide insight into the need for skilled care.

Comorbidities (Complicating or Precautionary Information). In many cases additional information regarding the patient's overall health and functional status is not documented. If included, the data may justify a longer period of coverage. Patients with factors such as severe shortness of breath that require continuous oxygen or patients who experience angina may be viewed as requiring skilled care because of unsafe ambulation, dizziness, and/or loss of balance. Phillippi personally saw the reversal of denials during the appeal process for COPD and CHF patients who were unsafe for nursing staff or a caregiver to ambulate because of the factors just listed. Although the initial documentation did not reflect these factors for the patients, and the safety risks, further information at the time of appeal provided evidence that skilled care was necessary. It is therefore important to provide data that justify the need for the skills of a therapist, rather than nonskilled personnel, to safely perform and instruct patients in functional activities. Example 1 demonstrates proper communication of such information. It is clear that the potential for injury exists and that the skills of a therapist are required for teaching mobility skills to the patient and caregiver.

Example 1: Per order Dr. XYZ—orthosurgeon: LLE to be protected from unusual stress. To be nonweight-bearing. 1 attendant to be responsible for protecting LLE during transfers. (Case 16: Subacute, p. 193)

This concept can be transferred in principle to every practice setting. Therapists need to provide more detail in documentation regarding any specific complication preventing a patient from progressing to a higher level of functioning. It is easy to assume that the reviewer is as familiar with the patient as the therapist. Therefore, the therapist tends to omit important items that are easily accessed from direct observation, nursing notes, and physician orders, such as the presence of a catheter, oxygen, weight bearing restrictions, or orthotic use. Omission of these items or other factors make it difficult for the reviewer to agree that initiation or extended treatment is justified.

Physical Therapy Intake/History

Reviewers find it challenging when patient identifying information such as date of birth, age, and gender is inadvertently omitted. These data, as well as the start of care date and the patient's primary complaint, help complete the patient history. The start of care date and the date of birth are also important for billing claim submission, as billing forms need to accurately correspond to the therapist's documentation of patient data. Inaccurate data may delay the processing of a claim.

Date of Birth, Age, and Gender.   These data are often accurate when provided. However, reviewers frequently find them missing. From a reviewer's perspective date of birth, age, and gender may influence rehabilitation potential. Such data help to identify the proper third-party payer such as the age for Medicare eligibility.

Date of birth is especially needed, as data retrieval is frequently based on this information. As electronic claims submissions will undoubtedly increase, with health care reform and advances in technology, accuracy of initial data entry will grow in importance.

Start of Care.   An accurate start of care date is needed. It is the basis for determining the length of coverage and the reasonableness of the duration of treatment with respect to the functional progress documented. It is also necessary for billing. Reviewers will often compare the start of care date to the onset date of the diagnosis. If there is a delay in the initiation of treatment, a reviewer may seek additional clarification. Depending on the diagnosis, a reviewer may also question any extended delay between the date of the physician referral and the start of care. If there is an unreasonable delay (i.e., weeks or months) the documentation should support the present need for skilled intervention. If this point is not documented, the question may arise that if the patient could wait for care, then is it really medically necessary?

Primary Complaint.   The patient's primary complaint is often not documented or is vague, as demonstrated in Example 1. This example of vague data lacks the location of pain and the functional deficits experienced by the patient.

Example 1: Right pain. (Case 7: Outpatient, p. 130)

As emphasis on documenting functional deficits is increasing, further attention to the patient's primary complaint needs to be considered by therapists. The patient's insight into his or her own functional deficits is needed. When documented correctly, these data provide the reviewer with insight into the patient's functional goals, barriers to progress, and the need for skilled care. In Example 2 this is adequately described.

Example 2: Both pain and dysfunction continues in hands bilaterally, but he states that there has been improvement since his last surgery. He stated that his goal is to return to work in a modified capacity as a Finish Carpenter. (Case 6: Industrial Health—Work Hardening, p. 118)

Referral Diagnosis

The establishment of the diagnosis is relevant to the reviewer for determining the patient's rehabilitation potential and need

for skilled care. Two areas for consideration are the mechanism of injury and prior diagnostic imaging/testing.

Mechanism of Injury.   Although frequently overlooked or stated vaguely by therapists, the mechanism of injury can be helpful in two ways to the reviewer. First, it may provide valuable data regarding the primary and secondary payer. For example, is the injury due to an accident or is it work-related? This is important and the reviewer will assess the appropriateness of coverage based on the plan's guidelines. Example 1 demonstrates a vague description that is not helpful to the reviewer for determining the mechanism of injury.

Example 1: Gradual onset. (Case 5: Industrial Health—Workers' Compensation, p. 110)

Second, the mechanism of injury provides valuable clinical insight into rehabilitation potential and often identifies an area of potential concern. Reviewers find it helpful to determine the need for skilled care when the mechanism of injury is documented. This is demonstrated in Example 2, where safety during transfers will need to be evaluated.

Example 2: Pt. fell at home 03-15-95 while transferring from bed to commode. (Case 16: Subacute, p. 193)

Prior Diagnostic Imaging/Testing.   Relevant data are often lacking in the area of diagnostic imaging and testing. Therapists often overlook the fact that the reviewer does not have access to this data in most circumstances. Omission of the data makes it difficult for the reviewer to determine the patient's rehabilitation potential and the medical necessity of treatment.

Example 1: X-rays were taken which indicate lumbar degenerative disc disease. (Case 9: Outpatient—Managed Care, p. 147)

In Example 1 the patient presented with complaints of low back and leg pain. The evaluation data provided indicates an x-ray was performed. This aids the reviewer in determining the patient's rehabilitation potential.

Prior Therapy History

The patient's prior therapy history for treatment of the same or a similar diagnosis is often missing or incomplete in an initial evaluation. Reviewers as well as payers want to know what types of therapeutic intervention have been received in the past, especially if it is for the same diagnosis. If a patient has been seen for physical therapy prior to the present evaluation, this needs to be noted. In addition, an explanation of the need for initiation of additional therapeutic intervention needs to be addressed in the body of the evaluation to justify treatment. Example 1 illustrates incomplete data.

Example 1: Had prior PT at ABC Care Center. (Case 14: Skilled Nursing Facility, p. 175)

In Example 1 the reviewer is unable to determine why or when the patient received prior physical therapy. Furthermore, what intervention was received and whether it was successful are unknown. If prior intervention was unsuccessful at the site of the same or a different provider of service, the reviewer may limit services, deny authorization, or ensure that another treatment approach is attempted. On the other hand, if intervention was successful, it may be authorized and an explanation for the reoccurrence/regression examined, as a change in the plan of care may be necessary to foster extended carryover.

An accurate prior therapy history containing details pertaining to function is also helpful to the reviewer in determining the need for skilled care. In situations where the patient is discharged to another location for physical therapy service, it assures the reviewer that continuity of care exists. In an environment of controlling costs, continuity is important. Example 2 illustrates a transition of skilled care to another location that is documented adequately.

Example 2: Referred to XYZ for IP rehab for deconditioning/ steroid myopathy. By D/C from IP rehab had weaned from oxygen except for night use, was ambulatory walking 250 ft behind W/C and could walk on treadmill 0.7 mph for 25 minutes. (Case 8: Outpatient, p. 138)

Example 2, although adequate, would be enhanced if the dates of service were defined and emphasis was placed on the functional deficits or barriers to independence that still exist. This approach would strengthen the justification for skilled care.

Sometimes in reviewing the medical history or patient record or in interviewing the patient, there is no evidence of previous therapy treatments. At a minimum, the therapist should document *no evidence of previous therapeutic intervention available*, or *none reported* in order to provide the reviewer with the reassurance that the area was addressed and not overlooked during the evaluation process.

Baseline Evaluation Data

From a reviewer's perspective baseline evaluation data are often inadequately described to allow future comparisons or are missing. Without an adequate foundation reviewers are unable to justify the authorization of treatment or determine future progress and medical necessity.

Cognition. Data pertaining to cognition are often lacking. Reviewers closely examine data to ensure that the patient is able to participate in an intensive skilled physical therapy program. This is especially true for patients with cognitive deficits. Documentation for patients with cognitive deficits is closely scrutinized because of the often limited ability for functional carryover of learned skills to activities of daily living. Depending on the diagnosis and the modalities performed, cognition may or may not be a factor. Example 1 is one situation where cognition is not a deterrent to the progress associated with wound healing because of caregiver availability.

Example 1: Facility: Skilled Nursing Facility

Diagnosis/onset date: L-Malleolus decubitus ulcer/12-03-96

Secondary diagnoses: S/P CVA, progressive dementia

Cognition: Alert/oriented to person; disoriented to place/time; able to follow commands; Slurred speech. Patient does not have knowledge of disability. (Case 14: Skilled Nursing Facility, p. 175)

Example 2: Oriented to person, not to place or time; alert; motivation—good; directives ability—good, follows 3 step commands. Poor short-term memory. (Case 16: Subacute, p. 193)

Cognitive deficits can be documented in a positive manner to display the patient's ability to benefit from skilled intervention. In Example 2 the therapist describes the ability to follow directions. However, poor short-term memory is documented. Although it is unclear how poor short-term memory was evaluated or the effect on functional activities and safety, the ability to participate in rehabilitation is described. The documented ability to follow commands and directives may help to determine initial coverage as the patient can participate. In this case the reviewer may limit the treatment authorization or request additional data during the course of intervention to monitor the patient's progress and rehabilitation potential. The reviewer will also consider other essential elements described in the evaluation, including the patient's prior level of function and the availability of supportive services.

Many payers establish guidelines or local medical review policies that pertain to specific diagnoses that affect cognition and limit coverage for patients with impaired cognition. Therefore, it is important, when skilled care is felt to be medically necessary for the cognitively involved patient, that the reason for the skills of a therapist be clearly described. Reviewers are finding that functional gains and anticipated carryover are not documented. As a result coverage is often limited, as the cost of obtaining the outcome is not justifiable. Reviewers tend to encourage the increased role of caregivers. Fostered are shorter durations of skilled care with more frequent evaluations to reestablish individualized programs.

Cognitive data are not needed in cases where cognition is obviously not relevant to the patient's participation in rehabilitation. This is often true for outpatient orthopedic and industrial health patients.

For patients with good cognitive ability who have a diagnosis that may affect cognition, such as the diagnosis of cerebrovascular accident, it is recommended that data be provided. Doing so assures the reviewer that cognition deficits will not affect rehabilitation.

Vision/Hearing. Reviewers find that vision and hearing deficits are not documented for most patients. This data can be relevant and may extend the duration of skilled care if the deficits affect participation in rehabilitation and/or safety. In the presence of multiple diagnoses (such as diabetes, hypertension, cerebrovascular accident) and/or when ambulation is unsafe, balance deficits exist, and safety is a concern, it is reasonable to expect baseline vision data. If visual deficits do not affect function, this should be documented as well.

Impaired hearing should also be documented. Often the skills of a therapist are required to evaluate the best approach to care, and the duration of care may be affected. For instance, does the patient respond best to physical cues in order to perform functional tasks? If so, it may be determined that teaching and training will occur at a slower rate.

Vital Signs. Reviewers find that routine clinical considerations are not documented, such as monitoring pulse rate and blood pressure. When clinically necessary, as is the case with most cardiopulmonary conditions, baseline data are relevant. The interpretation of the data require the skills of a therapist to ensure patient safety. If data are lacking at evaluation, then a reviewer is unable to make future progress comparisons.

Example 1: Oxygen saturation 87, pulse 120 at rest, dec. to 85, 119 after 3 minutes 24 seconds on treadmill at .8 mph. (Case 8: Outpatient, p. 138)

In Example 1 it is reasonable to expect additional data regarding blood pressure and respiratory rate at rest, during, and after activity. Obtaining baseline data to monitor the patient for safe performance of a functional activity would demonstrate another need for the skills of a therapist.

Example 2: Blood pressure (resting): 134/100, Target measure: 120/80. Cardiovascular MET level: 5.4. (Case 6: Industrial Health—Work Hardening, p. 118)

It is also helpful for the reviewer to be provided with a clear understanding of the resulting functional deficit. In Example 2 a consistent and understandable format is used to describe vital signs. However, a reviewer may not understand the significance of this data unless the functional deficits are described, such as the inability to perform job duties full-time.

Vascular Signs. When clinically appropriate to evaluate, vascular signs presented in documentation are often vague. Lacking most often is the location of the body part examined, as demonstrated in Examples 1 and 2.

Example 1: No discoloration noted distally. Skin in good condition other than healing incision. (Case 3: Hospital, p. 92)

Example 2: Skin appears in good condition. Circulation appears intact. (Case 4: Hospital, p. 101)

It is always helpful to demonstrate that potential complicating factors have been eliminated. In Example 2 the reviewer is able to determine that vascular signs have been addressed. This is important because if impairments exist they may affect rehabilitation. It also seems appropriate to state "Circulation *appears* intact," as often a doppler test is not used for this determination. However, it is recommended that this approach be avoided and the word *appears* not be used. Instead, documenting objectively the evaluation findings would be appropriate. For example, to provide an objective statement describing the location examined, skin color and temperature, and girth measurements or stating that the skin is intact would be more acceptable.

Sensation/Proprioception. Reviewers find that this area lacks description. The impact sensory and proprioceptive deficits have on rehabilitation is not customarily found in documentation. It is helpful to the reviewer if the effect on skilled intervention is described.

For instance, in Example 1 the documentation indicates that an ankle foot orthosis (AFO) is used and the patient has a diagnosis of a hip fracture and a cerebrovascular accident. Under these circumstances it is reasonable to evaluate sensation and proprioception because of the potential skin integrity and ambulation challenges that may exist. If deficits exist, they need to be described.

Example 1: Diagnosis: Left Femur fracture, CVA with left hemiplegia.

Sensation/proprioception: Intact pinprick right and left soles of feet; Light touch intact R and LLE, position sense intact R and L great toes.

Orthotic/prosthetic use: Uses left AFO.

(Case 17: Subacute, p. 203)

Reviewers also find that the relationship of deficits to function or the need for evaluation of sensation and proprioception is not described. What are the functional deficits or challenges to rehabilitation? In Example 1 the reviewer with a rehabilitation background may recognize the challenges diminished sensation presents to a patient wearing an AFO. However, it would be better to clearly state the effect sensation and/or proprioception have on skin integrity and gait quality, as not all reviewers may recognize the challenges.

Edema. Documentation frequently lacks description when edema is present. Reviewers find that the location of edema, circumference measurements bilaterally, whether edema is pitting or nonpitting, and the effect on function are lacking. These inadequacies are evident in Example 1.

Example 1: Edema: Moderate to maximal edema of. (Case 2: Home Health, p. 83)

Example 1 exemplifies the challenge faced by a reviewer for rendering a coverage decision when evaluation data are lacking. The description is incomplete and not measurable. The extent of involvement is unknown to the reviewer. What is *moderate* edema? How many centimeters is moderate? Where is the edema? Lastly, how does edema affect function? Without these data it is difficult for a reviewer to determine a realistic duration of treatment or the need for skilled care.

Posture. The importance of postural deficits in relationship to function is helpful in determining the need for skilled care. Reviewers find that posture is frequently not addressed or lacks description. When evaluating a patient's functional ability, posture can have a direct effect on vital signs (e.g., respiration), bed mobility, balance, transfers, ambulation, wheelchair use, and activity tolerance.

Example 1: Lies supine with LLE externally rotated. Standing—flexed hips and R knee—does not come to full standing. (Case 16: Subacute, p. 193)

Example 2: Standing posture presents with decreased weight bearing right lower extremity and flat lumbar spine. Patient is also noted to have forward head and C-curving of spine (thoracic area). Sitting posture is remarkable for C-curving of spine and sacral sitting. (Case 9: Outpatient—Managed Care, p. 147)

For instance, Example 1 describes supine and standing posture. Without knowing the patient's diagnosis, the reviewer can ascertain that posture affects standing and ambulation potential. Although the description could be enhanced for future comparisons, by including measurable terms, the functional deficit is clear. However, in Example 2 the functional relationship is unclear, yet the description of posture is more detailed. In Example 2, the description is not measurable. The lack of measurable terms will hinder the ability to demonstrate any future functional progress.

Active Range of Motion/Passive Range of Motion (AROM/ PROM).   Range of motion is commonly measured by physical therapists. However, data are frequently lacking and *do not relate to function*. In order for the reviewer to determine future improvement, baseline data are necessary. Specifically helpful are the body part measured, opposite limb measurements, the differentiation of passive and active range of motion, and the relationship to function.

Example 1: BUE and RLE WFL. L knee and ankle ROM limited approximately 50% secondary to increased edema and pain. (Case 3: Hospital, p. 92)

Example 2: WFL except left sh. abd 90°, left sh. E.R. 0°, left elbow ext. –20°, left sup. 65°, left hip flex 88°, left hip abd 10°, left knee flex 70°, Left leg length discrepancy; 5 cm. (Case 17: Subacute, p. 203)

In Example 1 specific measurements such as the degree of loss are not provided. Range of motion measurements require the skills of a qualified therapist. From a reviewer's perspective the percentage of loss indicated (i.e., approximately 50%) could by determined by nonskilled personnel. Therefore, it is important to document evidence that skilled care was provided.

In Example 1 it is also difficult for the reviewer to determine if a realistic range of motion goal is established, as opposite limb measurements and norms are not defined. Also, the documented factors of edema and pain are helpful, but the effects on function are lacking. Example 2 includes a vague description of opposite limb measurements (WFL) and demonstrates that the skills of a therapist were used to obtain specific range of motion measurements. However, once again the effect of the range of motion deficits on functional activities is not defined, nor does the reviewer know if the measurements were obtained actively or passively.

Documentation that lacks baseline data make it difficult for a reviewer to make future progress comparisons and determine the need for skilled care. For instance, are the established treatment strategies reasonable for improving range of motion? The reviewer must consider this in order to determine if the evaluation and recommended modalities are reasonable and necessary. If baseline data are lacking, then authorization of the need for skilled intervention is unlikely.

It is helpful to the reviewer if baseline data for range of motion are presented in terms of norms. Not all reviewers know the normal degree of movement. Therefore, to provide data in terms of norms, or determined target measures that will allow the patient to perform functional activities are needed. One such example is presented in Example 3.

Example 3:

Assessed area	Current measure	Target measure
ROM/Wrist Right Flexion	35°	80°
ROM/Wrist Left Flexion	30°	80°
ROM/Wrist Right Extension	35°	70°
ROM/Wrist Left Extension	30°	70°
ROM/Wrist Right Ulnar Deviation	20°	30°
ROM/Wrist Left Ulnar Deviation	20°	30°
ROM/Wrist Right Radial Deviation	25°	20°
ROM/Wrist Left Radial Deviation	15°	20°

(Case 6: Industrial Health—Work Hardening, p. 118)

Example 3 clearly presents an organized list of range of motion, and the reviewer is able to understand the degree of loss. Once again, though, passive and active range of motion are not differentiated, nor is the degree of loss related to function, which puts the reviewer at a disadvantage.

Strength.   Documentation regarding strength tends to lack data for determining the need for skilled care. Reviewers find general observations rather than skilled descriptions reflecting that manual muscle testing was performed. The relationship of the muscle grade to a functional deficit is often lacking as well. These inadequacies are demonstrated in Example 1. However, Example 1 does provide the reviewer with the grade in terms of the norm (i.e., 3+/5). Documenting the normative value helps reviewers who are unfamiliar with the grading scale to understand the amount of loss.

Example 1: General strength is at a 3+/5 level. (Case 1: Home Health, p. 74)

Reviewers find it helpful to demonstrate the skilled aspect of the testing. Documentation that manual muscle testing was performed and an objective summary of the pertinent findings are helpful. Reviewers are often frustrated by large quantities of unnecessary data that are not clearly presented. A description of the necessary objective findings that are pertinent to the reason for rehabilitation is welcomed for future progress comparisons. The relationship of strength deficits to function is also needed.

Pain.   Pain is often a factor in determining the need for skilled care. A description of the pain scale used, the location of pain, and its effect on function are needed. However, reviewers find that not all of these components are described in evaluations. In fact, as in Example 1, pain is often vaguely described and therefore is not helpful in determining the need for skilled care.

Example 1: Patient has consistent c/o LLE pain and edema. (Case 3: Hospital, p. 92)

Example 2: Pain: 10 on a 0 to 10 scale. Activities that increase pain include upper extremity activities, work, repetitive lifting and reaching. Pain decreases after patient rests for 15 minutes. Pain more severe during work and after activity. (Case 5: Industrial Health—Workers' Compensation, p. 110)

In Example 1 the reviewer does not know the influence pain has on function, nor is the severity of the pain known. The reviewer will therefore have difficulty determining if pain has diminished in future reports because of the limited data. In Example 2, data are measurable and allow for future comparison. The functional relationship is also clear, and only the location of pain is lacking.

Coordination. The relationship of deficits in coordination to the safe and efficient performance of functional activities is often lacking in documentation from a reviewer's perspective. When clinically applicable, documentation of coordination should be functional and measurable.

Example 1: Gross/Fine: R = G. L = 0. (Case 15: Skilled Nursing Facility, p. 184)

Example 2: He demonstrates "Parkinson's" type problems with initiation of activity. Movement is rigid and jerky. (Case 1: Home Health, p. 74)

In Example 1 data are vague and lack description. The reviewer may not understand what good (G) coordination entails. Is it coordination of the upper or lower extremities? How does a lack of coordination affect function? Example 2 provides more description; however, the reviewer does not know the impact on safety or function. What activity is the therapist referring to? Are the activities performed with the upper extremities or lower extremities? What are the "Parkinson's type problems?"

Reviewers may not be familiar with how coordination can affect mobility. That relationship must be documented in an objective way so that progress can be monitored. To describe coordination in terms of safety and function is helpful.

Bed Mobility. Reviewers find that documentation pertaining to bed mobility frequently lacks measurable and descriptive data. It is important to describe the amount of assistance and verbal cuing to complete bed mobility safely. This is helpful to determine the need for skilled care. The data are also necessary for future progress comparisons.

Example 1: Requires assist for bed mobility. (Case 4: Hospital, p. 101)

Example 2: Rolling R/L, moving sideways and bridging requires Max A; Sit to/from supine requires Max A. (Case 14: Skilled Nursing Facility, p. 175)

In Example 1 the description of bed mobility is vague and not measurable. A reviewer needs to know and understand how much assistance the patient requires and what is contributing to the loss of mobility. Documentation to answer these questions will help justify the need for evaluation and subsequent treatment.

Example 2 provides baseline data for the amount of assistance. However, it does not provide insight into the potential cause of immobility (e.g., pain, range of motion limitations) or complications that may arise (i.e., skin breakdown, contractures). These relationships are often lacking. They are especially necessary when the reviewer is not familiar with rehabilitation.

Balance (Sit and Stand). From a reviewer's perspective, balance deficits are relevant to the patient's rehabilitation potential. Descriptions are reasonably expected when cognition, vision, posture, ambulation, or transfers are a problem. Commonly reviewers find this area is not addressed or vague data are provided.

Example 1: Requires minimal/moderate assistance for balance. (Case 1: Home Health, p. 74)

Example 1 demonstrates a vague description. Although the documentation is measurable, further data are need to help the reviewer determine the need for skilled care. How does the loss of balance affect safety? When does balance loss occur and in what direction? For instance, patients may exhibit balance deficits without an assistive device on elevated or uneven surfaces, yet may be independent in the community with a device.

For patients with a high level of functioning (i.e., contact guard assist, supervision, independent) the reviewer will look for why the skills of a therapist are needed. If the patient is functioning at a high level or is free of falls, then goals to improve balance alone may be deemed unnecessary. It is important that the functional outcome be considered and the deficits documented.

Transfers. There are many types of transfers that may be described in documentation. Reviewers find that evaluation data may lack the type of transfer, amount of physical assistance, verbal cuing needed for safety, and posture during the transfer. Reviewers look for the need for skilled teaching and training, complicating factors, and safety issues. To demonstrate skilled intervention for transfer training, the documentation needs to reflect that the skills of a therapist rather than nonskilled personnel are needed. Examples 1 and 2 provide insight into transfer descriptions.

Example 1: Mr. ABC requires assist for transfers and gait. Patient relates 90% independence for ADL's. (Case 3: Hospital, p. 92)

Example 2: Max. assist of 3. (2 assists for sliding board transfer plus 1 assist to support and align LLE, bed to and from w/c.) (Case 16: Subacute, p. 194)

In Example 1 the documentation lacks measurability and complicating factors that demonstrate the need for skilled care. The description is vague and does not allow for future progress comparisons. A statement describing the level of assistance and the activities of daily living that are limited is needed.

Transfers are better described in the evaluation data presented in Example 2. This description includes the level of assistance and alludes to concerns regarding lower extremity alignment. From a reviewer's perspective the need for teaching and training is evident.

Ambulation (Level and Elevated Surfaces). Evaluation data pertaining to ambulation are important. Reviewers find that gait descriptions are lacking in measurability for future comparisons. Often the type of assistive device, use of an orthotic or prosthetic device, weight bearing restrictions, ambulation distance, gait quality, and safety issues are missing.

Example 1: He does not come to stand independently, but requires moderate assistance with this movement. He attempts to use his right UE for major weight bearing assistance when in the upright position. Can stand independently for brief periods by using his right hand on the parallel bars. The major impediment to standing is knee flexion contracture of about 60 degrees bilaterally. (Case 11: Pediatric, p. 155)

To establish the need for skilled care, evaluation data must describe the deficits that exist. Gait analysis is skilled. In Example 1 the skills of a therapist are evident in obtaining the data for future comparison. Only the data, "Can stand for brief periods. . ." should be specified with a defined time frame.

If data pertaining to gait analysis are lacking, then the skills of a therapist may be viewed as unnecessary. This is demonstrated in Example 2.

Example 2: WBAT with 2 crutches. (Case 7: Outpatient, p. 130)

In Example 2 the need for skilled care is not described. A reviewer could reasonably determine that the patient is functional. These data would be enhanced if they included a description of the gait deficits, ambulation distance, the amount of assistance needed (if any), complicating factors such as pain, and/or the patient's ability to safely negotiate stairs/elevated surfaces.

Orthotic/Prosthetic Devices. Reviewers are often concerned regarding duplication and overbilling of services for orthotic or prosthetic devices. Reviewers find it helpful if the need for the device and the specific role of the therapist in the process (e.g., gait training) are defined in the evaluation.

Example 1: Diagnosis: Torn medial/lateral meniscus and ACL/ 05-25-96

Medical history: Surgery 06-23-96. Underwent arthroscopic repair to the meniscus and ACL.

(Case 7: Outpatient, p. 130)

Reviewers find that orthotic and prosthetic devices may be present but are not documented. In Example 1 the patient presents with a diagnosis of a torn medial/lateral meniscus and ACL. The medical history indicates that surgery was performed. However, an orthotic device is not mentioned. In this case it is reasonable to expect that with this type of surgery a brace is used. The presence of the device would be evidence to the reviewer of joint instability and therefore would reinforce the need for skilled care.

Wheelchair Use. The patient's ability to safely negotiate in his or her living environment and community is important to a reviewer. Reviewers often find that baseline data regarding wheelchair or scooter use are lacking. Frequently missing are data pertaining to the type of wheelchair, special adaptation/ seating systems, ability to propel, amount of physical and verbal assistance, safety factors, and functional limitations.

Example 1: Unable. (Case 2: Home Health, p. 83)

Example 2: W/C position: Head control—forward flexion; Trunk control—leans left, but mostly forward; has lap buddy which prevents severe forward flexion. (Case 14: Skilled Nursing Facility, p. 175)

In Example 1 the reviewer is provided with no data. The term "Unable" does not provide insight into the reason for limited wheelchair use. In this case the reviewer may find it helpful to know why the patient is unable to use the wheelchair. Also, do the data provided mean that the patient is unable to propel the wheelchair, or that the patient is unable to be positioned in it? Further description would help justify the evaluation and possible need for skilled care.

Unlike Example 1, the documentation provided in Example 2 describes the patient's wheelchair positioning. However, whether the patient can propel the wheelchair is unclear, and how positioning affects functional activities is not included.

Wheelchair evaluations may be scrutinized depending on the practice setting and payer. Often reviewers will determine if the skills of a therapist are needed or those of a vendor. Generally the therapist's role involves facilitating improvement in range of motion, strength, and muscle tone to allow proper wheelchair positioning with a goal of improving function. Reviewers will seek to ensure that duplication of service is avoided. Therefore, proper documentation in the plan of care and/or assessment is important.

Durable Medical Equipment (DME) (Used or Required). Reviewers find that documentation regarding DME is often lacking. Although not always provided for in a separate area, DME use needs to be listed. Reviewers want to know that the equipment is used safely. Evaluation data describing safety deficits or the need for equipment are another indication of the need for skilled care. One example of an oversight is failure to document patient use of a wheelchair. Another may be the omission that the patient owns and/or uses an assistive device such as a standard walker, cane, and/or hemiwalker.

Activity Tolerance. Activity tolerance is the functional way to document endurance. Reviewers find that endurance is often improved during normal activities. Therefore, endurance building does not require the skills of a therapist under normal circumstances. With this in mind, it is helpful to view endurance as activity tolerance.

Baseline data for activity tolerance is best incorporated into functional activities. Example 1 provides a functional description of a patient's limited activity tolerance for a reviewer. The functional deficits are presented and reinforce the need for skilled care.

Example 1: Patient states she cannot tolerate walking upright and needs to walk slightly bent over for relief. Patient states she has difficulty with ADL activities, such as making dinner. Patient states she cannot tolerate reaching overhead into cupboards to make dinner. Patient also has difficulty straightening up to take a shower. Patient states she can only walk a short distance (approximately 80 feet) before she has to sit and relax. Patient states she can only grocery shop if she leans forward onto cart. (Case 9: Outpatient—Managed Care, p. 147)

Reviewers frequently find statements regarding activity tolerance that do not relate to a functional activity, as in Example 2.

Example 2: Standing endurance 10 sec. (Case 16: Subacute, p. 194)

In Example 2 the reviewer would not know whether standing is important as a functional activity. Is ambulation important or is the patient wheelchair dependent? Is standing tolerance important for transfers or grooming? The functional significance is unknown to the reviewer without additional baseline data. Example 2 could be improved by stating *in preparation for gait training.*

Wound Description, Including Incision Status. Baseline data for wounds and incisions are essential for future progress comparisons. Reviewers often find that the evaluation data are brief. As a healing incision site may affect functional progress, it is important that the size of the incision and its status be documented as in Example 1.

Example 1: Patient presents with healing incision approximately 15 inches in length over the medial aspect of the lower extremity approximately mid-thigh to distal knee. (Case 3: Hospital, p. 92)

In regard to wounds, it is essential that a thorough description be given for the reviewer to determine the need for skilled care. Example 2 demonstrates a detailed account of baseline data that will allow for future progress comparisons.

Example 2: Wound evaluation: L-lateral malleolus Stage IV, oblong in shape 2.6 cm inferior–superior x 1.9 cm, depth at anterior border 0.3 cm at midpoint with tunneling and green drainage; Depth at posterior border 0.1 cm, at superior border 0.2 cm, at middle of ulcer 0 depth. 25% of wound inferior aspect meaty red tissue, remaining of ulcer marbleized w/green-ish yellow necrotic tissue (10% of red/pink tissue). No odor noted. Drainage on dressing noted with slightly brownish red drainage at inferior aspect and dime-size amount of greenish drainage. Inflamed pink area around periphery approximately 1 cm; Wound debrided to 50% clean; Foot purplish with decreased circulation; Appeared to be Stage IV inflammatory stage. (Case 14: Skilled Nursing Facility, p. 175)

Depending on the payer guidelines the reviewer will determine whether the size and/or stage of the wound meets the payer's coverage criteria. Also, the reviewer may determine if treatment was performed at the time of evaluation and if it is properly documented. If not, payment for treatment on the day of evaluation may be denied because of insufficient documentation.

The reviewer will also review the treatment strategies defined in the plan of care to ensure that they meet coverage criteria. Experimental treatments or methods not defined in the standards of practice for wound healing are not covered by most payers.

Special Tests. Special tests are frequently performed by therapists during the evaluation process. When these tests are used, reviewers often find that the clinical relevance is not explained. As reviewers may not understand the need for special tests, it is important to document the reason for testing and the significance of the testing results. For the reviewer, data pertaining to relevant special tests reinforce the need for a qualified physical therapist.

Architectural/Safety Considerations. Emphasis on return to home is always a common patient goal. Despite this emphasis, reviewers find that architectural barriers and safety issues are not addressed at the time of evaluation. At a minimum, reviewers hope to find documentation pertaining to a discussion with the patient, family, or caregiver regarding architectural barriers in order to help establish goals that will foster safe return to home.

Baseline data regarding architectural considerations provide the reviewer with insight into the patient's functional limitations and the need for skilled intervention. Example 1 demonstrates helpful data in the review process.

Example 1: Lives in 1 story home with 1 step at entrance. (Case 16: Subacute, p. 194)

Requirements to Return to Home, School, and/or Job. Reviewers are unable to determine if skilled care is reasonable when the requirements to return to home, school, and/or job are not defined. Often the data are not included in an evaluation. When the data are described, as in Example 1, the reviewer can determine the need for skilled care, if the long-term goal is realistic, and can later identify an appropriate duration of treatment based on the functional progress reported.

Example 1: Daughter can assist Pt. with transfer and amb. (no lifting) post. discharge. (Case 16: Subacute, p. 194)

Prior Level of Function

Prior level of function is one area reviewers find lacking or vaguely stated. The reviewer and payer need to know the status of the patient prior to injury, or the onset of the exacerbation or disease/disability. Without these data the reviewer is unable to determine if the plan of care is realistic. The prior level of function may be specific to mobility (home and community), employment, and/or school.

Mobility (Home and Community).   Reviewers find that the prior level of function does not reflect the presence or amount of caregiver support, adaptive equipment, and/or community supportive services that patients require. The goal of most payer sources is to return the patient to the level of function prior to illness or to achieve maximal functional ability based on the patient's diagnosis. If the therapist is specific in describing the prior level at the time of the evaluation, the reviewer will be able to assess the progress, direction, and appropriateness of the treatment plan.

Example 1: Was independent in driving, cooking, active/social outings. (Case 8: Outpatient, p. 138)

Example 2: Pt. lived with 91 yr. old husband and daughter. Ambulated with walker indep. level surfaces. Negotiated steps with rail and SBA. (Case 16: Subacute, p. 194)

In Example 1 the prior level of function is documented; however, it is not related specifically to the provision of physical therapy service. Many patients are independent in driving, cooking, and active in social outings. These data are not helpful to the reviewer as they are not specific to the reason for physical therapy treatment. More specific documentation is presented in Example 2. This description is specific to functional areas (e.g., ambulation, stair climbing) that often require skilled teaching and training.

Employment.   Prior level of function pertaining to employment is often found by reviewers to be vaguely stated as in Example 1. Example 1 does not provide the reviewer with the functional duties previously performed. This makes it difficult to determine if the plan of care and goals are reasonable.

Example 1: ABC Electronics. Off of work. (Case 5: Industrial Health—Workers' Compensation, p. 110)

Reviewers look for an accurate and specific description of the patient's functional abilities prior to the onset of injury. As payers frequently do not know the employment status of the patient during treatment, it is important to include this information. Also, it may assist in the appeal process.

School.   Reviewers find that the prior level of function does not incorporate the child's ability to participate in all areas of the educational experience. Often documentation does not address mobility, self-help, and play skills. It is important for the reviewer to understand the level of independence in the school environment. Expectations are to achieve age-appropriate skills or to maximize function based on the patient's diagnosis.

Example 1: Gross motor skills are at the 11 to 12 month level. (Case 13: Pediatric—Individualized Education Program, p. 173)

In Example 1 the present level of gross motor skills is reported in terms of months. These data do not provide the reviewer with information regarding functional deficits that may affect educational performance. However, documentation that includes functional terms, such as that presented in Example 2, provides a clear picture to the reviewer of the patient's mobility levels.

Example 2: Gross motor skills are at the 11 to 12 month level. Patient sits in and transitions out of a variety of positions independently on the floor. The patient crawls independently and can pull up to standing on a stable object. The patient walks holding on to objects or with one hand held for 400–500 feet. (Case 13: Pediatric—Individualized Education Program Worksheet, p. 173)

Treatment Diagnosis

The treatment diagnosis reflects what is actually being treated. It may be different from the diagnosis. When documentation is reviewed, the treatment diagnosis is often missing or vague. Example 1 demonstrates a vague treatment diagnosis.

Example 1: Pain and instability. (Case 9: Outpatient—Managed Care, p. 147)

In Example 1 the location of pain and where joint instability are occurring are lacking. It is helpful for the reviewer to determine the need for skilled care when the treatment diagnosis is specified. This is especially helpful when the patient has multiple diagnoses that may affect rehabilitation.

Example 2 demonstrates an appropriate treatment diagnosis.

Example 2: Diagnosis/onset date: COPD exacerbation/04-07-95.

Treatment diagnosis: Decreased functional activity. (Case 8: Outpatient, p. 138)

In Example 2 the diagnosis is COPD exacerbation. As this diagnosis is the medical reason for skilled care, it is primary. However, the patient treatment diagnosis, decreased functional activity, is the diagnosis for which physical therapy services are rendered.

Assessment

The therapist's clinical impressions of the patient at evaluation are helpful to the reviewer for determining the reason for skilled care. Frequently, expectation statements, which help justify the need for treatment, are lacking.

Reason for Skilled Care.   Reviewers find that it is important at the time of the evaluation to provide expectation statements.

Expectation statements reflect the personal judgment of the therapist in regard to the patient's potential to respond to therapeutic intervention. Specifically, that the therapist believes the treatment strategies chosen will improve the patient's ability to function. By using expectation statements, the therapist enhances the reviewer's ability to discern the appropriateness of physical therapy intervention.

Often the therapist's insight into the patient's functional limitations and expectations for improvement is missing or inadequate. If absent, the reviewer is left to decide whether skilled intervention is required. For example, has skilled intervention been helpful in the past and could a similar outcome be expected? Why are the skills of a therapist required rather than those of nonskilled personnel?

Example 1: In summary, patient appears to be a good candidate for skilled P.T. services with emphasis on closure of wound and prevention of additional skin breakdown; will continue with whirlpool to increase circulation. (Case 14: Skilled Nursing Facility, p. 175)

In Example 1 the reason for skilled care could be more effectively stated by focusing on why the skills of a therapist are needed, what risk factors are present that may affect healing, and what outcome is expected.

Example 2: Fair progress. Improved use of arm. Decreased pain. Increased function. Slow improvement. Progress limited by the number of PT visits. (Case 10: Outpatient—Managed Care, p. 152)

All too often the reviewer will not have an adequate picture of what the overall expectations or outcomes from therapy will be. Descriptions are frequently found to be inadequate, as in Example 2, and are not objectively based. They may not describe the patient's functional deficits and need for skilled care. As a result, it is challenging for the reviewer to approve treatment. Therefore, it is important to define why the skills of a therapist are needed to justify skilled intervention.

Problems

It is helpful to determine the patient's problems in order to focus treatment. Each problem identified should correspond to a subsequent short-term goal. Often reviewers find that the problems are not listed or are vaguely stated. This makes it difficult to determine the appropriateness of goals and treatment strategies. Reviewers find it helpful when the problems are clearly identified.

Example 1:

1. *Reduced balance with walking.*
2. *Reduced strength.*
3. *Stiffness.*

(Case 1: Home Health, p. 74)

In Example 1 three problems are identified. Problem 1 relates the balance deficit to function (walking). This functional relationship is helpful to the reviewer. Problem 2 lists the deficit without identifying a location or a functional relationship. This problem is not optimally stated. However, Problem 3, "Stiffness," is vague.

Another common deficit in documentation is that the problems established are not justified with baseline data. In Case 5 (Industrial Health—Workers' Compensation, p. 110) this is evident. The problems identified include descriptions that pain exists and that palpation was performed and tenderness reported. However, objective data are not present to substantiate these conclusions. Therefore, how can the problems exist?

It is important to focus treatment through the establishment of a problem list, as reviewers will frequently determine whether the problems identified are justified in relationship to the baseline data presented. Although multiple problems may exist for many patients, it is important to determine those of highest priority. Specifically, which problems have the highest impact on function? A maximum of five problems are recommended in order to focus treatment.

Plan of Care

There are eight areas in the plan of care that reviewers find important. They provide the reviewer with the therapist's insight into what is needed for a successful functional outcome. These areas include specific treatment strategies, frequency, duration, patient instruction/home program, caregiver training, short-term goals and achievement dates, long-term goals and achievement dates, and rehabilitation potential.

Specific Treatment Strategies. The specific treatment strategies (i.e., procedures and modalities) are important to a reviewer. The reviewer will determine whether the strategies chosen are effective for treatment of the diagnosis or diagnoses provided and whether they are within the coverage guidelines of the payer. In general, the reviewer will not evaluate the therapist's choice among one or more appropriate strategies. However, experimental or unproven strategies will customarily be denied.

Reviewers often find undefined modalities. This is a concern to the reviewer who wants to know what is specifically needed to achieve a functional outcome. Reviewers also find that it is helpful when the rationale for use is provided.

Example 1:

1. *Modalities as needed for pain and swelling.*
2. *NMES to right quad to increase quad contraction.*
3. *Therapeutic activity/exercise to increase ROM, strength.*
4. *HEP.*

(Case 7: Outpatient, p. 130)

In Example 1 the reviewer is provided with the relationship between the treatment strategies selected and the patient's physical limitations. This rationale is helpful, especially for reviewers who may be unfamiliar with rehabilitation. However, to indicate "Modalities as needed . . ." is not acceptable (Example 1, number 1). It is common for therapists to provide general statements such as this rather than specifically listing each modality. The reviewer wants to know the purpose of each modality, and if more than one is utilized, the need for multiple modalities must be justified.

The treatment strategies provide the reviewer with information to help determine the appropriateness of intervention. Reviewers find that use of a single modality is usually nonskilled or inappropriate. For example, listing hot packs as the only strategy may be viewed as nonskilled, as it could be applied independently by the patient. To be skilled, and considered for coverage, another treatment strategy such as exercise or home program instruction needs to be included. Also, why the skills of a therapist are needed for safe application should be documented. The authors recognize that circumstances do exist that allow for coverage of one modality. However, it is always important from a reviewer's perspective to closely analyze the need for additional strategies to facilitate functional carryover.

Reviewers expect that treatment strategies will be listed in the evaluation and that they correspond to the services billed. Example 2 is an adequate list of treatment strategies, although they could be enhanced if the relationship to function was described.

Example 2: Patient to be seen for LLE ROM, strengthening, transfer and gait training with walker. Instruction in a HEP. (Case 3: Hospital, p. 92)

Depending on the payer's guidelines, reviewers may determine if the plan of care (i.e., primarily the treatment strategies, frequency, duration, and goals) has been approved by a physician. Certain payers will only reimburse for those services approved by a physician. If this is the case, documentation must reflect an accurate list of treatment strategies and demonstrate that the physician's signature was obtained. The process for achieving the physician's approval may vary depending on the payer. Example 3 demonstrates a direct relationship between the specific treatment requested by the physician and treatment strategies established by the therapist. This assures the reviewer of proper physician approval. If additions to the treatment strategies existed, the reviewer might seek clarification of the physician's involvement.

Example 3: Specific treatment requested: PT to see patient 2x/ wk for 2 wks for gait and balance training and to resume home exercise program.

Specific treatment strategies: PT for gait and transfer training and resumption of home exercise program.

(Case 1: Home Health, p. 74)

In conjunction with establishing the appropriateness of the treatment strategies, the reviewer will determine the reasonableness of the frequency and duration.

Frequency.   The frequency of treatment is important to the reviewer. There are no set frequency standards for diagnoses or patient groups. This is largely left to the discretion of the thera-

pist and physician. Certainly the severity of the functional decline and the deficits the patient exhibits will affect the determination of the frequency. However, regardless of the patient's level of disability, realistic frequencies need to be determined by the anticipated progress, by how much can be taught as a home program, and by the constraints imposed by the third-party payer. These limitations can be policy guidelines or prospective approval of visits allowed.

Reviewers often have trouble determining the patient's treatment needs when the frequency presented is variable, as demonstrated in Example 1.

Example 1: 6x/wk, 7 as tolerated. (Case 16: Subacute, p. 194)

When the frequency is variable, a reviewer may question whether the service is reasonable and necessary. In this example, does the patient need intervention six or seven times a week to achieve the stated goals?

The reviewer will also consider if the frequency established is reasonable and necessary based on the patient's expected improvement. Documentation in areas such as the diagnosis, history, and rehabilitation potential help in determining an appropriate frequency. Considerations must include the long-term impact of rehabilitation on health care costs. For example, would it be more cost-effective for the patient to receive more frequent intervention (five times or more per week) for a shorter duration or less frequent intervention (three times or less per week) for a longer duration? What are the long-term benefits of rehabilitation? Although these and other related questions are not easily answered, payers and providers seek data to ensure cost-effective care delivery through outcome studies. Therefore, the duration of service is equally important.

Duration.   In addition to the frequency, the duration of therapy receives especially close scrutiny from the reviewer. Often, vague or excessive durations are found by reviewers. At times, durations are even missing.

Example 1: Hospitalization. (Case 3: Hospital, p. 92)

Example 1 demonstrates a vaguely documented duration. The reviewer would be unable to determine the amount of therapy needed to achieve the established goals. Therefore, it is important to indicate the estimated duration in terms of days, weeks, or a number of visits. The duration should be nonvariable. Example 2 demonstrates an appropriately written duration.

Example 2: 4 weeks. (Case 7: Outpatient, p. 130)

Too often reviewers find what is referred to as the "until death do us part" duration. Example 3 demonstrates one such example.

Example 3: Indefinite. (Case 2: Home Health, p. 83)

It is unrealistic to expect a payer to cover the cost of a skilled rehabilitation program indefinitely. Although Example 3 is an extreme example, reviewers find that therapists do not provide enough focus on carryover of learned activities, and therefore durations may be considered excessive at times. As changes continue in the health care industry, emphasis will remain on providing skilled care for short durations. Indeed, the patient's progress, complicating factors, and diagnosis all affect decisions regarding duration. Therefore, a realistic duration, justified through objective data, must be established.

Patient Instruction/Home Program. Frequently reviewers find that home program instruction and/or restorative nursing recommendations are not initiated at the time of evaluation. As payers are interested in controlling costs, patients' involvement in their own wellness becomes important. Patients must be actively involved in their own wellness through education. With the focus on self-management, reviewers find that initiation of a home program and patient instruction are important components of treatment and should be initiated at the time of evaluation.

Documentation pertaining to the initiation of a home program and the relevance of the exercises to improving function needs to be described. If these details are lacking, the reviewer may not understand the functional importance for the patient.

Example 1: Instructed in towel roll. (Case 5: Industrial Health—Workers' Compensation, p. 110)

In Example 1 home programming is initiated and the therapist describes an activity involving a towel roll. However, the significance of that activity is not described. It is reasonable to expect that most reviewers may not understand the need for this exercise.

Example 2: Restorative nursing recommendations: Will need to provide Max assist w/all functional mobility, but encourage him to assist. Reposition every two hours to retain skin integrity. (Case 15: Skilled Nursing Facility, p. 184)

In Example 2 recommendations are established to foster carryover from rehabilitation. In this case the reviewer can ascertain that nursing involvement will help in practicing functional skills learned in rehabilitation, and the significance of the activities is known. The other essential element that justifies skilled care, and is related to home programming, is training the caregiver.

Caregiver Training. The one area most commonly omitted in documentation is evidence of family, patient, caregiver, nursing, and employer training. This is true regardless of the patient care setting, clientele seen, or diagnosis being treated. Often there is no mention as to what, if any, training was performed. This is crucial in justifying the reason for skilled care.

The other finding is that although training may be mentioned, there is no indication that training was actually performed. This is clear in Example 1.

Example 1: Patient positioning in bed and chair will be discussed with nursing. (Case 4: Hospital, p. 101)

In Example 1 the reviewer does not know who specifically will be trained (e.g., certified nursing assistants, licensed nurses,

or registered nurses), when or if they were actually trained, and what positioning needs were addressed. If training is not properly documented, the reviewer assumes it was not done, and another justification of the need for skilled care is lacking in the evaluation. It is important to document that caregiver training has occurred.

Short-Term Goals and Achievement Dates. Reviewers are often challenged by poor goal writing. Short-term goals often lack one or more of the three necessary components (i.e., measurable, functional, and time specific), are not justified with baseline data, and do not relate to the problems identified in an organized manner.

Example 1:

Problems:
1. Patient is dependent on scooter.
2. Spared quadriplegic.
3. Dependent edema of both lower extremities.

Short-term goals and achievement dates:
1. Decrease edema of lower extremities.
2. Increase mus. activities of lower extremities.
3. Increase circulation of lower extremities.

(Case 2: Home Health, p. 83)

Reviewers are frequently frustrated with goals such as those provided in Example 1. The short-term goals in Example 1 are lacking all goal components. The goals do not correspond to the order of the problems and, as the reader will find in Case 2 (Home Health, p. 83), baseline data are lacking to objectively justify the problems and goals listed.

Another problem occasionally seen at the time of evaluation is that the goals established may not be realistically achieved within the time frame specified or are more appropriate for the long-term goal area. For instance, it would not be appropriate to establish a short-term goal that states *will be independent with pivot transfer in two weeks* when the patient presents with a hip fracture that requires maximal assistance of two for transferring safely and the anticipated duration of treatment is eight weeks. It is always better to establish short-term goals in the evaluation that can be achieved in a short duration and then upgrade goals in future reports to demonstrate functional progress.

Reviewers expect goals to be properly written. If the therapist does not document what will be achieved, then why would the payer want to reimburse the provider for the services rendered? As goals are a very important part of documentation success, the reader is encouraged to refer to the case studies presented in Chapter 4 for additional goal examples.

Long-Term Goals and Achievement Dates. Reviewers do not customarily expect a long-term goal for every short-term goal established. Instead, they find it helpful when a statement containing measurable and functional components is provided. (The reader is reminded that a time frame is encouraged. However, reviewers will usually infer that the duration is the estimated achievement date.) An appropriate long-term goal is provided in Example 1.

Example 1: Return to work as a Finish Carpenter with defined return-to-work guidelines. (Case 6: Industrial Health—Work Hardening, p. 122)

Unfortunately, reviewers find that the long-term goal often is vague and lacks goal components, as in Example 2.

Example 2: Facilitate better tissue length and muscle strength to enhance development. (Case 12: Pediatric, p. 165)

In Example 2 the reviewer does not have a clear picture of what development is or how it is being enhanced. The goal lacks measurability. Therefore, how would the reviewer know when it is achieved? It is important that the long-term goal be measurable and functional.

Rehabilitation Potential. Reviewers find that rehabilitation potential is often missing in documentation. It is important to indicate the rehabilitation potential, as it helps in assessing the reasonableness of care. It is commonly indicated as a one-word response such as *excellent*, *good*, *fair*, or *poor*. Reviewers consider many essential elements in documentation for determining a patient's rehabilitation potential. The patient's potential for achieving the established goals influences the frequency and duration of treatment approved by the reviewer.

Essential Elements Lacking in a Progress Report

Attendance

Documenting attendance reflects the patient's compliance and participation in rehabilitation. It is helpful to the reviewer in several ways. First, it helps identify barriers to progress that may require an extended treatment duration. For example, an extended illness may impede functional progress. Second, it allows the reviewer to compare dates of service (or the number of visits) with the dates of service (or number of visits) submitted to the third-party payer for accuracy.

Often reviewers find that attendance is missing in documentation or is vaguely stated, as in Example 1.

Example 1: Good. (Case 7: Outpatient, p. 134)

It is helpful when attendance includes the number of visits scheduled and any reasons for absence.

Example 2: Mr. ABC was seen daily 12-05-95 and 12-06-95 for gentle range of motion, transfer training, gait training and home exercise program instruction. Mr. ABC was evaluated 12-05-95 and was discharged 12-06-95. (Case 3: Hospital, p. 97)

Example 2 provides a thorough description of attendance. Although the treatment strategies described are helpful in the review process, they are not required elements for attendance from a reviewer's perspective.

Current Baseline Data

The reviewer expects baseline data for the essential elements of documentation that affect the patient's ability to achieve a functional outcome. From a reviewer's perspective, comparative data related to function are needed to demonstrate the need for skilled care. What is found are that comparative data, objective measurements, the functional deficits of the patient, and the functional outcomes of treatment interventions are often lacking.

Readers should note that the reviewer findings presented for the essential elements in current baseline data for a progress report are the same as for a discharge report. The only notable exception is that the comparative data presented in a discharge report should include comparisons since the last formal report *and* from the start of care. With this in mind, examples that are used may be from either progress report or discharge report data found in the case studies presented in Chapter 4.

Cognition. Cognition is often not addressed in progress reports. However, when cognitive deficits are identified in an evaluation, it is important to document for the reviewer any changes in cognition that may affect safety and participation in rehabilitation. The reviewer often is unable to determine the reasonableness of skilled care when data are not provided and may question if the patient can achieve the established goals.

Vision/Hearing. The reviewer finds that vision and hearing are often not addressed in documentation. This may be a concern, especially when balance and safety issues are identified. Any deficits in vision and hearing that may affect rehabilitation need to be documented. Vision and hearing deficits may provide another reason for skilled care.

Vital Signs. Vital signs such as respirations per minute, pulse rate, and blood pressure are often not applicable or lacking in documentation. Reviewers can reasonably expect data in the presence of cardiopulmonary diagnoses. If vital signs are monitored during therapy intervention to ensure the patient's safety, this would reinforce the need for the skills of a therapist and should be documented.

When applicable, the data presented should be in comparative form and related to function.

Example 1: Performs at 7.6 METS. (Case 6: Industrial Health—Work Hardening, p. 126)

In Example 1, data are provided; however, the functional importance may not be understood by the reviewer and comparative data are lacking. What can the patient do now that he or she could not do before? This needs to be stated to demonstrate functional progress and the need for skilled care.

Vascular Signs. Data pertaining to vascular signs and their effect on function are expected by the reviewer when clinically applicable. What is commonly found is that this area is not addressed when it could help in justifying the need for skilled care. For example, when a short-term goal is established relating to improving circulation, it is reasonable to expect comparative data (Case 2: Home Health, pp. 83–91).

Data pertaining to vascular signs such as girth measurements, skin color, and skin temperature help the reviewer to understand the complications experienced by the patient. Documented improvements reinforce the benefits from intervention. Conversely, regressions may justify the need for continued skilled care or the need to evaluate the use of alternative treatment strategies.

Sensation/Proprioception.   Reviewers find that sensation and proprioception are frequently not addressed or are vaguely stated. Data in this area are often helpful in identifying potential challenges to rehabilitation and reinforce the need for skilled intervention. For instance, neglect of an extremity, diminished sensation, or tactile defensiveness may have a direct effect on patient function. Teaching and training to ensure patient safety is skilled service. Insight into sensation and proprioceptive deficits and their relevance in terms of function and safety help the reviewer understand the need for skilled care.

Vague data for sensation and proprioception that lack comparatives are often found by reviewers, as demonstrated in Example 1.

Example 1: Intact. (Case 7: Outpatient, p. 134)

It is important to provide comparative data for the reviewer. In Example 1 the reviewer would need to search through the documentation provided to know the patient's previous status and the location of deficits. Any effects on function and rehabilitation would be unknown, as they are not described. Documentation of sensation and proprioceptive deficits provide the reviewer with information about the need for continued skilled care.

Edema.   Data pertaining to edema are often vaguely described and the effect on functional progress lacking. Reviewers are challenged to provide coverage decisions for patients without measurable comparative data. Commonly the reviewer finds vague data, as in Example 1.

Example 1: Minimal edema. (Case 2: Home Health, p. 88)

Data that lack measurability or a relationship to functional performance are confusing to a reviewer. In Example 1, how much is *minimal* edema? Where is the edema? Was there improvement in function? What skilled treatment was performed? From a reviewer's perspective, data described in this vague manner demonstrates nonskilled care.

A reviewer would be more inclined to consider comparative descriptive data as skilled. For instance, it would be helpful to include the location of edema and comparative data regarding circumference measurements of the involved and uninvolved extremity, whether the edema is pitting or nonpitting, the skilled services provided to decrease edema, and the resulting functional changes.

Posture.   Comparative data regarding the effects of posture on functional activities are often missing. When appropriate, data pertaining to instruction and patient performance of proper body mechanics or postural analysis measurements are helpful in demonstrating skilled care. How improvements in posture are facilitated by the therapist and the resulting effects on ambulation, transfers, and bed mobility are also helpful.

AROM/PROM.   Reviewers find that sequential objective measurements for range of motion need to be recorded *and related to functional deficits*. Data describing the skilled treatment techniques provided are frequently lacking. In addition, data may appear repetitive and nonskilled, and may lack a relationship to function.

Documentation often lacks objective comparative measurements. In Example 1, passive range of motion data are provided, yet the reviewer is left with many unanswered questions.

Example 1: PROM—Flex 95°, Ab 90°, ER 35°, IR 60°. (Case 10: Outpatient—Managed Care, p. 152)

The reviewer would find it helpful if additional data were provided. To demonstrate that skilled intervention was rendered, data are needed regarding the skilled treatment techniques performed (i.e., contract/relax, proprioceptive neuromuscular facilitation, joint mobilization, or static stretch), the patient's response as indicated by comparative measurements, expected normative values, and the resultant functional changes. Any complications such as pain or edema would be helpful in demonstrating why the skills of a therapist are needed.

Range of motion documentation often is repetitive and may not reflect improvement, as in Example 1.

Example 1: Initially, ROM R-extremities WFL's, LLE: Hip ext –20°, Knee extension –20°; Presently, R-extremities ROM WFL's; LLE –20° hip extension (S), –20° knee extension (S). (Case 14: Skilled Nursing Facility, p. 179)

In Example 1, comparative data are provided and it is clear that range of motion has not improved. Retrospectively, from a reviewer's perspective, the frequency and duration of treatment as well as the treatment interventions will need to be assessed in this case. If range of motion is addressed as a problem, it will need to be reviewed in terms of whether the service provided was reasonable or necessary. It would have been helpful to the reviewer for the documentation to include barriers to progress and why the skills of a therapist were needed. For instance, was pain a complicating factor, and what functional activities were affected?

Strength.   Manual muscle testing requires the skills of a physical therapist when the objective measurements are recorded and specifically related to functional deficits. A reviewer relies on objective data to help determine the need for skilled care. The relationship of the data to the patient's functional limitations is a key element in seeking reimbursement. Often reviewers find that strength grades are missing, vaguely stated, lacking comparisons, not related to function, and at times clinically inappropriate.

Example 1: In mid and lower trapezius is 4-/5. (Case 5: Industrial Health—Workers' Compensation, p. 115)

Example 1 is vaguely stated. The reviewer does not know the site being tested. Is it the left or right extremity? Also, progress comparisons and their relationship to functional deficits are lacking. Additionally, it would be helpful if the techniques used to improve strength were described to demonstrate a skilled approach to care (e.g., progressive resistive exercise, isometric exercises, vibration, or manual resistive exercise). However, despite these shortcomings the therapist does provide the strength grade in terms of a norm (4-/5). This is helpful to the reviewer, especially one who is unfamiliar with manual muscle test grades.

At times reviewers find that strength grades are not clinically appropriate. For example, manual muscle testing may not be appropriate in the presence of abnormal tone (Case 12: Pediatric, p. 170). However, the documentation should reflect strength limitations in functional areas such as bed mobility, balance, transfers, or ambulation. Another finding that is not understood by the reviewer involves the use of percentages as in Example 2.

Example 2: Performs fingering/handling at a FREQUENT level. Grip strength is at the LIGHT PHYSICAL DEMAND level. Overall average strength of left and right extremities have increased 8% since May 96. (25% since start of program.) (Case 6: Industrial Health—Work Hardening, p. 126)

In Example 2 comparative data are provided. The reviewer is able to ascertain that progress has occurred. However, objective data are not provided to substantiate this result. What is an "8%" increase?

Finally, reviewers find strength grades briefly summarized and inappropriate as presented in Example 3. When documented in such a manner, the validity of one strength grade for one or all extremities may be questioned.

Example 3: BU/LE strength poor. (Case 4: Hospital, p. 106)

Reviewers often are concerned that the strengthening exercises performed in rehabilitation are nonskilled and repetitive. As examples, riding a bike, walking on a treadmill, or using a Cybex™ may be questioned by a reviewer if the documentation is vague. Another common finding is that the patient has increased the amount of resistance tolerated during progressive resistive exercise (e.g., "Now tolerates three pounds for ten repetitions of knee extension, previously two pounds"). Therapists need to document the complicating factors involved that require their skills. In essence, they must document why the goals established for strength cannot be achieved through a home program. For instance, are pain, muscle spasm, joint instability, muscle substitution, or cardiopulmonary deficits present, thus necessitating skilled care? To describe a protocol or provide bar graphs and strength grids is objective and important. However, the functional relevance of the data needs to be explained for the reviewer to determine the need for skilled care.

Explanation of the functional significance of skilled care when strength grades are near a normal range (e.g., Good) is often lacking. If the functional deficits of the patient are not described, reviewers will often scrutinize the need for skilled care. What, if any, functional goals will be accomplished by improving strength from Good to Normal? If clearly described, this information will help the reviewer determine the need for skilled care.

Pain. Pain is frequently a complicating factor that influences patient progress. Documentation of pain helps the reviewer assess the patient's potential to progress or maintain mobility. However, despite its importance in determining the need for skilled care, the reviewer regularly finds it missing or vaguely stated in documentation.

When pain is present, it is important to document the location of pain, include comparative data, describe treatment intervention, and identify activities that increase or decrease pain. Reviewers are then challenged to determine the impact pain has on participation in rehabilitation and functional performance. For example, is pain monitored to ensure safe performance of range of motion? Is it a complicating factor that is affecting performance of bed mobility, transfers, gait, or activities of daily living? Is it affecting job performance? When pain is not documented, another reason for justifying skilled care is missing.

Although most often documentation of pain is missing, when present it regularly lacks description. Example 1 is a common finding.

Example 1: Decreased subjective complaints of lower extremity pain. (Case 3: Hospital, p. 97)

Vague terms such as *decreased* or *increased* are commonly found in documentation. In Example 1 the reviewer cannot reasonably be expected to know if pain is absent or has improved, as no data are provided to justify this conclusion. Comparative ratings are needed, as well as a description of what functional activities have improved. It would also be helpful to describe the treatment strategies performed to further justify why the skills of a therapist are needed. In the situation where a patient is unable to use a pain rating scale, as when communication or cognitive barriers exist, it is helpful to describe observations of pain. Observations may include facial grimacing or muscle substitution during treatment.

Reviewers will also question the reasonableness of a treatment strategy if functional progress is limited. Reviewers expect documented progress or a reason for the lack of progress when determining the effectiveness of intervention. It is challenging to justify long durations of treatment with limited functional outcomes. In such a case, alternative treatment strategies may be necessary, and the reviewer will seek data pertaining to the patient's involvement in a home program.

Coordination. Reviewers find that coordination is often addressed at the time of evaluation but data are missing in subsequent reports. If deficits exist, comparative data are needed because of the potential effects on mobility and safety. The treatment strategies used to improve coordination should also be described.

Bed Mobility. Bed mobility is frequently addressed in therapy reports. However, the reviewer finds the data lack description. Often comparative data and the amount of verbal cuing for safety are missing. This is the case in Example 1.

Example 1: Rolls L independently; R w/CGA and VC. Sit to supine w/Mod assist. Supine to sit w/Min assist and VC. (Case 15: Skilled Nursing Facility, p. 189)

Although the levels of assistance are provided in Example 1, the reviewer would be unable to determine what, if any, deficits exist that affect safe performance. Why are the skills of a therapist required? Is the therapist providing instruction? Why is assistance needed? Are there complicating factors such as pain, balance deficits, or limited trunk mobility? Further description would help the reviewer determine the need for skilled care.

Balance (Sit and Stand). Balance deficits, when documented, are helpful to the reviewer in determining the need for skilled care. However, the reviewer frequently finds that data are vaguely presented and lack description, as in Example 1.

Example 1: Increased trunk stability. (Case 2: Home Health, p. 88)

Vague terms such as *increased* or *fair* are not helpful to the reviewer. They are meaningless unless objective comparative data are provided such as the direction of balance loss, the amount of assistance to correct the loss, and the effect of balance on functional activities. As balance deficits affect safety, they are important to the reviewer.

Transfers. Reviewers seek comparative data regarding transfers and that the skills of a therapist are required. In essence, does the documentation describe skilled care and transfer training, or does it describe practicing? What reviewers often find is that data are brief and usually include only the level of physical assistance. The data lack description of the type of transfer training provided (e.g., tub, shower, toilet, car, wheelchair, floor), the amount of verbal cuing, the type of assistive device, and posture. Example 1 represents a common finding.

Example 1: He requires moderate assistance of one for both balance and weight bearing to get to and maintain standing. (Case 11: Pediatric, p. 160)

In lieu of any additional data, the reviewer does not know whether the transitional activity is from sit to stand or from floor to stand. However, balance and weight bearing appear to be complicating factors that require the skills of a therapist. Evidence of training or cuing for safety, the presence of an assistive device if applicable, and a description of posture may be helpful for determining the need for skilled care.

Ambulation. Documentation pertaining to ambulation often lacks skilled terminology and an adequate description of deficits. Reviewers frequently find that therapists correlate an increase in ambulation distance with functional progress that requires skilled care. This is not necessarily so.

Example 1: Distance is improved from 30 feet to 200 feet x 3 in hallway. Walks around apartment every hour. (Case 1: Home Health, p. 79)

Example 1 provides comparative data describing an increase in walking distance. However, these data alone do not justify the need for skilled care. They instead reflect nonskilled care and an endurance problem that may be resolved through practice and repetition. A reviewer may reasonably deny gait training or request an additional description of the gait deficits and the need for skilled training. However, if the distance provided (200 feet) is the distance between the patient's bedroom and the bathroom, and the patient must perform this safely in order to return to or remain in the home environment, then it may be considered reasonable and necessary.

Vague data that lack objective progress comparisons are also common findings.

Example 2: In standing, he is improving with his UE weight bearing and he will tolerate standing without back support and the support in his LE's for 30 seconds. (Case 12: Pediatric, p. 169)

In Example 2, standing time is measured. However, comparative data and the device used for "UE weight bearing" are not provided. The addition of these data would help explain the improvement reported.

Gait should be described in terms of instruction in the safe use of an assistive device, the amount of physical assistance, and verbal cuing. Also, the presence of complicating factors such as balance deficits or pain, gait deficits, and the need for training on level and elevated surfaces to ensure safety are helpful. Without the proper description, *walking* can improve without the skills of a physical therapist.

Orthotic/Prosthetic Devices. Documenting the presence of or need for orthotic/prosthetic devices is helpful to the reviewer in determining the need for skilled care. Reviewers frequently find that devices are present, but their use is not documented. When a device exists, the amount of use and/or need for adjustments should be described. Is the therapist analyzing the gait pattern and providing data to the orthotist or prosthetist when adjustments are needed? Is skin integrity a concern, and is the skin examined before and after activity by the therapist? Is the patient safe when using the device? Comparative data and evidence of training are needed.

Complicating factors—for example, the impact a diagnosis such as peripheral vascular disease or data related to diminished sensation have on safe use of the device—need to be clearly described. Documentation of any consultations, any adjustments to the orthosis or prosthesis, and their impact on function is needed. Therapists often assume that a reviewer will understand this relationship, but depending on the reviewer's medical background, that may not be the case.

Wheelchair Use. Data regarding wheelchair or scooter use are frequently missing in documentation. Details as to how a patient negotiates within his or her living environment and in the community are important to the reviewer. Comparative data regarding the level of wheelchair propulsion skills and the patient's safety are relevant. Teaching and training is evidence of skilled care, especially in the presence of challenges such as postural deficits, neurological involvement, abnormal muscle tone, diminished strength, and/or range of motion deficits.

DME (Using or Required). DME is overlooked in most reports. Reviewers find it helpful for determining skilled care and for understanding the patient's functional limitations when the use of or need for equipment is documented as in Example 1.

Example 1: Equipment has been ordered—hospital bed. Pt. has own walker and commode. (Case 16: Subacute, p. 199)

Activity Tolerance. Reviewers find that comparative data for activity tolerance are commonly reflected in other essential elements such as ambulation (i.e., distance), balance, or vital signs. This is helpful to the reviewer for understanding the patient's functional limitations and determining the need for skilled care. However, reviewers are watchful for repetitive endurance-building activities that do not reflect the need for a physical therapist. If data are present that reflect endurance-building, the reviewer may deny coverage with the expectation that a home program could have been established.

Wound Description, Including Incision Status. Reviewers frequently find that the status of an incision is not described except in the initial evaluation. It is important to provide comparative data regarding the status of an incision, especially if there are soft tissue restrictions, pain, or challenges to healing that may affect functional progress.

A common area of concern for a reviewer is in patients requiring wound care. Frequently, comparative data of wound measurements and descriptions are less than adequate. Reviewers evaluate documentation for a demonstration of wound healing within a reasonable time frame based on the patient's complicating factors. The treatment strategy will be assessed and must be within the payer's guidelines. If findings reveal no descriptive or comparative data to demonstrate healing, coverage may be denied or an alternative treatment strategy expected. Example 1 is an adequate wound care description, except that the data pertaining to modality parameters are not defined.

Example 1: Initially, L-lateral malleolus Stage IV, 2.6 cm x 1.9 cm x .3 cm, 25% of wound meaty, red tissue remaining marbleized with greenish yellow necrotic tissue. No odor/drainage noted. Presently, wound measures as of 01-24-97, 2.1 cm x 2.0 cm x .3 cm after debridement, serous drainage, yellow eschar tunneling noted; Patient receiving whirlpool to L malleolus along with HVPC, 5x/week. (Case 14: Skilled Nursing Facility, p. 180)

Special Tests. Reviewers find that special tests are documented at the time of initial evaluation and are lacking in subsequent reports. When applicable, comparative data and the relevance of the test to rehabilitation would be helpful to the reviewer for identifying the patient's functional progress. If the special test will be administered or performed in the future, then the last formal testing date and anticipated retesting date should be indicated.

Architectural/Safety Considerations. Architectural and safety considerations are frequently missing elements in documentation. Reviewers find it helpful when potential barriers are identified that may affect functional carryover to the job site, home, community, or school. For example, barriers may be stairs, curbs, ramps, or carpeting. Also, a home or job site assessment may identify activities that require consideration, such as lifting or reaching. The date of the assessment and a summary of the findings and recommendations are needed. Identifying architectural and safety concerns helps the reviewer determine the need for skilled care.

Treatment Diagnosis

The treatment diagnosis for which physical therapy services are rendered is important to the reviewer, as it may change during the course of intervention. Reviewers find that the treatment diagnosis is frequently not addressed or may not be a diagnosis that reflects the need for skilled physical therapy service.

Reviewers also find that treatment diagnoses may not be supportive of the need for skilled care. As examples, the treatment diagnoses "Debility" (Case 15: Skilled Nursing Facility, p. 184) and "Weakness" (Case 4: Hospital, p. 101) are not diagnoses for justifying the need for skilled physical therapy service. From a reviewer's perspective, they may imply that the patient will recover mobility through the course of routine daily activities with nonskilled personnel. Therapists should use the most appropriate treatment diagnosis that reflects the reason for service and seek education from third-party payers regarding specific guidelines for diagnosis coding to ensure accuracy.

Assessment

From a reviewer's perspective, the therapist's clinical impressions of the patient's progress and insight into the expected outcomes from intervention are helpful. Focusing on the reason for skilled care helps the reviewer in determining the appropriateness of continued intervention.

Reason for Skilled Care. Often the reason for skilled care is present, but is vaguely stated and does not justify the need for intervention. Expectation statements regarding future progress are also frequently lacking. These inadequacies are evident in Example 1.

Example 1: Fair progress. Improved use of arm. Decreased pain. Increased function. Slow improvement. Progress limited by the number of PT visits. (Case 10: Outpatient—Managed Care, p. 152)

The need for continued skilled care is not provided to the reviewer. What is *fair* progress? Improvement is subjectively and vaguely reported with the terms such as *improved* and *increased*. It would appear from the data in Example 1 that a home program would be sufficient, as the patient is doing well.

It is important to define why the skills of a therapist are needed if continued treatment is requested. The reviewer finds it helpful to determine if continued treatment is reasonable when the barriers to progress are explained. This is demonstrated in Example 2.

Example 2: Resident initially made G progress, then was placed on Haldol, because of severe agitation on the nursing unit. PT was not informed of this, but did note a regression and documented as such. As this regression continued, we discussed this w/nursing and learned of the medication change. Nursing is now in the process of decreasing the Haldol, and we anticipate improvement as the medication decreases. Family continues to want to take resident home. Resident is regular in attendance and family is supportive. Resident remains impulsive, but less so than documented previous month. Is showing somewhat better judgment. Has begun to progress again, now that medication has been reduced. (Case 15: Skilled Nursing Facility, p. 189)

The explanation provided in Example 2 is helpful to the reviewer, as the regression is justified by the medication change. The reviewer is reassured that progress is occurring and expected. Therefore, consideration for coverage may be given, as the reviewer has an adequate picture of the patient's recent challenges. It is important that the reason for skilled care be clearly described.

Problems

The problem list helps to focus treatment. Despite its importance, the problem list documented at the time of evaluation is frequently not provided in subsequent reports. Reviewers often find that problems are absent, are revised without justification, and do not directly correspond to the short-term goals.

Reviewers may question problem revisions that occur without explanation. It is important that an explanation for the revision and the date it occurred be documented, as the reviewer may not have access to all previous reports. It is also helpful when the order of the problem list corresponds to the short-term goals. An organized report eases the review process.

Example 1:

1. *Decreased strength.*
2. *Max assist to perform bed mobilities.*
3. *Max w/ability to perform transfers.*
4. *Inability to walk.*

(Case 15: Skilled Nursing Facility, p. 189)

Problems are customarily stated in vague terms such as *decreased* and *inability* as demonstrated in Example 1, numbers 1 and 4. However, in numbers 2 and 3 it is noted that a measurable component is present (Max). Unfortunately, even when problems are stated in measurable terms, reviewers find that they are not subsequently revised to take into consideration the

patient's progress. This may be confusing to a reviewer if the problems are not rewritten to reflect that progress.

Plan of Care

The plan of care includes the following essential elements: specific treatment strategies, frequency, duration, patient instruction/home program, caregiver training, short-term goals and achievement dates, long-term goals and achievement dates, and the rehabilitation potential. Reviewers find that these areas are important in determining if physical therapy services are reasonable and necessary.

Specific Treatment Strategies. The specific treatment strategies used provide the reviewer with information to help determine the appropriateness of treatment intervention. Reviewers find that treatment strategies (e.g., modalities and procedures) are not addressed, are not appropriately revised based on the patient's progress, and do not always correspond to the services billed for.

Reviewers are watchful as to whether the treatment strategies described are effective for treatment of the patient's diagnosis, treatment diagnosis, and functional deficits. If a lack of progress is evident, the reviewer will expect alternative strategies to be attempted within a reasonable time frame. Depending on the payer's guidelines, the changes in treatment strategies will be reviewed to ensure compliance regarding physician approval. If recertifications are lacking or untimely, a technical denial of payment may occur.

Reviewers occasionally report that the treatment strategies are missing or do not correspond to the services billed. It is an expectation of third-party payers that the modalities rendered be described and correspond to the services billed. It is also expected that the strategies be within the coverage guidelines of the payer as recognized billable services. Experimental procedures are customarily denied.

Frequency. Documentation needs to provide a frequency to help the reviewer determine the reasonableness of the therapy services rendered in relationship to the functional progress reported. It can also help when analyzing documentation and the corresponding service billed. However, reviewers find that the frequency is sometimes missing or stated in variable terms and may be unrealistic based on the functional progress reported.

When the frequency of therapy is not stated or is variable, the reviewer is confused as to what is necessary. Example 1 illustrates this.

Example 1: 6x/wk, 7 as tolerated. (Case 17: Subacute, p. 208)

In Example 1 the reviewer may reasonably conclude that seven times a week is not necessary. It would be more appropriate to indicate a treatment frequency of seven times per week and describe the reason for any absence in the attendance section of upcoming reports.

The reasonableness of the established frequency is not so easily explained. Reviewers expect that as the patient progresses, a lesser frequency may be reasonable to achieve the stated goals in the established time frame. To enable the reviewer to ascertain the need for skilled intervention, the therapist needs to identify specific functional deficits and how these deficits will be addressed in the goals and treatment plan.

If the therapist presents information regarding a patient's treatment plan that appears unskilled, repetitive, or maintenance, it is unlikely that coverage for that therapy will continue; it may even be retrospectively denied. The therapist needs to consider whether it appears that a caregiver, nursing assistant, or individual patient could perform these exercises without the skills of a therapist.

There is no cookbook formula to make it easy for the reviewer or the therapist to determine frequency. Even a specific number of visits ordered by the physician is not proof of medical necessity. Clinical judgment and documentation are needed. The end result is, if the skills can be justified, then the frequency will follow suit. If the patient is doing more and more without help and/or others can be trained to do the activity/activities, then either the frequency of therapy is decreased or the therapy is discontinued.

Duration. The anticipated duration of therapy service is helpful to the reviewer. The reviewer will analyze the patient's functional progress and goals to determine if the treatment is reasonable and necessary. What the reviewer often discovers is that durations are frequently missing or vaguely stated.

When the duration is missing, the reviewer is left without an indication of the length of treatment. As it is unrealistic that treatment be provided indefinitely, the duration would need to be defined, and requesting this information is reasonable. The duration may also be requested when it is vaguely stated as in Example 1.

Example 1: Through the summer. (Case 11: Pediatric, p. 160)

As with the established frequency, the reasonableness of the duration is not easily explained. Reviewers expect that as the patient progresses, the duration will decrease based on the ability of the patient to achieve the stated long-term goal. To enable the reviewer to ascertain the need for skilled intervention, the therapist needs to identify specific functional deficits. If the therapist presents information regarding a patient's treatment plan that appears unskilled, repetitive, or maintenance, coverage for that therapy may be discontinued or even retrospectively denied. Once again, the therapist needs to consider in reading the documentation whether it appears that a caregiver, nursing assistant, or individual patient could perform these exercises without the skills of a therapist.

Patient Instruction/Home Program. There are three commonly weak areas in the documentation of home programs: an ill-defined home program; limited progression of the program; and lack of evidence of training and self-management of pain, activity tolerance, or entry into community-based activity programs.

The easiest example to present from a reviewer perspective is when the home program is ill-defined. Often there is no mention of the home program at all—the therapist does not even mention its existence. Or the therapist will provide a statement such as in Example 1 that does not provide a detailed account of the home program.

Example 1: Mom is carrying out a ROM program at home. (Case 12: Pediatric, p. 169)

Rarely does the therapist define the home program, the goals, the patient/caregiver understanding of the program, or how this home program will evolve into the discharge plan with a focus on self-management. It is important that the patient be totally independent with the program and aware of health prevention and wellness goals to avoid future reoccurrences of the problem/disability.

Limited progression of a home program is another shortcoming found by reviewers. Documentation often does not reflect additions or deletions to the home program. Carryover of functional gains and the establishment of a home program are necessary and skilled components of rehabilitation. When emphasizing carryover, therapists need to be mindful of the various community resources available for patients. It is essential for therapists to participate in cost-effective treatment approaches and accept the growing influence of managed care. Therapists have an increasing responsibility to refer patients to aquatic programs, local fitness gyms, and other resources once they have received maximal benefit from rehabilitation. Referral to community resources can transition a patient from short-term intervention to a lifelong self-management program.

Caregiver Training. Evidence of ongoing patient education and training provided to the patient, family, caregiver, teacher, nurse, and/or employer helps justify the need for skilled care. There is often no mention of what, if any, training was performed or the amount of training still needed. Third-party payers are particularly interested in communication regarding the carryover of functional activities. It is important to document the dates of training, who was trained, and safe performance of the exercises or functional activities.

Short-Term Goals and Achievement Dates. To most therapists, goals may seem mundane and simple to write. However, from a reviewer's perspective, the need to improve functional goal writing is essential. Frequently one or more of the three goal components are missing. That is, the goals lack a measurable, functional, or time-specific component, as demonstrated in Example 1.

Example 1:

1. *Decrease edema.*
2. *Increase circulation.*
3. *Facilitate muscle activity both lower extremities.*
4. *Increase sitting balance.*

(Case 2: Home Health, p. 88)

In this example, all three goal components are missing. This being the case, the reviewer is unable to determine if the goals are achieved.

Reviewers find that a documented goal progression helps to justify functional progress and the need for continued skilled care. Example 2 illustrates a goal progression that is helpful to the reviewer. This example would be enhanced if the date the goal was met was provided.

Example 2: 2c. Child will tolerate tall kneeling with minimal assist for 3 minutes. Goal met. NEW GOAL: Child will maintain a 4-point position for 1 minute independently. (Case 12: Pediatric, p. 169)

Functional goal writing is essential for reimbursement. To document goal achievement and the establishment of new goals demonstrates the functional progress achieved from skilled intervention.

Long-Term Goal and Achievement Dates.   The long-term goal is another area that is vaguely documented or missing. It is established at the time of evaluation and any subsequent revisions need to be clarified in the assessment. Reviewers find that a vaguely stated long-term goal or one that is omitted demonstrates a lack of treatment focus.

Example 1: Maintain ROM and prevent joint contractures secondary to muscle tightness. (Case 4: Hospital, p. 106)

In Example 1 the long-term goal is maintenance and does not demonstrate the need for the skills of a physical therapist.

Rehabilitation Potential.   The rehabilitation potential is customarily documented as a brief one-word response. It helps the reviewer determine the reasonableness of skilled care in relationship to the stated goals. The therapist's insight into the patient's rehabilitation potential is important. However, often this area is not addressed in documentation.

Essential Elements Lacking in a Discharge Report

The essential elements lacking in a discharge report are similar to those for a progress report. The attendance, treatment diagnosis, and problems are documented as for a progress report. However, the current baseline data differ: the comparisons include not only data since the last formal report, but an overall comparison since the start of care.

Reviewers frequently find that data are lacking in discharge reports to justify the need for skilled care since the last formal report. As a result, unfavorable coverage decisions may occur. Patients are often at a higher level of functioning near the time of discharge. Therefore, it is important that the current baseline data clearly provide the reviewer with the reason skilled care was provided, the deficits that existed, and the functional progress made.

To avoid redundancy, the next section pertaining to discharge reports emphasizes the areas that differ from the findings in progress reports. The focus is on the essential elements that are lacking in the assessment and plan of care.

Assessment

It is helpful to the reviewer to know the therapist's clinical impressions of the patient and the outcomes achieved from skilled intervention. This is achieved by focusing on the reason for skilled care.

Reason for Skilled Care.   Reviewers find that data to support the effectiveness of the treatment provided since the last report are lacking in discharge reports. Documentation of the complications that were present, an explanation of why goals were not met (if applicable), the need for skilled care, the reason for discharge, and an expectation statement of the therapist's insight regarding successful carryover to home, school, and/or work are helpful items to consider in the reason for skilled care. Example 1 illustrates a vague description that does not help the reviewer in determining if the care provided was medically necessary and skilled.

Example 1: The short-term goals were achieved. (Case 5: Industrial Health—Workers' Compensation, p. 115)

In Example 1 the functional outcome is not clear. Could the goals have been achieved without skilled intervention? What was the effect of the modalities rendered on the functional outcome? It is important to describe for the reviewer why the skills of a therapist are needed, as provided in Example 2.

Example 2: Patient has made significant functional progress since WBAT LLE was initiated last month. Pt. has reached full benefit of inpatient P.T. She is being discharged home 6-20 to live with daughter (who will assist pt.) and Pt's husband. Home P.T. recommended to instruct and train pt. and family in the home environment, continue functional training, etc. (Case 16: Subacute, p. 199)

Example 2 describes the progress that was made, the discharge plan, and recommendations for continued physical therapy intervention. Further description of why the patient is a candidate for continued skilled care would be helpful. It would provide the reviewer with insight into the remaining functional deficits.

Plan of Care

For the reviewer to determine if therapy services were reasonable and necessary, it is helpful to provide information regarding the plan of care. The plan of care includes specific treatment strategies, frequency, duration, patient instruction/home program, caregiver training, short-term goals and achievement dates, long-term goals and achievement dates, and the discharge prognosis.

Specific Treatment Strategies.   The specific treatment strategies are often not documented in a discharge report. It is common for a reviewer to find a statement like the one in Example 1.

Example 1: Discontinue PT. (Case 1: Home Health, p. 79)

As this is a discharge report, it is true that the obvious plan is discharge. However, this information does not allow the reviewer to determine the reasonableness of the plan of care in relationship to the functional progress reported. For instance, were the treatment strategies changed as the patient progressed?

Reviewers usually have access to the evaluation and the reports for the period in question. Depending on the duration of treatment and patient progress, the treatment strategies listed in the evaluation may not be the same strategies used through discharge. Therefore, it is helpful to provide a summary of the treatment strategies used, as illustrated in Example 2.

Example 2: Treatment utilized: Hot pack, ultrasound, soft tissue mobilization, therapeutic exercise, instruction in HEP and electrical stimulation. Discharge patient from PT this date. (Case 5: Industrial Health—Workers' Compensation, p. 115)

A summary helps the reviewer determine the reasonableness of care. It also helps when analyzing the documentation and the corresponding services billed. In essence, if billing occurred for the strategies, is there documentation that they were performed?

Frequency. In a discharge report the frequency of further care is not applicable. Therefore, this area is usually not addressed. However, to provide a summary of the frequency helps the reviewer determine the reasonableness of care in relationship to the functional progress reported. It also allows the reviewer to analyze documentation and the corresponding services billed.

Reviewers usually have access to the evaluation and the reports for the period in question. As the patient progresses, it is common to find that the frequency decreases. Therefore, the frequency listed in the evaluation may not be the same at the time of discharge. Therefore, it is helpful to provide a summary of the frequency (e.g., "Was seen three times per week").

Duration. At the time of discharge there is not an anticipated duration of care. Therefore, this area is usually not addressed. However, to provide a summary of the duration helps the reviewer determine the reasonableness of care in relationship to the functional progress reported (e.g., "Was seen for eight weeks"). It also allows the reviewer to analyze the documentation and the corresponding services billed.

Patient Instruction/Home Program. Emphasis on prevention and self-management is increasing in health care. Despite this emphasis, reviewers find that home and restorative nursing programs are vaguely described, as in Example 1.

Example 1: Home exercise program updated and reviewed on date of discharge. (Case 6: Industrial Health—Work Hardening, p. 127)

As revisions of home and restorative nursing programs require the skills of a therapist, it is important to include a summary of the activities that were performed, the frequency of per-

formance, and the dates training and/or changes to the program occurred. Evidence of home programming needs to be ongoing and not initiated on the day of discharge.

Example 2: Exercise program 1–2x daily with supervision. Tolerates 2 sets of 10 reps of each exercise. (i.e., Straight leg raising, hip abduction, hip/knee flexion, TKE, LTR, bridging, marching, standing balance exercise at counter and upper extremity cane exercises.) Client to walk in hallway 2–4x daily. (Case 1: Home Health, p. 79)

Example 2 contains a detailed program description. However, it does lack evidence of revision. As this program was probably initiated earlier in the course of rehabilitation. The lack of data regarding the patient's previous program and the need for skilled training may be of concern to the reviewer.

Caregiver Training. Reviewers find that evidence is lacking of training to the patient, family, caregiver, teacher, nurse, and/or employer, although what the patient can perform is listed. However, equally important to the reviewer is why the skills of a therapist were needed.

Example 1: Patient learned to take pulse accurately. (Case 8: Outpatient, p. 143)

In Example 1 the description is brief and lacks skilled terminology. A reviewer may question why the skills of a therapist are needed. Was the patient instructed in energy conservation techniques in order to safely perform functional activities?

It is helpful to the reviewer when the documentation indicates that the patient, family, caregiver, teacher, nurse, and/or employer have demonstrated learned skills. Safety and carryover of learned activities are important in self-management.

Short-Term Goals and Achievement Dates. In discharge reports reviewers frequently find that one or more of the three goal components are missing. That is, the goals may not be measurable, functional, and/or time-specific. Omission of the measurable and functional components makes it difficult for the reviewer to determine the extent of goal achievement and the reasonableness of care.

Reviewers find it helpful when goal comparisons and the status of the goals at discharge are documented. Instead, they find that goals may be stated in a vague and objective manner as in Example 1.

Example 1:

1. *Ambulates with rolling walker 200 feet in hallway 2x's daily with supervision. (Surpassed goal: Doing this 3–4x's daily.)*
2. *Home exercise completed daily with wife with home health aide.*
3. *Returned to level of functioning when last d/c'd by PT on 07-92. (Case 1: Home Health, p. 79)*

All three goals in this example are statements of status. This approach is not helpful to the reviewer. It would be better to state the previous goals and their status at discharge, such as *goal achieved* or *not achieved*. If the goals were revised since the last report, this also needs to be reflected (e.g., "Goal revised __/__/__").

In Example 1, number 1, the reviewer is provided with comparative data. This is always helpful. However, the statement in number 3, "Returned to level of functioning when last d/c'd . . ." is vague. Unless the reviewer has access to the evaluation or a previous report that indicates the prior level, the status of this goal will be unknown. Challenges relating to vague data and the unknown status of goals are common.

Long-Term Goals and Achievement Dates. To determine the success of the skilled services provided, the reviewer finds the status of the long-term goal important. Often the long-term goal is vaguely stated, as in Example 1, or not addressed.

Example 1: Pt. will be discharged home. (Case 16: Subacute, p. 199)

Example 1 lacks a measurable and functional component. Discharge to home in itself is not helpful to the reviewer in determining what functional progress has occurred. Does the patient have good strength? Is the patient safe? Are there supportive services at home? Is assistance or an assistive device required for ambulation?

Equally important is the status of the long-term goal. Was it achieved? If not achieved, was it revised? If revised, when and why would be helpful to the reviewer. (Readers note that the reason for discharge should be provided in the assessment.) A positive functional outcome is helpful in justifying skilled care. However, when it does not occur, documentation must describe the skilled care provided and how the professional judgment of the therapist was needed to arrive at the decision for discharge. The discharge report must reflect the circumstances that led to a reasonable expectation of progress, and why has the patient been discharged.

Discharge Prognosis. The discharge prognosis is frequently not addressed. From a reviewer's perspective, it is helpful to know how successful the patient will be if he or she adheres to the recommendations made by the therapist. This one-word response (e.g., *excellent*, *good*, *fair*, *poor*) is helpful to the reviewer for assessing the success of skilled intervention.

Essential Elements Lacking in an Individualized Education Program (IEP)

Present Levels of Educational Performance. Reviewers find that the present levels of educational performance are briefly stated as in Example 1.

Example 1: Gross motor skills are at the 11 to 12 month level. (Case 13: Pediatric—Individualized Education Program, p. 173)

As demonstrated in Example 1, reviewers frequently find the skill level is defined by age equivalency. It is helpful to review-

ers, and to the team members, to describe the functional skills observed in the school environment. The use of measurable and descriptive functional terms helps to provide a clear picture of the child's skill level.

Annual Goal. The annual goal, like the present level of educational performance, is frequently vaguely defined by age equivalency as illustrated in Example 1.

Example 1: John will increase his gross motor skills to 18 month level. (Case 13: Pediatric—Individualized Education Program, p. 173)

It is important to the reviewer when determining the need for skilled care that the annual goal be measurable and that it focus on functional outcomes.

Short-Term Objectives. Reviewers often find that the short-term objectives described in an IEP lack functional and objective terms that both parents and teachers can understand. The objectives also are often not related specifically to the school environment. These documentation deficiencies are evident in Example 1.

Example 1:

1. *John will develop balance reactions in standing.*
2. *John will ambulate 100 feet independently.*
3. *John will increase weight shift and transitional skills necessary for transitions from sitting to standing.*
4. *John will ascend and descend stairs with one railing and minimal assist.*

(Case 13: Pediatric—Individualized Education Program, p. 174)

Schedule. The schedule is the time frame anticipated for achievement of the short-term objectives. The time frame defined in IEPs is often described in terms of "annually." Reviewers find that a quarterly or more frequent review is more reasonable. It is also a requirement in many states.

Specific Special Education and Related Services That Will Contribute to Meeting This Goal. Reviewers often find that therapy documentation is too compartmentalized by specialty and reflects a narrow vision of who will help to meet educational goals. For an IEP to be effective, it is important that all staff who will be involved in facilitating one or more goals be identified, such as the occupational therapist, classroom teacher, classroom aides, and parents.

Summary

The role of the reviewer in determining coverage is challenging in light of the areas frequently lacking in documentation. The reviewer often finds that essential elements are omitted or inadequate details are provided. When presented with such limited information regarding the patient's overall functional deficits and the treatment plan, the reviewer questions why support staff, nursing assistants, or caregivers could not perform the program.

To justify the need for skilled care, therapists need to incorporate the essential elements defined in Chapter 1 and avoid the commonly found deficiencies described in this chapter. Indicating complicating factors, using expectation statements, providing comparative data, and documenting evidence of skilled care help the reviewer to determine if physical therapy services are medically reasonable and necessary. The key criterion for the justification of coverage is to provide evidence that the skills of a professional are required to effectively treat an individual patient.

Chapter 3 explores documentation tips that help ease the review process. Emphasis is placed on functional phrase alternatives, descriptive terminology, the professional appearance of documentation, and a proactive approach to appeal processing.

References

1. Morrissey-Ross M. Documentation: if you haven't written it, you haven't done it. *Nurs Clin North Am* 1988; 23(2): 363.
2. American Physical Therapy Association. Guide to Physical Therapist Practice. *Phys Ther* 1997; 77(11): 1625–1633.
3. Department of Health and Human Services, Health Care Financing Administration. *Medicare Skilled Nursing Facility Manual*, Laurel, Maryland: Government Printing Office, Publication 12, Revision 262, Section 214.3, 1987, 2-17.3–2-17.4.
4. American Physical Therapy Association. *Guidelines for Peer Review Training*. Alexandria, VA: 1997.
5. Wisconsin Physical Therapy Association. *Guidelines for WPTA Peer Review*. Madison, WI: 1994, 10–11.
6. Kane R. Looking for physical therapy outcomes. *Phys Ther.* 1994; 74(5): 56/425.
7. Stewart DL, Abeln SH. *Documenting Functional Outcomes in Physical Therapy*. St. Louis: Mosby—Year Book, Inc., 1993, 38.
8. Baeten A. Documentation: The Reviewer Perspective. *Top Geriatr Rehabil* 1997; 13(1): 15.

Review Questions

1. The need for medical review of physical therapy services has increased with the rising cost of health care. To achieve a positive functional outcome, there are four players involved in the review process. List the four players and a unique responsibility they each have in the review process.
2. Although there is a lack of national standards for medical review of physical therapy services, there are some general guidelines that may be used. List the resources for information that may provide general guidelines for reviewers of physical therapy services.
3. Explain who defines "medical necessity."
4. According to the Wisconsin Physical Therapy Association (WPTA), in their *Guidelines for WPTA Peer Review*,[5] medical necessity review could be used to determine what five considerations?
5. What are the credentials of reviewers of physical therapy documentation for third-party payers?
6. List the four purposes of physical therapy peer review.
7. Why is being a reviewer of physical therapy claims challenging?
8. Describe in general terms two common documentation deficiencies that are found by reviewers.
9. Is the statement "Decreased subjective complaints of lower extremity pain" appropriately written from a reviewer's perspective? Explain why or why not.
10. Explain why the statements "Distance is improved from 30 feet to 200 feet x 3 in hallway. Walks around apartment every hour" are not appropriately written from a reviewer's perspective. Also, rewrite the statements to reflect the need for skilled care.

Review Question Answer Sheet

1. The four players and their responsibility in the review process:

   (i) The provider of physical therapy service. Responsible for clinical, legal and ethical practice. Standards are outlined by the American Physical Therapy Association.

   (ii) The insured (the patient). Responsible for providing insurance information and any copayments or deductibles.

   (iii) The third-party payer. Responsible for ensuring that the patient receives medically necessary and reasonable services that are within the scope of the insurance plan's coverage criteria. This helps to control costs for the patient and the payer.

   (iv) The reviewer. Responsible to the provider of service and the payer for providing an opinion regarding the need for or appropriateness of the physical therapy intervention.

2. There are several resources that provide general guidelines for reviewers. One is summarized in the Medicare Part A physical therapy coverage guidelines. Although designed primarily for skilled nursing facilities, the guidelines apply to most settings. The American Physical Therapy Association also provides a written document, entitled *Guidelines for Peer Review Training,* to promote standardization for peer review training and performance. Last, state association guidelines and the third-party payer's coverage criteria are other sources of review criteria.

3. Medical necessity is defined by the third-party payer based on the language found in the patient's insurance policy. This is usually a vague definition that requires the reviewer of physical therapy documentation to provide an opinion regarding the services based on the data provided.

4. The five considerations that could be used to determine medical necessity review as defined by the WPTA include the following:

   (i) The appropriateness of planned/delivered procedures for the treatment of the identified diagnosis and/or deficits identified in the initial or subsequent evaluations.

   (ii) If treatment has resulted in progressive improvement as demonstrated by objective comparative clinical findings of physiological and/or anatomical changes in the patient's status that correlate with functional improvements in the area of activities of daily living, mobility, pain and/or safety.

   (iii) If the active physical therapy intervention at the frequency and duration indicated in the plan of care is required for progressive improvement of the patient's condition.

   (iv) If duplicated services are being delivered by multiple providers.

   (v) If the patient had a beneficial response to any previous physical therapy treatment for the same diagnosis.

5. The reviewers of physical therapy documentation for third-party payers are usually registered nurses, physicians, peers, and nonmedical personnel. They may or may not be familiar with rehabilitative services.

6. The four purposes of physical therapy peer review include the following:

   (i) An opportunity to network with insurance companies.

   (ii) An opportunity to offer education regarding the field of physical therapy.

   (iii) To display a commitment to monitoring the profession and ensuring that the highest standards for delivery of care are being followed.

   (iv) To interact with third-party payers and be in a position to make recommendations and/or review coverage for services, modalities, treatment techniques, and equipment.

7. Being a reviewer of physical therapy documentation can be challenging as documentation is often insufficient for determining skilled need.

8. Two common documentation deficiencies include:
   - Lack of measurable data (i.e., data are vague or omitted).
   - Data are not related to function (i.e., how is the patient affected?).

9. The statement "Decreased subjective complaints of lower extremity pain" is not appropriately written from a reviewer's perspective. This statement regarding pain is vague. Objective data are needed such as a pain rating. A description of what functional activities have improved is missing.

10. The statements "Distance is improved from 30 feet to 200 feet x 3 in hallway. Walks around apartment every hour" are not entirely complete for documentation from a reviewer's perspective. Comparative data regarding distance are present and helpful for a reviewer. However, walking distance alone does not justify the need for the skills of a physical therapist. The activity described reflects endurance building. It lacks description of the gait deficits and the need for skilled care. For example, it is better to include data that may answer the following questions: Was gait training performed? Does the patient use an assistive device and, if so, is it used safely? Are gait deficits present? Does balance loss occur during gait training? As an example: Gait training with rolling walker and supervision of 1 for 200 feet x 3. (Previously 30 feet with minimal/moderate assistance for balance.) Base of support and stride length within normal limits without verbal cuing. (Previously moderate verbal cuing required.)

<u>**SECOND OPINION PROVIDER**</u>

PHYSICAL/OCCUPATIONAL/SPEECH THERAPY CONSULTANT
REVIEW

DATE REFERRED FOR REVIEW: _____   REVIEW TIME: _____

SENT TO: _____

DATE COMPLETED:_____

Patient's Name _____   File # _____

Subscriber Number _____

<u>CRITERIA FOR DECISION</u>

1. IS THE PATIENT BENEFITTING FROM THE THERAPY?
2. IS THE THERAPY EXCESSIVE FOR THE DIAGNOSED CONDITION?
3. WHAT IS LACKING IN THE DOCUMENTATION?
4. IS THE THERAPY APPROPRIATE FOR THE CONDITION?
5. HAS THIS THERAPY MET WITH WIDE USE BY OTHER PROVIDERS FOR THIS CONDITION
    AND IS IT SUPPORTED BY PUBLISHED MEDICAL LITERATURE (PERIODICALS, TEXTBOOKS).
6. DO THE DIAGNOSIS AND THERAPY RENDERED CORRELATE?
7. IS THERE IMPROVEMENT OR IS THIS MAINTENANCE THERAPY?

DATES OF THERAPY PREVIOUSLY PROCESSED FOR PAYMENT
                                        FROM _____ THROUGH _____

DATES OF THERAPY PREVIOUSLY DENIED AS NOT MEDICALLY NECESSARY
                                        FROM _____ THROUGH _____

DATES OF SERVICE PREVIOUSLY DENIED, MEDICAL DOCUMENTATION NOT RECEIVED
FROM PROVIDER
                                        FROM _____ THROUGH _____

PLEASE REVIEW DATES OF SERVICE _____ THROUGH _____
WHICH DATES OF SERVICE, IF ANY, SHOULD BE DENIED?
                                        FROM _____ THROUGH _____

WHICH DATES OF SERVICE, IF ANY, SHOULD BE ALLOWED:
                                        FROM _____ THROUGH _____

ANY SPECIFIC SERVICES THAT SHOULD BE DENIED
                            FINDINGS AND RECOMMENDATIONS

Figure 2.1 Sample form a reviewer may use. (Reprinted with permission of Meridian Managed Care.)

CIGNA MANAGED CARE
(Fax to CIGNA: 414-266-8030)

INITIAL Request For PT, OT, And ST Authorization

Please complete the following:

1. Patient Name _____

2. Patient Cigna ID# (include member suffix, ie. 01, 02, 03)_____

3. Patient date of birth:_____

4. Patient Diagnosis: Date of onset _____ ICD-9 and description _____

5. Date of initial evaluation_____

6. Is this a work related injury?_____

7. Has patient been treated for this condition previously?_____

8. Type of therapy: PT   OT   ST   (circle)

9. Number of visits and duration of treatment requested. _____
   _____

10. Treatment procedures/strategies (including documentation as appropriate of what is medically interfering with the patient's ability to be independent in a home exercise program).
    _____
    _____
    _____

11. Therapy provider clinic name: _____

12. Therapist name and professional designation: _____

13. Provider phone #: _____ Fax: _____

(Below for office use only)

14. # of visits authorized:_____

15. Date of authorization: From _____ to _____

16. Authorization number:_____

17. Comments: _____
    _____
    _____

18. Reviewer: _____

19. Membership status: _____

20. Benefit level:_____

Please note: This plan has a short-term rehabilitation benefit versus a conventional physical therapy benefit. In general, the benefit is limited to sixty days and is for the acute phase of acute conditions only.

NOTE: If you wish to re-verify eligibility (not coverage) at any time during the course of treatment, you may call 1-800-832-3211.

Figure 2.2 Sample form a reviewer may use. (Reprinted with permission of CIGNA Managed Care.)

CIGNA MANAGED CARE
(Fax to HealthReach 414-780-0717)

<u>**EXTENSION Request for PT, OT and ST Authorization**</u>

Please complete the following:

1. Patient name: _____

2. Patient Cigna ID# (including member suffix ie. 01, 02, 03) _____

3. Additional number of visits/duration of treatment requested: _____

4. Send written justification of need for further treatment, and copy of initial Cigna Authorization Form (including documentation of what is medically interfering with patient's ability to be independent in a home exercise program).

5. Type of therapy: PT   OT   ST   (circle one)

6. Therapy Provider Clinic name: _____

7. Therapist name and professional designation _____

8. Provider phone # _____   Fax: _____

(Below for office use only)
_____

9. Additional number of visits authorized _____ for a total of _____ visits.

10. Date of authorization _____ to _____

11. Authorization number: _____

12. Comments: _____

_____

13. Reviewer: _____

14. Membership Status_____

15. Benefit level _____

Please note: This plan has a short-term rehabilitation benefit versus a conventional physical therapy benefit. In general, the benefit is limited to sixty days and is for the acute phase of acute conditions only.

Note: If you wish to re-verify eligibility (not coverage) at any time during the course of treatment, you may call 1-800-832-3211.

Figure 2.3 Sample form a reviewer may use. (Reprinted with permission of CIGNA Managed Care.)

Chapter 3
Documentation Tips

Introduction

Physical therapy documentation is the primary means of communication with the reviewer. Chapter 2 highlighted common documentation findings and the resulting challenges faced by reviewers in rendering coverage decisions. This chapter explores helpful documentation tips, from a reviewer's perspective, that enhance the skilled nature of physical therapy service and ease the review process. Emphasis is placed on commonly used terms and their functional phrase alternatives, descriptive versus non-descriptive terminology, the professional appearance of documentation, and a proactive approach to appeal processing.

Functional Phrase Alternatives

Documentation is a routine professional expectation. As a result, documentation may follow certain patterns that are specific to the physical therapist, such as the order in which data are recorded and the use of common terms. These patterns are culminations of the therapist's experiences that may include a variety of practice settings and exposure to numerous documentation formats and third-party payer guidelines. In the review process, the pattern of using common terms may not reflect the skilled service delivered to the patient and may result in a claim denial or limit authorization for further treatment.

There is a tendency for therapists to develop documentation patterns using common terms that are nonskilled. Common terms frequently surface because they are used in daily conversation with patients or peers. For example, it is common to report to a family member or caregiver, "He *walks* with a rolling walker." (Case 1: Home Health, p. 74) *Walks* describes a functional outcome. However, when documented or dictated using the same words, this statement does not provide the reviewer with a perspective on the skilled therapy service rendered, such as gait training or gait analysis. To enhance the skilled nature of common terms, functional phrase alternatives should be considered in therapy documentation.

Functional phrase alternatives are terms or phrases that convey to the reviewer the skilled nature of the service provided. It is important that the functional phrase alternative chosen by the therapist be professional and easily understood by the reviewer. Using a functional phrase alternative describes the skills of the physical therapist and the patient's status accurately for the reviewer, rather than being assumed as with a common term. Use of functional phrase alternatives is helpful to the reviewer in determining the need for skilled care. Table 3.1 provides some examples of this concept.

The concept of using functional phrase alternatives can be expanded to all practice settings. To develop an awareness of documentation patterns, therapists can audit and analyze their own documentation, analyze documentation of peers within their practice setting (internal chart review), or develop a rapport with peers outside their practice setting (external chart review). Professional publications pertaining to the therapist's practice may also provide valuable insight into functional phrase alternatives. Incorporating this alternative will enhance the quality and skilled nature of documentation from a reviewer's perspective.

Nondescriptive versus Descriptive Terminology

While remaining aware of the patterns that can develop relating to common terms, therapists can strengthen their documentation by using descriptive terminology. In fast-paced clinical settings, documentation may lack the description necessary to paint a clear picture of the patient so the reviewer can render a positive coverage decision. Providing descriptive objective data makes the functional deficits evident to the reviewer.

The following are five examples of nondescriptive terminology:

1. Poor quad contraction. (Case 7: Outpatient, p. 130)
2. Patient unable to balance unsupported in sitting. (Case 16: Subacute, p. 193)
3. Ambulation: Distance is improved from 30 feet to 200 feet x 3 in hallway. (Case 1: Home Health, p. 79)
4. Patient currently complains of a constant ache in the low back radiating into the right lateral leg, right anterior thigh and right shin. (Case 9: Outpatient—Managed Care, p. 147)
5. Initially, ROM R-extremities WFL's, LLE: Hip ext –20°, Knee extension –20°; Presently, R-extremities ROM WFL's; LLE –20° hip extension (S), –20° knee extension (S). (Case 14: Skilled Nursing Facility, p. 179)

The reviewer is left with many questions when the medical record contains nondescriptive, objective data like those shown

Table 3.1 Functional Phrase Alternatives (Reprinted with Permission from Table Adapted from: Baeten A. Documentation Tips. Focus: Skilled Terminology. *Gerinotes* Summer 1995; 2(3): 4.)

Common Terms	Functional Phrase Alternative
Ambulated/walked	Gait training
Confused	Attention span deficit
Debility/deconditioned	Functional strength deficit
Declined	Functionally regressed
Did not appear to understand	Following ___ minutes of training demonstrated inconsistent . . .
Difficulty walking	Gait deviation
Endurance	Functional activity tolerance
Helped	Facilitated
Improved	List comparative data such as: "Presently ____. (Previously ____.)"
Observed/monitored	Evaluated/analyzed
Pacing of activity	Instructed in energy conservation techniques
Patient unable to . . .	Patient exhibits . . . (describe)
Performs lower extremity exercise	Performs an individualized lower extremity strengthening program emphasizing . . .
Poor gait	Gait abnormality or gait disturbance
Practiced	Instructed
Reminders	Verbal cues
Some drainage	Indicate specific amount
Stable	Beginning to respond
Stays in bed	Bed confined
Strengthening	Progressive resistive exercise
Walked	Ambulated or gait trained
Water-pik™	High pressure irrigation
Weakness	Strength deficit
Went to doctor	Transported for physician's appointment

in these five examples. The most important question is, "What are the patient's functional limitations?" Unfortunately, data are frequently presented in this brief fashion, as will be illustrated in the case studies presented in Chapter 4.

Documenting in descriptive terms provides the reviewer with the functional limitations and justifies the necessity for skilled physical therapy intervention. This is accomplished by documenting specific objective measurements and attaching a functional component. Table 3.2 compares nondescriptive and descriptive terminology.

The use of descriptive terms is important in identifying function from a reviewer's perspective. It provides the basis for comparisons and displaying the overall functional progress of the patient. The type of documentation format used by the therapist can influence descriptive writing. For instance, the use of checklists and flowsheets, although concise and expedient from a managed care perspective, should be analyzed by the therapist to ensure functional content for justifying the need for skilled care.

Developing a descriptive and yet concise writing style can be challenging. It requires a commitment to excellence by the ther-

Table 3.2 Nondescriptive versus Descriptive Terminology

Nondescriptive	Descriptive
1. Poor quad contraction.	Per manual muscle test right quadriceps strength is poor. Neuromuscular electrical stimulation applied to facilitate strengthening exercises. Patient uses one crutch for safe gait due to knee buckling.
2. Patient unable to balance unsupported in sitting.	Patient exhibits sitting balance loss to the left and posteriorly when reaching for objects and requires contact guard assistance to correct.
3. Ambulation: Distance is improved from 30 feet to 200 feet x 3 in hallway.	Gait training with rolling walker and supervision of 1 for 200 feet x 3. (Previously 30 feet with minimal/moderate assistance for balance.) Base of support and stride length within normal limits without verbal cuing. (Previously moderate verbal cuing required.)
4. Patient currently complains of a constant ache in the low back radiating into the right lateral leg, right anterior thigh and right shin.	Patient reports a 10, on a scale of 1 to 10, regarding pain in the low back radiating through the right lower extremity. Patient states difficulty falling asleep secondary to low back pain.
5. Initially, ROM R-extremities WFL's, LLE: Hip ext −20°, Knee extension −20°; Presently, R-extremities ROM WFL's; LLE −20° hip extension (S), −20° knee extension (S).	Static stretch performed within patient tolerance to improve hip extension for rolling. Pain monitored. Range of motion right lower extremity is within functional limits. Left hip and knee extension −20°. (Previously −20°.)

apist and is an ongoing endeavor. The results for the provider of service are reflected in a decrease in denials from third-party payers and the ability to analyze the effectiveness of service delivery.

The Professional Appearance of Documentation

The review process can be a challenging task. Depending on the third-party payer's documentation requirements, a reviewer may be faced with multiple providers using various documentation formats. The formats may even vary by diagnosis. With this in mind, the therapist can help the review process by ensuring that the documentation submitted to the third-party payer is legible, appropriately presented, and accurate.

One of the challenges reviewers face, in rendering coverage determinations, is the legibility of the documentation submitted. Can the reviewer read the therapist's handwriting? Illegible handwriting slows the review process and may even result in an unfavorable decision if essential elements cannot be deciphered.

Therapists need to ensure that documentation is legible, as it communicates patient care. Scott[1] suggests that managers take the necessary steps to ensure legibility or provide alternative documentation systems. This is also important because documentation serves multiple purposes, including reimbursement and legal. Legible documentation is expected by the reviewer and, although the legal aspect is not explored in this text, it must not be forgotten.

Appropriately organizing and presenting requested documentation is helpful to the reviewer. Third-party payers customarily request specific information for case review that may include items such as physician orders, the initial evaluation, progress reports (monthly, weekly, and/or daily entries), a discharge report, completed forms specific to the payer, and/or itemized statements. It is important that the billing provider, preparing the packet of information for submission, clearly understand the request. Submitting the correct documentation in an orderly and timely manner is essential to avoid a delay in authorization or a denial in a retrospective review process.

When preparing requested documentation, ensure that the documents being reproduced are of good quality. Frequently when documents are copied, quality is sacrificed, making the document difficult to read. It is also important to ensure that all requested documents are present and not inadvertently omitted. To avoid these pitfalls, the packet of documentation should be reviewed by the treating therapist before submission. This will help to ensure accuracy and provide an opportunity to highlight information that may help the reviewer in determining the need for skilled care.

A systematic approach for submitting documentation is needed. Submit the documentation requested in a logical order. The order may be specified by the third-party payer. If not, an internal procedure for submission should be developed for consistency. For example, the provider may wish to submit documentation with a copy of the initial request for information from the third-party payer (and possibly a cover letter), fol-

lowed by the requested documents in chronological order, and finally the itemized statements and billing information. The reviewer will welcome consistency in the order of the documentation packet submitted.

The accuracy of the documentation submitted is essential. It is helpful to the review process to ensure that information is consistent. Do the dates of billing coincide with the dates of service reported in the therapy documentation? Does the plan of care correctly reflect the modalities and procedures billed? Is the number of treatment visits accurately listed? If physician certification is required for rehabilitation, are the necessary signatures in place? Attention to such details is important to ensure that the claim is reviewed for medical necessity and not technically denied because of discrepancies. Reports should be carefully proofread before they are signed by the therapist, and should also be reviewed before the request for information is submitted.

Attending to the details involved in submitting documentation to the reviewer that is legible, organized, and accurate makes clear the professionalism of the provider. Although adjudication of claims is based on clinical content, appearance plays an important role in helping the reviewer determine the need for skilled care. It also is a positive reflection on physical therapy as a health care profession.

A Proactive Approach to Appeal Processing

Receiving a denial from a third-party payer is often a terrifying experience for therapists. The need to justify skilled physical therapy services may initially result in a defensive posture. The fact that reimbursement may be denied or further services will not be authorized can be detrimental financially to the rehabilitation provider and upsetting for patients, depending on how frequently it occurs. What is commonly overlooked is that appeal processing can be a positive experience.

Providing documentation tips for pursuing claim denials begins in understanding the rationale for initiating the appeal process. By participating in this process the therapist serves not only the clinical needs of the patient, but the financial needs as well. Indeed, health care is a business, and a proactive perspective encompassing both the clinical and financial needs of the patient is a necessity for the delivery of quality care.

So why appeal a claim denial? There are many reasons. The first is to be an advocate for the patient. Patients are not always aware of their appeal rights. By involving the patient in the appeal process, therapists provide consumer education. Not all patients understand the coverage limitations or the process necessary to secure authorizations for skilled physical therapy services. The voice of the consumer in health care reform is important; therefore, education is essential.

Second, appeal processing allows the therapist to validate the use of the treatments chosen and to pave the way for others. Therapists have a professional responsibility to their patients and third-party payers to provide reasonable and necessary service. Reviewers commonly are not peers; therefore, an appeal will help educate reviewers and third-party payers regarding the practice and benefits of physical therapy services. Thus, pursuing an appeal may inadvertently help others who are submitting similar claims.

To appeal a denied claim is also a right that allows the provider of physical therapy services and the patient to better understand the third-party payer's expectations and coverage limitations. The knowledge gained from the appeal experience will assist in preventing similar situations from occurring. Therapists often discover the deficiencies in their documentation during this process.

Finally, the ability to recover payment is also beneficial to the provider and often to the patient. Liability for payment will vary depending on the third-party payer's guidelines. It is often best to pursue claims to the highest level to achieve success. As a provider, the ability to recover costs will help in preventing eventual cost of service adjustments and changes to the professional staffing plan, both of which may directly affect the consumer.

The decision to appeal a denied authorization or claim needs to be carefully considered by the billing provider and the patient. The reason for denial and an analysis of the specific patient situation needs to be performed. To begin the appeal process unprepared may result in an unpleasant experience.

First, the provider must have working knowledge or obtain information regarding the third-party payer's guidelines. In certain situations the provider, according to the provider agreement, is aware of coverage limitations. For example, certain health maintenance organizations may only allow a certain number of visits. Others payers may allow therapy visits to be extended with prior authorization, and some may have defined amounts of payment allowed per year.

Understanding the guidelines and exploring any options for extraordinary circumstances must be done *prior* to appeal. Third-party payers customarily have resources or provider representatives available for educational purposes. Other potential resources include the state insurance commissioner, the department of labor and insurance, the workers' compensation bureau, private attorneys, professional organizations, and/or advocacy organizations.

Also to be considered is the support of the patient and family, the deadlines for submission of an appeal, and the availability of supportive documentation. Appeal rights vary and often may not be initiated by the provider. However, in certain circumstances, a patient may appoint the therapist as his or her representative, allowing the provider to initiate an appeal. Patient involvement is important for both consumer education and the establishment of medical necessity.

Deadlines for appeal submission are important to know. Timelines are defined by the payer and may vary from days to months. However, in the event prior authorization for treatment is denied, prompt response to the acute needs of the patient is helpful. To delay initiation may demonstrate to the reviewer that intervention is not medically necessary, as the patient is functioning without service. In a retrospective case denial, a delay in appeal submission may slow case resolution and payment. In either case, a prompt response is the best approach, as supportive documentation is then the most accessible and the treating therapist is available.

Finally, an examination of the therapy documentation and supportive evidence is needed. Therapists must analyze their documentation, the coverage decision, and the data provided by other health care professionals. Is the plan of treatment realistic? Is the duration reasonable as a standard of practice? Are the skills of a therapist required? The American Physical Therapy Association's *Guide to Physical Therapist Practice*[2] is one reference that may help in this process. Through documentation analysis, a decision to pursue either a full or partial reversal can be determined. Even if the therapy documentation appears nonsupportive, key points may exist upon which an appeal can be developed.

Identifying key points in documentation that appears nonsupportive is challenging, but is an important part of developing a successful appeal. These points may include highlighting the presence of multiple complicating diagnoses, describing the treatment strategies used and why nonskilled personnel could not safely perform them, identifying complicating factors, and finding key words that relate to the need for the skills of a therapist. For example, a key word such as "dizziness" may indicate why the skills of a therapist are needed to safely provide mobility training when a cardiopulmonary diagnosis exists.

Often prior authorizations for treatment and retrospective denials occur because the need for skilled care is not well documented. The therapist should try to isolate the reason for denial and to provide additional evidence to support the appeal process. To supply the reviewer with the same information will not justify medical necessity. It is helpful to submit supportive evidence from sources such as the referring physician, nursing, social services, other rehabilitation professionals, the patient, and/or family members/caregivers. Highlighting pertinent data can also help the reviewer in determining the need for skilled care.

The representing therapist should display confidence in his or her decision making during the appeal process and should pursue the appeal to the highest level. The ability to remain calm and professional and to pursue with tact is helpful. Remember, the patient is the third-party payer's customer. The payer wants to ensure the customer's well-being. The payer is not an adversary, but a partner in overseeing and assuring effective and reasonable rehabilitation service. Therefore, if therapists understand appeal rights, know the guidelines, and review the case closely, a positive appeal process is likely.

How to Write an Appeal Letter

When the need to request a reconsideration for coverage occurs, an appeal letter is recommended. The letter is often submitted with other supportive patient data and, in certain instances, with standardized forms required by the third-party payer. The appeal letter provides a patient profile, summarizes for the reviewer the need for skilled care, and identifies additional data that may have been lacking in the documentation initially received by the reviewer. The outline in Table 3.3 highlights essential components for writing an effective appeal letter.

Table 3.3 Essential Components for Writing an Appeal Letter (Outline adapted with permission of MJ Care, Inc., Racine, Wisconsin.)

I. Specify the letter's intent. Include dates denied and patient identifying data such as the health insurance claim number.

II. Provide a summary of data accompanying the referral.
   A. Diagnosis/onset date and reason for referral.
   B. Pertinent secondary diagnoses and/or complicating treatment diagnoses/conditions.
   C. Medical history, including dates of hospitalization, as indicated.
   D. Complications that have contributed to the duration of care.
   E. Prior level of function. Be specific!

III. Briefly summarize pertinent baseline data from the initial evaluation and the relationship to functional deficits. Establish the reason for skilled care. Why were skills of a therapist needed? Data should focus on the problems identified and may include the following:
   A. Cognition
   B. Vision/hearing
   C. Vital signs
   D. Vascular signs
   E. Sensation/proprioception
   F. Edema
   G. Posture
   H. AROM/PROM
   I. Strength
   J. Pain
   K. Coordination
   L. Bed mobility
   M. Balance (sit and stand)
   N. Transfers
   O. Ambulation (level and elevated surfaces)
   P. Orthotic/prosthetic devices
   Q. Wheelchair use
   R. DME (using or required)
   S. Activity tolerance
   U. Wound description, including incision status
   V. Special tests
   W. Architectural considerations

IV. Provide specific functional comparisons of progress and skilled service for the dates in question. Address each problem area, as appropriate. Include home program instructions, if appropriate, and whenever possible, highlight any program upgrades.

V. Address as appropriate:
   A. References to attached additional evidence, such as a copy of the home program, letter from the physician and/or patient/family supporting the need for your care, nursing notes, diagnosis and/or medication sheets, nursing flowsheets, social service notes, physician entries, consultation reports, and/or specialized test score sheets from the patient file.
   B. Nursing and family inservices (list specific dates).
   C. Discharge planning meetings.
   D. Specific complications that arose, or particular needs unique to the patient.
   E. Discharge status or level of independence achieved.

VI. Conclusion
   A. State why the skills of a therapist were/are needed for the patient to achieve stated goals.
   B. Indicate the reason, according to the third-party payer's guidelines, that reconsideration is warranted.

The following sample letter applies the essential components for writing an effective appeal letter. This letter was written following a retrospective request for information that resulted in a denial. The reason for denial indicated that the physical therapy service provided was not reasonable or necessary based on the chronic diagnosis of chronic obstructive pulmonary disease. The data corresponding to this letter are presented in Chapter 4, Case 8: Outpatient, pp. 138–146.

Sample Appeal Letter

(Date)
(Address of third-party payer)

Dear Reviewer,

This letter is to formally appeal the physical therapy denial on Mrs. ABC, HICN 000-00-0000, from 00/00/00 thru 00/00/00.

Mrs. ABC was hospitalized 00/00/00 for an exacerbation of chronic obstructive pulmonary disease. Upon discharge from the acute care hospital and inpatient rehabilitation hospital on approximately 00/00/00, the patient presented with balance and functional strength deficits and insufficient activity tolerance for independence in the community. The therapeutic exercises and skilled activities employed required a qualified therapist to ensure treatment effectiveness and patient safety. Mrs. ABC's condition required monitoring of the oxygen saturation rate during functional activities. Prior to this illness the patient was independent in the community without an assistive device.

Upon initial evaluation on 00/00/00 (not 00/00/00 as the claim denial indicated), the patient was assessed to be at a moderate risk for falling based on the Tinetti Balance/Gait Assessment Tool. Please see attached. Mrs. ABC was also dependent on an assistive device for ambulation that she had not been required to use prior to hospitalization.

This patient demonstrated poor functional activity tolerance evidenced by ability to ambulate on the treadmill 3 minutes and 24 seconds at .8 mph with a decline in oxygen saturation from 87 to 85. Mrs. ABC was referred to physical therapy specifically to monitor oxygen saturation in conjunction with progressing functional strength, balance, and activity tolerance to return to and remain independent in the community.

Mrs. ABC progressed steadily in therapy until placed on hold 00/00/00 thru 00/00/00 secondary to a decline in condition after sustaining a lower extremity laceration when she fell at home on 00/00/00. Patient returned to therapy 00/00/00 displaying a decline in Tinetti from 20/28 initially to 19/28 on 00/00/00, indicating poor functional balance for any activities in standing.

By discharge on 00/00/00, the patient's Tinetti score had increased to 27/28 placing her at a low risk for falling. Continued therapy beyond the date of denial was necessary as the patient had been demonstrating progress and had not reached her highest level of functional independence and safety. The 10 minute treadmill ambulation on 00/00/00 was the patient's maximal ability which was a decline from 15 minutes from the previous month prior to the patient's fall at home. The patient also continued with poor oxygen saturation levels documented on 00/00/00, 00/00/00 and 00/00/00. See attached.

It was indicated in the reason for denial that the patient was ambulatory without an assistive device on 00/00/00, which is correct, however only for ambulation indoors on level surfaces and only for 110 feet. This patient is a community ambulator and at that point was not tolerating ambulation out of doors or on steps.

Also, by discharge, the patient's single limb stance improved significantly from 3 seconds to 11–19 seconds, indicating a higher functional level as the patient was now able to pick objects off the floor and walk while carrying objects without loss of balance.

It is our mission to provide quality therapy services to our patients. I strongly urge you to reconsider this case. This patient benefited highly from our services and as a result is independent in her community and continues to maintain her functional strength and activity tolerance through performance of a home exercise program within safe pulmonary parameters.

Thank you for your time and consideration. I welcome any questions you may have concerning this case. I can be reached Monday through Friday from 8:00 a.m. to 4:00 p.m. at (000) 000-0000.

Sincerely,

Writing an effective appeal letter is often challenging and at times humbling for the documenting therapist. When the letter is completed accurately, deficiencies in the original documentation become evident. Depending on the circumstances and availability of additional evidence, this process can be frustrating and time-consuming. Therapists need to keep in mind that appeal processing is an opportunity for learning that leads to improved functional documentation skills and reimbursement. Pursuing appeals to the highest level allowed will often result in a successful outcome.

A pitfall to this process is apathy. To take a defensive posture and quickly complete an appeal letter without understanding the guidelines will result in frustration. The therapist must be willing to analyze denials, understand functional writing, and remain proactive in health care reform.

For example, the following appeal letter is poorly written. It was received by a peer physical therapist reviewer (Lynn Phillippi, MS, PT) at the request of a third-party payer. This appeal letter is the treating physical therapist's response to the third request for information issued by the payer:

(November)
(Address of third-party payer)

Dear Reviewer,

This letter is to provide the missing information to personnel at ABC Insurance on subscriber Mrs. X. It will address information from June to present, as this is where questions start.

The diagnosis has remained the same throughout the course of therapy. It remains rotator cuff tear.

Functional goals have been continuously set, starting from Mrs. X's initial therapy date of January 25, which was her first appointment after her January 20th surgical rotator cuff repair. On June 4th, a goal of active flexion 115° was set. On June 23rd the goal was addressed and found not to have been met. On that date a new goal of active shoulder flexion to 120° was set. On July 15th a new goal was set to increase active shoulder flexion to 130°. On August 3rd that goal was found to be met and a new goal was set. The new goal was that Mrs. X would be able to perform her standing flexion/abduction progressive resistive exercises with a four pound dumbbell. On September 7th that goal was addressed and found to have been met so a new goal was set and addressed on a regular basis.

Another question was the patient's status and how she was improving. Throughout the time period from June there are both subjective and objective notes pertaining to this.

06-20   S - "Pt. states she continues to progress with ROM."
06-29   S - "Little pain, but c/o weakness."
        O - Fatigues quickly with PNF.
07-02   S - "Feel strong as long as she stays below her head."
07-05   O - Improved tolerance to PNF manual resistance.
07-12   S - "Feeling stronger and notices increased mobility."
        O - Making progress with ROM and improving with manual resistive exercise.
07-18   S - "Feeling good."
07-19   S - "Hiking with ROM."
07-21   O - Strength improving with manual resistance.
07-26   O - Improved strength. Continues to demonstrate shoulder hiking with AROM.
08-04   S - "Feels good."
08-08   O - Gaining strength.
08-22   S - "Frustration with inability to do reaching activities with her arm."
08-25   S - "Able to perform all activities functionally except overhead reaching."
09-06   S - "Feels ROM has plateaued."

I hope this will answer any remaining questions in regards to Mrs. X's continuing need for physical therapy services from June to present.

Please call me direct if there are any remaining questions.

Professionally,

This poorly written appeal letter is, unfortunately, real. A lack of clinical insight and skilled services is evident, as is limited knowledge of functional documentation. The letter indicates that a goal of active shoulder flexion of 115° was upgraded to 120° when the previous goal had not been achieved. It also defines functional activity as the performance of progressive resistive exercises. Patient quotes appear inaccurate, as it would be unusual for a patient to refer to herself as "she" (e.g., "Feel strong as long as *she* stays below *her* head"). Descriptive terminology justifying skilled care is also lacking.

As health care reform evolves, therapists need to take a proactive approach. Apathy must be avoided. To be successful in the appeal process, therapists must be realistic in decision making. Emphasis on positive functional outcomes, objective data (not subjective), and establishing the need for skilled care are needed.

Conclusion

Demonstrating that physical therapy services are reasonable and necessary can be accomplished through descriptive terminology and emphasizing positive functional outcomes. Accurately documenting physical therapy services gives the therapist the opportunity to validate the efficacy of treatment intervention. Involvement in appeal processing, within reasonable clinical boundaries, allows therapists to be active participants in health care reform.

Involvement in the state and national physical therapy associations will help therapists understand the changes in reimbursement strategies. As managed care advances, so must rehabilitative services. To believe change will never happen is unrealistic. Therapists in all settings will do best to adapt to changes in ways that allow quality care. As documentation is streamlined for cost efficiency, functional writing skills must continue to improve.

Functional writing skills are not easily developed without attention to the essential elements of documentation. To enhance the reader's understanding of the essential elements, it is helpful to analyze documentation from the perspective of the reviewer. This opportunity is provided in Chapter 4.

Chapter 4 explores and analyzes documentation from a reviewer's perspective. The challenges reviewers face in rendering coverage decisions become evident. The documentation tips presented to this point are used to help justify skilled physical therapy intervention.

References

1. Scott RW. *Legal Aspects of Documenting Patient Care*. Gaithersburg, Maryland: Aspen Publishers, Inc., 1994, 45.
2. American Physical Therapy Association. Guide to Physical Therapist Practice. *Phys Ther* 1997; 77(11): 1163–1650.

Review Questions

1. What are functional phrase alternatives?
2. Explain why descriptive terminology is helpful to the reviewer of physical therapy documentation.
3. List the three things that a therapist can do regarding the appearance of documentation submitted to a third-party payer that can help the review process.
4. List four reasons for appealing a physical therapy claim denial.
5. When a claim denial is received, the billing provider and/or the patient needs to carefully consider if an appeal is warranted. Explain what the provider should consider and/or know before appealing a denied claim.
6. Why is an appeal letter from a therapist important when a request for reconsideration (i.e., an appeal) is submitted?

Review Question Answer Sheet

1. Functional phrase alternatives are terms or phases that convey to the reviewer the skilled nature of the service provided. Using a functional phrase alternative describes the skills of the physical therapist and the patient's status accurately for the reviewer, rather than allowing assumptions based on a common term. As an example, it is better to use the term *gait training* than *walk*.

2. Descriptive terminology is helpful to the reviewer of physical therapy documentation for several reasons. It helps to paint a clear picture of the patient. The reviewer can then render a positive coverage decision. Example: *Poor quad contraction* is better stated as *Per manual muscle test right quadriceps strength is poor. Neuromuscular electrical stimulation applied to facilitate strengthening exercises. Patient uses one crutch for safe gait due to knee buckling.*

3. The therapist can help the review process through the professional appearance of the documentation submitted to the third-party payer. Ensuring that documentation is legible, appropriately presented (i.e., in a logical and consistent order), and accurate facilitates the review.

4. Reasons for appealing a claim denial include:

   (i) To be an advocate for the patient, as not all patients are aware of their appeal rights. Consumer education is important.

   (ii) To allow the therapist to validate the use of the treatments chosen and pave the way for others. This provides a means of educating the third-party payer.

   (iii) To allow the provider of physical therapy service and the patient to better understand the third-party payer's expectations and guidelines.

   (iv) To recover payment.

5. Before appealing a denied claim, the provider should consider several things. First, the provider must understand the third-party payer's guidelines. Is the provider in compliance with coverage limitations? Also to be considered is the support of the patient and/or family, the deadlines for submission of the appeal, and the availability of supportive documentation.

6. It is helpful to include an appeal letter when submitting for a reconsideration of a claim denial. The appeal letter provides a patient profile, summarizes the need for skilled care, and identifies additional data that may have been lacking in the documentation initially received by the reviewer.

Chapter 4

Case Studies: Analyzing Documentation from a Reviewer's Perspective

Introduction

The ability to analyze physical therapy documentation from a reviewer's perspective fosters the development of skilled writing techniques. In the preceding chapters the essential elements for documentation were defined, areas of insufficient data were presented, and strategies to foster skilled writing were provided. Based on that information, the case studies in this chapter serve as learning tools for refining documentation skills to facilitate the payment process and demonstrate the efficacy of skilled physical therapy intervention.

The following case studies represent a variety of settings and patient types:

- Home health
- Hospital
- Industrial health
- Outpatient
- Pediatric
- Skilled nursing facility
- Subacute

The case studies are displayed in a consistent format to help in identifying the essential elements of documentation within the boundaries defined in this text. They are not specific to any third-party payer, review process, or facility documentation format. However, the data entry for the initial evaluation, the progress or discharge report, and the individualized educational program closely reflects the verbiage and abbreviations used by the original documenter to best demonstrate what a reviewer encounters. (Refer to Appendix 8 for abbreviations.)

The cases are intended to display a reviewer's perspective and foster discussion. There will be room for interpretation, as there are limited standards and guidelines for the review process. The comments provided in the worksheets represent the opinions of the authors and stress the basic principles for documentation

success. Analyzing documentation from a reviewer's perspective will help the reader develop an appreciation for the challenges faced in rendering coverage decisions.

General Instructions

1. Choose a case study that best represents your practice setting or area of interest.
2. Read the patient data presented in the initial evaluation and complete the corresponding case study worksheet. Compare your worksheet and comments with those provided by the authors. (See Directions for Worksheet Completion, pp. 65–72.)
3. Read the patient data presented in the progress or discharge report, as applicable. Complete the corresponding case study worksheet. Compare your worksheet and comments with those provided by the authors. (See Directions for Worksheet Completion, pp. 65–72.)
4. If possible, compare comments and answers with a peer or group of peers. The variety of responses may be surprising!

Directions for Worksheet Completion

Step 1. Following a review of the patient data, please select the corresponding case study worksheet:

- Initial Evaluation Worksheet (pp. 66–67)
- Progress or Discharge Report Worksheet (pp. 68–69)
- Individualized Education Program Worksheet (p. 70)

Permission for reprinting is not required for the three worksheets provided on pp. 66–70 when used for the sole purpose of analyzing the case studies in *Documenting Physical Therapy: The Reviewer Perspective*.

Initial Evaluation Worksheet

1. Are the "essential elements" (defined in Chapter 1) for documentation present?

Essential Element	Y, N, or N/A	Comment(s)
Referral		
Reason		
Specific treatment requested		
Data Accompanying Referral		
Diagnosis/onset date		
Secondary diagnoses		
Medical history		
Medications		
Comorbidities (complicating or precautionary information)		
Physical Therapy Intake/History		
Date of birth		
Age		
Gender		
Start of Care		
Primary complaint		
Referral Diagnosis		
Mechanism of injury		
Prior diagnostic imaging/testing		
Prior Therapy History		
Baseline Evaluation Data		
Cognition		
Vision/hearing		
Vital signs		
Vascular signs		
Sensation/proprioception		
Edema		
Posture		
AROM/PROM		
Strength		
Pain		
Coordination		
Bed mobility		
Balance (sit and stand)		
Transfers		
Ambulation (level and elevated surfaces)		

Essential Element	Y, N, or N/A	Comment(s)
Orthotic/prosthetic devices		
Wheelchair use		
DME (using or required)		
Activity tolerance		
Wound description, including incision status		
Special tests		
Architectural/safety considerations		
Requirements to return to home, school and/or job		
Prior Level of Function		
Mobility (home and community)		
Employment		
School		
Treatment Diagnosis		
Assessment		
Reason for skilled care		
Problems		
Plan of Care		
Specific treatment strategies		
Frequency		
Duration		
Patient instruction/home program		
Caregiver training		
Short-term goals and achievement dates		
Long-term goals and achievement dates		
Rehabilitation potential		

2. Is the overall history of the patient adequate?

3. Is there evidence of the need for skilled intervention?

4. Are there adequate baseline data to develop future comparisons?

5. Are the objective data related to functional deficits?

6. Are comparative statements and data clearly outlined?

7. (A) Are the three components for goals present (measurable, functional, time frames)?

(B) Are the goals realistic for the individual case?

8. Do you feel the proposed treatment is reasonable and necessary?

Progress or Discharge Report Worksheet

1. Are the "essential elements" (defined in Chapter 1) for documentation present?

Essential Element	Y, N, or N/A	Comment(s)
Attendance		
Current Baseline Data		
Cognition		
Vision/hearing		
Vital signs		
Vascular signs		
Sensation/proprioception		
Edema		
Posture		
AROM/PROM		
Strength		
Pain		
Coordination		
Bed mobility		
Balance (sit and stand)		
Transfers		
Ambulation (level and elevated surfaces)		
Orthotic/prosthetic devices		
Wheelchair use		
DME (using or required)		
Activity tolerance		
Wound description, including incision status		
Special tests		
Architectural/safety considerations		

Essential Element	Y, N, or N/A	Comment(s)
Treatment Diagnosis		
Assessment		
Reason for skilled care		
Problems		
Plan of Care		
Specific treatment strategies		
Frequency		
Duration		
Patient instruction/home program		
Caregiver training		
Short-term goals and achievement dates		
Long-term goals and achievement dates		
Rehabilitation potential or discharge prognosis		

2. Is there evidence of the need for skilled intervention?

3. Are there adequate baseline data to develop future comparisons?

4. Are the objective data related to functional deficits?

5. Are comparative statements and data clearly outlined?

6. (A) Are the three components for goals present (measurable, functional, time frames)?

   (B) Are the goals realistic for the individual case?

7. Do you feel the treatment was reasonable and necessary?

Individualized Education Program Worksheet

1. Are the "essential elements" (defined in Chapter 1) for IEP documentation present?

Essential Element	Y, N, or N/A	Comment(s)
Present levels of educational performance		
Annual goal		
Short-term objectives		
Schedule		
Specific special education and related services that will contribute to meeting this goal		

Step 2. The case study worksheet includes three columns. After each essential element, indicate the following:

Y   Yes, data are present. If incomplete, provide comment.

N   No, not addressed. Provide comment.

N/A   Not applicable in this case. No comment required, as the essential element is not pertinent to the patient because of the setting or clinical profile.

N/A   Not applicable at this time. Data are reasonably expected in a subsequent report or were addressed previously and are not longer pertinent to the case. Provide comment.

Comments should do the following:

- Describe the documentation deficit(s)
- Indicate why additional data would be helpful to the reviewer and/or describe what data are needed to assist in determining a coverage decision

Step 3. Answer the remaining worksheet questions.

Readers should note that Question 2 in the Initial Evaluation Worksheet (i.e., "Is the overall history of the patient adequate?") refers to the medical history and the prior therapy history.

Worksheet Completion Samples

Use Y to indicate yes, if data are present for the essential element listed. If the data provided are incomplete, provide comments describing the deficit(s), why additional data would be helpful to the reviewer, and/or what data are needed to assist in determining a coverage decision.

For example, the reason for referral in the initial evaluation for Case 1, Home Health, p. 74, is described as "The patient wants to regain balance, strength and to walk without someone holding onto them." Therefore, the Initial Evaluation Worksheet would be best completed as follows:

Essential Element	Y, N, or N/A	Comment(s)
Reason	Y	The reason for referral indicates, "The patient wants to regain balance, strength and to walk without someone holding onto them." Additional description of the patient's functional deficits in relationship to the long-term goal would be helpful. For instance, attaching the phrase *to decrease caregiver assistance and increase safety at home* would justify the need for skilled care.

Use N for "No," meaning that this essential element is pertinent to the case but is not addressed. Provide a comment describing why additional data would be helpful to the reviewer and/or what data are needed to assist in determining a coverage decision. For example in Case 1, Home Health, p. 75, medications are not addressed. The worksheet for this area would be best completed as follows:

Essential Element	Y, N, or N/A	Comment(s)
Medications	N	Not addressed. Based on the diagnosis of multiple cerebrovascular accidents, history of pain, and the balance deficits described in the evaluation, it would be helpful to know what medications, if any, are being administered that may affect rehabilitation, such as anticoagulants.

N/A is used to mean "Not applicable in this case." Based on the data presented, the essential element described is not clinically relevant to the case and is therefore appropriately left unaddressed. No comment is necessary.

For example in Case 1, Home Health, p. 77, the wound description, including incision status, is appropriately not addressed in the evaluation, as the patient data does not include a relevant diagnosis or history to require this essential element. The worksheet would be completed as follows:

Essential Element	Y, N, or N/A	Comment(s)
Wound description, including incision status	N/A	

N/A also means "Not applicable at this time." Based on the data presented, this essential element is not appropriate for evaluation or reassessment at this time. However, the element should be addressed in a future report. A comment is required.

For example, in Case 2, Home Health, p. 88, cognition was addressed in the initial evaluation and was not addressed in the progress report. The Progress Report Worksheet would be completed as follows:

Essential Element	Y, N, or N/A	Comment(s)
Cognition	N/A	Not applicable at this time, as the evaluation indicated that cognition was not impaired. Any changes since the evaluation that may affect rehabilitation should be documented.

Case Studies: Table of Contents

Case 1: Home Health, Initial Evaluation

Referral

Reason: The patient wants to regain balance, strength and to walk without someone holding onto them.

Specific treatment requested: PT to see patient 2x/wk for 2 wks for gait and balance training and to resume home exercise program.

Data Accompanying Referral

Diagnosis/onset date: S/P Multiple small CVA's/08-09-92
Secondary diagnoses: Recent decline in status.
Medical history: Patient was recently hospitalized from 08-09-92 to 8-14-92 for abdominal pains and nausea which has weakened him.

Physical Therapy Intake/History

Date of birth: 09-10-15
Age: 76
Gender: Male.
Start of care: 08-14-92
Primary complaint: Patient reports worse problems with walking over the last two weeks due to abdominal pains.

Prior Therapy History: He was seen in physical therapy, i.e., home visits from 03-92 through 07-92 with some breaks in service. He was discharged from therapy able to walk with a rolling walker with supervision around his apartment.

Baseline Evaluation Data

Posture: Postural muscles, i.e., trunk extensors, hip/gluteals, and quads, fatigue quickly, resulting in a forward flexed posture.
AROM/PROM: He has moderate stiffness throughout UE, LE, and trunk.
Strength: General strength is at a 3+/5 level.
Pain: No current complaints of pain.
Coordination: He demonstrates "Parkinson's" type problems with initiation of activity. Movement is rigid and jerky.
Bed mobility: Initiation of any mobility (i.e., rolling, supine to sit, transfers, walking) is difficult.

Balance (sit and stand): See Ambulation (level and elevated surfaces).
Transfers: Transfers and walking are unsafe to be done without supervision.
Ambulation (level and elevated surfaces): He walks with a rolling walker. Requires minimal/moderate assistance for balance. Distance 30 feet in apartment.
DME (using or required): Rolling walker, wheelchair, power wheelchair, scooter, bathtub equipment.

Prior Level of Function

Mobility (home and community): He required constant supervision due to poor judgment with safety.

Treatment Diagnosis: Gait dysfunction with ataxia.

Problems:

1. Reduced balance with walking.
2. Reduced strength.
3. Stiffness.

Plan of Care

Specific treatment strategies: PT for gait and balance training and resumption of home exercise program.
Frequency: 2x/wk.
Duration: 2 wks.
Patient instruction/home program: Has home health aide for bathing and lives with wife who does not appear to follow through with home exercise program with patient.
Short-term goals and achievement dates:

1. Ambulation with rolling walker with supervision distance to 50 feet in apartment every hour, 200 feet in hallway 2x's daily.
2. Follow through with home exercise program with wife's assistance.
3. Return to previous level of functioning at time of last PT discharge on 07-92.

Case 1: Home Health, Initial Evaluation Worksheet

1. Are the "essential elements" (defined in Chapter 1) for documentation present?

Essential Element	Y, N, or N/A	Comment(s)
Referral		
Reason	Y	The reason for referral indicates, "The patient wants to regain balance, strength and to walk without someone holding onto them." Additional description of the patient's functional deficits in relationship to the long-term goal would be helpful. For instance, to attach the phrase, *to decrease caregiver assistance and increase safety at home*, would justify the need for skilled care.
Specific treatment requested	Y	
Data Accompanying Referral		
Diagnosis/onset date	Y	The diagnosis of status post multiple cerebrovascular accidents with an onset of 08-09-92 requires clarification. A reviewer may question the accuracy of the onset date as the medical history indicates a hospitalization for abdominal pain and nausea on 08-09-92. No neurological deficits are described. It would seem reasonable that the diagnosis of abdominal pain and nausea resulted in the recent functional decline in gait. The status post multiple cerebrovascular accidents appears to be a secondary diagnosis.
Secondary diagnoses	Y	The secondary diagnosis is listed as "Recent decline in status." It is helpful to list specific diagnoses. The statement provided may be misinterpreted by the reviewer as a general decline that may not require the skills of a therapist.
Medical history	Y	The medical history needs to elaborate on the abdominal pain and nausea. Stating that these diagnoses "weakened him" is not sufficient. Elaborating on the facts, such as whether the patient was in bed for one week or more to facilitate this weakness, and history pertaining to the status post multiple cerebrovascular accidents would be helpful.
Medications	N	Not addressed. Based on the diagnosis of multiple cerebrovascular accidents, history of pain, and the balance deficits described in the evaluation, it would be helpful to know what medications, if any, are being administered that may affect rehabilitation such as anticoagulants.
Comorbidities (complicating or precautionary information)	N	Not addressed. It would seem reasonable that comorbidities (complicating or precautionary information) exist based on the documented status post multiple cerebrovascular accidents and the durable medical equipment listed. Are there changes in muscle tone, a history of seizures, or proprioceptive deficits? Documentation of these or other factors would justify the need for skilled care.
Physical Therapy Intake/History		
Date of birth	Y	Patient identifying information is important, as many physician offices and third-party payers file or trigger data retrieval based on date of birth.
Age	Y	
Gender	Y	
Start of Care	Y	
Primary complaint	Y	The documentation indicates, "Patient reports worse problems with walking . . . " This is an inadequate description of the functional deficits. How much assistance or what type of device is needed? Is safety a patient concern?

(continued)

Essential Element	Y, N, or N/A	Comment(s)
Referral Diagnosis		
Mechanism of injury	N/A	
Prior diagnostic imaging/testing	N	Not addressed. A description of the imaging/testing for the cause of abdominal pain could be relevant information in this case.
Prior Therapy History	Y	Data are present regarding dates of prior therapy service and ambulation ability. Additional information regarding transfers, activities of daily living, the primary diagnosis, and overall impact of therapy intervention on previously established goals would be beneficial to the reviewer in determining rehabilitation potential.
Baseline Evaluation Data		
Cognition	N	Not addressed. As poor judgment is indicated in the prior level of function, it would be helpful to know if cognition will affect participation in rehabilitation. Additional description of poor judgment in relationship to safety and functional deficits is needed.
Vision/hearing	N	Not addressed. This appears to be an important omission based on the history of multiple cerebrovascular accidents and the balance deficits described.
Vital signs	N	Not addressed. Again a notable omission, given the patient's history of multiple cerebrovascular accidents.
Vascular signs	N/A	
Sensation/proprioception	N	Not addressed. This appears to be an oversight by the therapist, as documentation indicates a history of multiple cerebrovascular accidents, balance deficits, and use of durable medical equipment. If sensation/proprioception deficits exist, they need to be documented.
Edema	N	Not addressed. Evidence of edema, if present, would demonstrate another need for skilled intervention to the reviewer.
Posture	Y	Postural deficits are not described except in relationship to fatigue; however, that relationship is unclear. Data pertaining to posture in the wheelchair, power wheelchair, and in standing would be relevant.
AROM/PROM	Y	The present data, "He has moderate stiffness throughout UE, LE, and trunk," do not provide objective measurable data for future comparison.
Strength	Y	The statement, "General strength is at a 3+/5 level," does not demonstrate a relationship to function and is not helpful to a reviewer in determining the need for skilled service. It is reasonable to expect strength discrepancies with a diagnosis of multiple cerebrovascular accidents.
Pain	Y	
Coordination	Y	Data are present and indicate, "Movement is rigid and jerky." However, further description of the coordination deficits in relationship to function (i.e., gait) is recommended to help a reviewer determine the need for skilled care.
Bed mobility	Y	Data indicates mobility is "difficult." Further objective data are needed for future comparisons. Is assistance or verbal cuing required? What is causing the difficulty?
Balance (sit and stand)	Y	The ambulation data indicate that the patient requires minimal/moderate assistance for balance. Further objective data are needed for future comparisons and to help the reviewer determine the need for skilled care. For instance, how often does the balance loss occur, and what is the direction of loss? Is balance influenced by postural, visual, or cognitive deficits?

Essential Element	Y, N, or N/A	Comment(s)
Transfers	Y	Transfers are documented as requiring supervision for safety. A reviewer may request further detail as to why the therapist documented transfers and walking as unsafe. The assistance level of supervision also appears inaccurate because of the minimal/moderate assistance level described for balance deficits during ambulation.
Ambulation (level and elevated surfaces)	Y	Ambulation is described. However, further description of safety and gait deficits are needed, such as step length and base of support. The term "walks" describes a functional outcome. However, it does not provide the reviewer with a perspective on the skilled therapy service rendered, such as *gait training or gait analysis.*
Orthotic/prosthetic devices	N	Not addressed. The use of an orthosis, if present, would help a reviewer in assessing the need for skilled care.
Wheelchair use	N	This appears to be an oversight, as a wheelchair and power wheelchair are documented in the evaluation. Based on the data indicating judgment and safety concerns, a reviewer could expect this area to be evaluated.
DME (using or required)	Y	It would be helpful to a reviewer to know what equipment is presently used by the patient and what equipment is required.
Activity tolerance	N	Not addressed. A description of the patient's level of fatigue during various functional activities would be beneficial.
Wound description, including incision status	N/A	
Special tests	N/A	
Architectural/safety considerations	N	Not addressed. This appears to be an oversight based on the patient's documented safety concerns and use of durable medical equipment.
Requirements to return to home, school, and/or job	N/A	
Prior Level of Function		
Mobility (home and community)	Y	Mobility is described as requiring constant supervision. It may be helpful to indicate for what functional activities.
Employment	N/A	
School	N/A	
Treatment Diagnosis	Y	
Assessment		
Reason for skilled care	N	Not addressed. Documentation indicating the physical limitations and their relationship to functional deficits as well as justification of the need for skilled care for a short duration are needed. A reviewer may question if the patient could continue with his previous home program to regain his strength, therefore not requiring skilled physical therapy intervention.
Problems	Y	Problems are listed. However, Problem 3, "Stiffness," is vague. It may be better described as *decreased coordination* or *increased lower extremity muscle tone.*
Plan of Care		
Specific treatment strategies	Y	
Frequency	Y	
Duration	Y	

(continued)

Essential Element	Y, N, or N/A	Comment(s)
Patient instruction/home program	Y	A description of the previous home program is needed. The therapist indicates the wife does not appear to follow through with the patient's home program. This appears to be an assumption and needs to be restated in a positive manner such as, *Wife (or patient) reports the home program is completed one time per week. The program was established for daily completion. Further education required.*
Caregiver training	N	See Patient instruction/home program. It is evident that, because of questionable home program compliance, caregiver training will need to be addressed. This requires the skills of a therapist.
Short-term goals and achievement dates	Y	Goals 2 and 3 lack functional and measurable components. All goals require a time frame.
Long-term goals and achievement dates	N	Not addressed. Because of the short duration of treatment (two weeks) it is acceptable not to have a long-term goal. This case, however, would be strengthened if a specific long-term goal was defined. For example, *Patient will regain strength and demonstrate independence in a home program for safe ambulation, bed mobility, and transfers with supervision of caregiver to maintain home placement.*
Rehabilitation potential	N	Not addressed. Rehabilitation potential is an essential element of documentation. It provides the therapist's insight into the potential success of the rehabilitation intervention for the stated goals. This helps the reviewer determine the reasonableness of skilled care.

2. Is the overall history of the patient adequate?

No, there needs to be more information regarding the effects of the abdominal pain, nausea, and history of multiple cerebrovascular accidents in relationship to the patient's present decline in mobility. Was the patient bedridden? Did the patient experience an increase in balance deficits after hospitalization?

3. Is there evidence of the need for skilled intervention?

This is not clearly stated, and not enough details of the patient's functional deficits are adequately presented. The reviewer is left with the question, why were the skills of a therapist needed? It would be helpful in justifying skilled intervention to describe the need for caregiver training and home program revision and to provide a description of the recent functional decline in mobility. Elaborating on challenges to the rehabilitation process, such as decreased proprioception, range of motion deficits, and tone influences, would also be helpful.

4. Are there adequate baseline data to develop future comparisons?

There are essentially no objective/measurable data, and what data are given, such as "Parkinson's type problems," do not adequately describe the patient's functional deficits. It is not clear how the patient is limited secondary to rigid and jerky movements, safety issues, and balance deficits.

5. Are the objective data related to functional deficits?

There are minimal objective data and the data that are provided are not clearly related to the patient's overall level of functioning. This is evident for range of motion, strength, bed mobility, and balance.

6. Are comparative statements and data clearly outlined?

Data are lacking or omitted for areas such as cognition, vision/hearing, sensation/proprioception, AROM/PROM, bed mobility, wheelchair use, and activity tolerance.

7. (A) Are the three components for goals present (measurable, functional, time frames)?

With the exception of Goal 1, there are no measurable data or defined functional components. Time frames are lacking for all goals. For example, Goal 2 states, "Follow through with the home exercise program with wife's assistance." This goal would be better stated as, *Patient will demonstrate independent and safe performance of the home program with wife's assistance in two weeks.*

(B) Are the goals realistic for the individual case?

Yes, but the goals themselves are unclear, and a reviewer must search the documentation in an attempt to find a measurable component such as with Goal 3. Goal 3 states, "Return to previous level of functioning at time of last PT discharge on 07-92." It is also noted that Goal 3 does not correspond to the identified problem of stiffness.

8. Do you feel the proposed treatment is reasonable and necessary?

Based on the decline in functional status (although the data are limited), it appears that evaluation and treatment are appropriate because of the short duration of skilled care requested, the apparent inconsistency in home program completion, and the acute decline in balance and ambulation.

Case 1: Home Health, Discharge Report

Attendance: 4 visits.

Current Baseline Data

Balance (sit and stand): Balance with gait is much improved. Initially he needed contact assist at all times, now needs only supervision.

Transfers: Requires supervision. Contact assist only on "bad days." Tub transfers with tub bench with supervision.

Ambulation (level and elevated surfaces): Distance is improved from 30 feet to 200 feet x 3 in hallway. Walks around apartment every hour.

Treatment Diagnosis: Gait dysfunction with ataxia; recent decline in status; hospitalized.

Assessment

Reason for skilled care: Gait dysfunction with ataxia improved. Improved since eval 08-14-92 from moderate to minimal/moderate level. Patient says that he is walking better.

Reason for discharge: Goals achieved.

Plan of Care

Specific treatment strategies: Discontinue PT.

Patient instruction/home program: Exercise program 1–2x daily with supervision. Tolerates 2 sets of 10 reps of each exercise (i.e., straight leg raising, hip abduction, hip/knee flexion, TKE, LTR, bridging, marching, standing balance exercise at counter, and upper extremity cane exercises). Client to walk in hallway 2–4x daily.

Caregiver training: Home exercise program completed daily with wife with home health aide assist. Patient is now receiving 4 hours of home health assistance care. When last discontinued by PT on 07-92 he had only 2 hours of care daily. The present aide (unlike the previous one) is excellent in following through with helping the patient exercise and walk.

Short-term goals and achievement dates:

1. Ambulates with rolling walker 200 feet in hallway 2x's daily with supervision. (Surpassed goal: Doing this 3–4x's daily.)
2. Home exercise completed daily with wife with home health aide.
3. Returned to level of functioning when last d/c'd by PT on 07-92.

Case 1: Home Health, Discharge Report Worksheet

1. Are the "essential elements" (defined in Chapter 1) for documentation present?

Essential Element	Y, N, or N/A	Comment(s)
Attendance	Y	Present information, "4 visits," does not provide the reviewer with the number of visits scheduled. It is helpful to list the number of scheduled visits and identify any reasons for absence.
Current Baseline Data		
Cognition	N	This area is not addressed in the evaluation or discharge summary. It would seem relevant to include data, as it relates to safety in negotiating within his surroundings, based on the judgment and safety issues identified in the evaluation, which acknowledged the need for supervised activities.
Vision/hearing	N	Not addressed in the evaluation or discharge report. A reviewer may have concerns as to whether there is a correlation between balance and safety deficits and vision/hearing.
Vital signs	N	Not addressed in the evaluation or discharge report. Once again, a reviewer may have concerns due to the history of multiple cerebrovascular accidents and balance deficits.
Vascular signs	N/A	

(continued)

Essential Element	Y, N, or N/A	Comment(s)
Sensation/proprioception	N	Not addressed in the evaluation or discharge report. If deficits exist, their impact on function needs to be documented to help demonstrate the need for skilled care.
Edema	N	Not addressed in the evaluation or discharge report. If edema is present, the impact on function needs to be documented to demonstrate the need for skilled care.
Posture	N	Not addressed. Postural deficits were described in relationship to fatigue in the evaluation. Comparative data in the discharge report would be important to a reviewer for determining progress.
AROM/PROM	N	Measurable data were not provided in the evaluation; however, moderate stiffness of the extremities and trunk was described. As "stiffness" was listed as a problem, comparative data are reasonably expected.
Strength	N	Although general strength is listed as 3+/5 in the evaluation, no data are given at the time of discharge. As emphasis is placed on a home program that focuses on strengthening, comparative measurable data are needed.
Pain	N/A	
Coordination	N	In the evaluation, the patient's movements were described as rigid and jerky with Parkinson type problems when initiating any activity. This needs to be described at the time of discharge. Do deficits still exist that influence gait?
Bed mobility	N	In the evaluation rolling and supine to sit are described as difficult, and yet no comparative data are presented to describe the patient's progress in this area.
Balance (sit and stand)	Y	The discharge report indicates that balance has improved, and a comparative statement is listed. The comparative statement indicates, "Initially he needed contact assist at all times, now needs only supervision." The data do not indicate the direction of balance loss and/or the relationship to safety. The statement is also inaccurate, as "minimal/moderate assistance for balance" was listed in the evaluation. A reviewer would find it helpful to know if strengthening and/or skilled activities improved balance.
Transfers	Y	There is no description of why transfers are difficult for this patient, and most reviewers would question what "bad days" actually means in terms of the patient's disabilities. The types of transfers and levels of assistance were not described in the evaluation. A reviewer would be unable to determine functional progress.
Ambulation (level and elevated surfaces)	Y	The discharge report provides comparative data for ambulation distance. This description alone does not justify the need for skilled physical therapy service. Was gait training performed? Does the patient use an assistive device and, if so, is it used safely? Are gait deficits present? Does balance loss occur during gait training? Descriptive terminology is needed such as: *Gait training with rolling walker and supervision of 1 for 200 feet x 3. (Previously 30 feet with minimal/moderate assistance for balance.) Base of support and stride length within normal limits without verbal cuing. (Previously moderate verbal cuing required.)*
Orthotic/prosthetic devices	N	Not addressed in the evaluation or discharge report. With a history of multiple cerebrovascular accidents, the use of an orthosis, if present, needs to be documented.
Wheelchair use	N	No details are given as to how the patient negotiates within his apartment or community in a wheelchair/scooter. A reviewer might ask about the patient's safety and/or how much assistance or cuing is required.

Essential Element	Y, N, or N/A	Comment(s)
DME (using or required)	N	The evaluation provided a list of durable medical equipment. Information about the patient's continued need for this equipment at the time of discharge would be helpful.
Activity tolerance	N	Activity tolerance is not addressed in the discharge report. Ambulation distance is the only reference. A description of the patient's tolerance for functional activities such as wheelchair propulsion and transfers would be beneficial.
Wound description, including incision status	N/A	
Special tests	N/A	
Architectural/safety considerations	N	Not addressed. More information regarding environmental barriers and potential safety concerns is needed.
Treatment Diagnosis	Y	
Assessment		
Reason for skilled care	Y	The reason for skilled care is inaccurate. It states, "Gait dysfunction with ataxia improved. Improved since evaluation 08-14-92 from moderate to minimal/moderate level," yet the evaluation listed a minimal/moderate level of assistance for balance and the discharge report does not specify an ambulation assistance level. Emphasis on why the skills of a physical therapist were needed is lacking. This area may be better stated as, *Patient has responded well to skilled intervention. Gait training with an emphasis on balance/safety and an individualized strengthening program have resulted in return to mobility at a supervised level. Training for safe performance of a revised home exercise program is completed.*
Problems	N	Not addressed. Problems are absent and the short-term goals do not relate to the problems established at the time of evaluation, except for goal 1.
Plan of Care		
Specific treatment strategies	Y	The plan of care describes the present treatment strategy as, "Discontinue PT." A summary of the treatment strategies used is needed. For example, *Patient was seen two times per week for gait, balance, and patient/caregiver training with emphasis on home program revisions.* This summary would help the reviewer determine the reasonableness of the plan of care in relationship to the functional progress reported. It can also help when analyzing documentation and the corresponding services billed.
Frequency	N	Not addressed. A summary of the frequency and duration is needed. For example, documenting that the patient *Was seen two times per week for two weeks* helps the reviewer determine the reasonableness of the frequency and duration in relationship to the functional progress reported. It can also help when analyzing documentation and the corresponding services billed.
Duration	N	See Frequency.
Patient instruction/home program	Y	There is a detailed description of the type of exercises and number of repetitions required. To determine if the skills of a therapist are required, a reviewer would find it helpful to know what revisions, if any, were made to the patient's previous home program. It is recommended that abbreviations that might not be familiar to a reviewer be written out in their entirety.

(continued)

Essential Element	Y, N, or N/A	Comment(s)
Caregiver training	Y	The data indicate that the home program is completed daily with wife and home health aide assistance. It is recommended that the negative statement, "The present aide (unlike the previous one) is excellent in following through with helping the patient exercise and walk." be avoided. It is more appropriate to state that the recently hired home health aide demonstrates follow-through.
Short-term goals and achievement dates	Y	The short-term goals are not restated from the evaluation; however, a statement describing each goal's status is provided. A reviewer may find it helpful if the goal from the evaluation is listed and followed by the goal status.
Long-term goals and achievement dates	N	Not addressed. It appears that the short-term goals reflect the long-term objective. Because of the short duration of treatment (two weeks), this is acceptable. This case, however, would be strengthened if a specific long-term goal was defined. For example, *Patient will regain strength and demonstrate independence in a home program for safe ambulation, bed mobility and transfers with supervision of caregiver to maintain home placement.*
Discharge prognosis	N	Not addressed. A discharge prognosis is an essential element of documentation. It helps the reviewer assess the patient's ability to maintain or improve physical mobility based on the skilled service and home program recommendations provided.

2. Is there evidence of the need for skilled intervention?

Yes, there is evidence of the need for skilled intervention. The evidence includes the involvement of the wife and caregiver in the home program and improvement in balance from minimal/moderate assistance to supervision.

3. Are there adequate baseline data to develop future comparisons?

Data are lacking, as several areas from the evaluation were not addressed in the discharge report: coordination, bed mobility, and posture.

4. Are the objective data related to functional deficits?

No, it is difficult to picture the deficits that this patient has because of the lack of descriptive data. For example, improvement in ambulation distance is described; however, was this progress related to improved judgment, gait quality, safety, and/ or strength? How does the patient function in activities of daily living, toilet transfers, bed to chair transfers, and wheelchair propulsion?

5. Are comparative statements and data clearly outlined?

Comparative statements are present for ambulation distance and balance. Overall comparative data from the evaluation to discharge are lacking. This is evident for range of motion, strength, bed mobility, posture, and coordination.

6. (A) Are the three components for goals present (measurable, functional, time frames)?

Time frames are lacking for all goals. Goals 2 and 3 lack functional components and are not measurable.

(B) Are the goals realistic for the individual case?

Yes, based on the limited data; however, if the treatment frequency and duration were longer, a reviewer might assess this differently.

7. Do you feel the treatment was reasonable and necessary?

Yes, as the patient did return to his prior level of function and there was more consistent compliance with the home program. From a managed care perspective, a reviewer may have only approved one or two visits based on the limited detail of the functional deficits.

This case is a good example of general debility. As health care reform advances, reviewers may hesitate to authorize treatment of this nature without further justification of the need for skilled care. A description of the need for home program revision, the presence of safety deficits, and complicating conditions such as abnormal tone or proprioception deficits is needed. Would this patient have achieved the same goals without skilled care? This is questionable.

Case 2: Home Health, Initial Evaluation

Data Accompanying Referral

Diagnosis/onset date: Syringomyelia x 20 years. Onset since birth. Exacerbation 10 years ago.

Secondary diagnoses: Chronic edema of the lower extremities.

Medical history: Surgical procedure(s) relevant to care include cystoperitoneal shunt 1982.

Comorbidities (complicating or precautionary information): Gets colds with upper respiratory infections 2–3x yearly.

Physical Therapy Intake/History

Age: 48
Gender: Female
Start of care: 06-16-91

Baseline Evaluation Data

Cognition: Oriented. Memory and ability to follow instruction—okay.

Vision/hearing: Okay.

Sensation/proprioception: Decreased sensation of heat with all 4 extremities, touch sensation 2 WWL.

Edema: Moderate to maximal edema of.

Posture: NA.

AROM/PROM: Not applicable.

Strength: Not applicable.

Coordination: Unable.

Bed mobility: None.

Balance (sit and stand): NA.

Transfers: Dep on assist 1 person, use Hoyer™ lift for shower.

Ambulation (level and elevated surfaces): Unable.

Wheelchair use: Unable.

Activity tolerance: Fair.

Prior Level of Function

Mobility (home and community): Homebound, lives alone. Family—summer vacation son present.

Assessment

Reason for skilled care: Patient will always be dependent on aide and PT to decrease edema of lower extremities. Patient is motivated and cooperative. Patient will require electrical stimulation to decrease edema and continue this activity indefinitely.

Problems:

1. Patient is dependent on scooter.
2. Spared quadriplegic.
3. Dependent edema of both lower extremities.

Plan of Care

Specific treatment strategies: Electrical stimulation to both lower extremities at 10 watts/cm^2 for about one hour.

Frequency: 3x weekly x inelop.

Duration: Indefinite.

Short-term goals and achievement dates:

1. Decrease edema of lower extremities.
2. Increase mus. activities of lower extremities.
3. Increase circulation of lower extremities.

Rehabilitation potential: Fair.

Case 2: Home Health, Initial Evaluation Worksheet

1. Are the "essential elements" (defined in Chapter 1) for documentation present?

Essential Element	Y, N, or N/A	Comment(s)
Referral		
Reason	N	The reason for referral is not stated. A statement of the reason for referral such as, *Patient referred by Dr. ABC for skilled physical therapy services to control lower extremity edema and promote circulation of the lower extremities* would help justify skilled therapy intervention.
Specific treatment requested	N	Not addressed. It is appropriate to indicate in the evaluation the physician's order and date. Reviewers find this helpful, as many third-party payers require the physician approve the plan of care.

(continued)

Essential Element	Y, N, or N/A	Comment(s)
Data Accompanying Referral		
Diagnosis/onset date	Y	The diagnosis and onset dates provided may be confusing to a reviewer. The diagnosis, "Syringomyelia x 20 years," is clear. However, the onset date is also listed as "Onset since birth" with a exacerbation date of "10 years ago." Despite the discrepancies, it is reasonable for a reviewer to assume this is a chronic condition. As a result, further explanation would be expected in the documentation to justify the need for skilled care.
Secondary diagnoses	Y	The secondary diagnosis is listed as "Chronic edema of the lower extremities," and data describing a recent exacerbation are lacking. It is reasonable for the reviewer to request additional evidence to justify the need for skilled care. Based on the data presented (which indicate that the focus of treatment is to decrease edema) it would be more appropriate to list edema as the treatment diagnosis, as it is the diagnosis for which physical therapy services are rendered.
Medical history	Y	The medical history indicates a "cystoperitoneal shunt 1982." Additional data would seem reasonable based on the limitations in mobility and the chronic diagnoses. A reviewer would find it helpful to understand the patient's past and/or present medical complications, caregiver support, surgical history, and/or prior therapeutic interventions associated with the need for physical therapy intervention.
Medications	N	The data presented do not address whether medications are being administered. As edema is indicated in the evaluation, it would be helpful to know if medications that may affect rehabilitation, such as diuretics or medications for a cardiac condition, are being used.
Comorbidities (complicating or precautionary information)	Y	The therapist appropriately documents the patient's susceptibility to respiratory infections. It would seem reasonable for a reviewer to find this information incomplete based on the patient's chronic diagnoses and functional limitations. Further data, such as shortness of breath if applicable, are needed to accurately determine the need for skilled care.
Physical Therapy Intake/History		
Date of birth	N	Not addressed. Patient identifying information is important, as many physician offices and third-party payers file or trigger data retrieval based on date of birth.
Age	Y	
Gender	Y	
Start of Care	Y	
Primary complaint	N	Not addressed. The patient's primary complaint helps the reviewer in determining the need for skilled care. Because of the chronic nature of the edema, it would seem reasonable that complaints of pain, immobility, and the potential for complications such as skin breakdown or circulatory deficits exist.
Referral Diagnosis		
Mechanism of injury	N/A	
Prior diagnostic imaging/testing	N	Not addressed. It is reasonable to expect that prior diagnostic testing was performed based on the chronic diagnoses and medical history of a cystoperitoneal shunt. A reviewer would find testing relevant if it is related to the patient's medical or functional limitations such as cardiac, pulmonary, and/or neurological status.

Essential Element	Y, N, or N/A	Comment(s)
Prior Therapy History	N	Not addressed. Based on the patient's chronic diagnoses and the apparent history of disability, it is reasonable to expect that prior therapeutic intervention has occurred. It is important for the reviewer to know what procedures were previously used and if they were successful. This data will help in determining the need for skilled care.
Baseline Evaluation Data		
Cognition	Y	Although briefly described as "Okay," this information is important to the reviewer as it demonstrates the patient's ability to participate in rehabilitation. A more professional term such as *intact* would be more appropriate.
Vision/hearing	Y	See Cognition.
Vital signs	N	Not addressed. Based on the "Moderate to maximal edema" indicated, it is reasonable to expect baseline data pertaining to respiration, pulse rate, and blood pressure. It may also be clinically indicated to assess vital signs in relationship to position changes.
Vascular signs	N	Not addressed. Data describing skin color and temperature of the lower extremities would be relevant to a reviewer in determining the need for skilled rehabilitation. This appears to be an oversight by the therapist, as data indicate the presence of edema and Goal 3 states, "Increase circulation of lower extremities."
Sensation/proprioception	Y	The safety issue of decreased sensation to heat is addressed. However, the description, "touch sensation 2 WWL," is not common terminology, nor is the impact on treatment or function clear.
Edema	Y	Edema is addressed as "Moderate to maximal edema of." This description is incomplete and not measurable. Baseline data are needed, such as the location of edema, circumference measurements, and is the edema pitting or nonpitting. These data are necessary for future progress comparisons and to determine the effectiveness of the treatment modalities provided. Does edema increase without skilled intervention, and how does it affect function?
Posture	Y	Posture is described as "NA." It would seem appropriate to address sitting posture and positioning.
AROM/PROM	Y	This area is listed as "Not applicable." Since lower extremity edema is the focus of treatment and Goal 2 is to increase muscle activity in the lower extremities, range of motion measurements (active and passive) are expected for future progress comparison.
Strength	Y	The data presented indicate, "Not applicable." Because of the presence of edema and the focus of Goal 2 on increasing muscle activity of the lower extremities, strength needs to be measured. Strength is a relevant functional area, as deficits may be contributing to positional limitations for edema control.
Pain	N	Not addressed. Data as to the presence or absence of pain should be documented. It is reasonable to expect that a patient with functional limitations and chronic edema may be experiencing pain.
Coordination	Y	The documentation provided indicates that this area could not be addressed. It would be helpful to describe the barriers to testing.
Bed mobility	Y	Bed mobility is assessed as "None." This is a vague term. It would be helpful for a reviewer to know the cause of this limitation (paralysis, edema, contractures, weakness) and what assistive devices are required to position/reposition the patient.

(continued)

Essential Element	Y, N, or N/A	Comment(s)
Balance (sit and stand)	Y	Balance is documented as "NA." As data indicate the use of a scooter and the patient transfers with assistance of one, an assessment of balance would be reasonable and necessary.
Transfers	Y	The patient transfers with assist of one and uses a Hoyer™ lift for the shower per the therapist's documentation. This infers that some functional abilities are present. A description of these abilities, such as the type of transfer performed, is needed.
Ambulation (level and elevated surfaces)	Y	Ambulation is described as "Unable." A reviewer would find it helpful to know the cause of this limitation, such as paralysis, edema, contractures, pain, and/or weakness. Can the patient stand?
Orthotic/prosthetic devices	N	Not addressed. The use of orthotics, if present, would help a reviewer in assessing the need for skilled care.
Wheelchair use	Y	The therapist indicated, "Unable." A reviewer may question what this means. For instance, is the patient able to propel or be positioned in a wheelchair or a scooter? It is reasonable for a reviewer to expect data as problem 1 lists the patient as "dependent on scooter."
DME (using or required)	N	Not addressed. It is reasonable to expect that the patient benefits from the use of durable medical equipment because of the functional deficits in bed mobility and ambulation. This information may be relevant to this case. For example, does the patient have a hospital bed that can be used to assist in lower extremity positioning for edema control?
Activity tolerance	Y	The therapist describes activity tolerance as "Fair." This is an incomplete description, and further data regarding the patient's ability to tolerate different positions that might assist in edema control would be helpful. For example, how long is the patient able to tolerate sitting?
Wound description, including incision status	N/A	
Special tests	N/A	
Architectural/safety considerations	N	As this patient is homebound, nonambulatory, and uses a scooter, it would seem relevant to identify architectural barriers and/or safety issues related to activities of daily living and positioning.
Requirements to return to home, school and/or job	N/A	
Prior Level of Function		
Mobility (home and community)	Y	The data describe the patient as "Homebound, lives alone." Documentation of homebound status is essential for home health care coverage. However, this description is incomplete. Information regarding the patient's prior mobility status, use of supportive services, strength, range of motion, edema, and/or positioning strategies are needed to identify the present functional regression calling for skilled care.
Employment	N/A	
School	N/A	
Treatment Diagnosis	N	Not addressed. It is important to identify the treatment diagnosis for which physical therapy services are rendered.
Assessment		
Reason for skilled care	Y	The reason for skilled care emphasizes that physical therapy will be required indefinitely and the patient will always be dependent on an aide to decrease edema in the lower extremities. It is not within the standards of physical therapy practice to provide any modality indefinitely. The need for the skills of a therapist rather than a registered nurse or aide needs to be described. Emphasis on long-term management of the lower extremity edema through a home program is needed.

Essential Element	Y, N, or N/A	Comment(s)
Problems	Y	The therapist lists three problems: 1. Patient is dependent on scooter. 2. Spared quadriplegic. 3. Dependent edema of both lower extremities. Problems 1 and 2 are not justified with objective baseline data.
Plan of Care		
Specific treatment strategies	Y	The authors deciphered the illegible documentation to read, "Electrical stimulation to both lower extremities at 10 watts/cm^2 for about one hour." It is important that documentation be legible, and the parameters for modalities need to be written out clearly to avoid misinterpretation. It would also seem appropriate to define other treatment modalities such as positioning, strengthening, range of motion, and/or patient/caregiver training.
Frequency	Y	The data indicates a frequency of "3x weekly x inelop." Three times weekly is a common description; however, "x inelop" is not understood. In this case, poor therapist penmanship resulted in the author's data interpretation of "inelop." Legible documentation is needed to ensure that data are interpreted correctly by other health professionals and third-party payers.
Duration	Y	The therapist indicates "Indefinite." This is a red flag for the reviewer, as it is inappropriate for any patient or payer source.
Patient instruction/home program	N	Not addressed. Patient education and the carryover of functional gains obtained through skilled rehabilitation are important to a reviewer. Omission of data in this area would be a concern, as the therapist has chosen to use one modality indefinitely. A reviewer would question why pressure garments or massage, which could be performed by nonskilled personnel, are not pursued.
Caregiver training	N	Not addressed. This appears to be an oversight by the therapist, as the patient is dependent on a caregiver.
Short-term goals and achievement dates	Y	The three goals described are not measurable, functional, or time-specific. The goals also do not correspond to the order of the problem list, nor are they objective and defined in the baseline evaluation data. For example, Goal 1 states, "Decrease edema of lower extremities" and Problem 1 states, "Patient is dependent on scooter." The functional relationship between edema and the scooter is not defined. Also, edema is defined as "Moderate to maximal," which is not measurable.
Long-term goals and achievement dates	N	Not addressed. A focus on caregiver training is absent and especially evident in the omission of a long-term goal.
Rehabilitation potential	Y	

2. Is the overall history of the patient adequate?

No. Minimal medical history or data regarding the patient's complications or comorbidities are given. Information regarding the patient's medications would also help the reviewer understand the patient's chronic edema. The patient most likely has severe functional limitations in basic activities of daily living as well as balance and transfers. These areas are not described or are minimally referred to. A reviewer would have difficulty interpreting why skilled therapy is justified.

3. Is there evidence of the need for skilled intervention?

No previous physical therapy history is provided. With a twenty-year duration of illness, it would seem evident that the patient has had previous therapeutic intervention. In addition, data regarding caregiver training for positioning, transfers, and range of motion exercises are absent. This makes it difficult for the reviewer to justify the skills of a physical therapist for training of the caregiver or to determine the need for skilled care.

4. Are there adequate baseline data to develop future comparisons?

Data are absent in all areas, except for cognition and transfers. The absence of specific data in the areas of edema and circumference measurements of the lower extremities, range of motion, pain, positioning, balance, durable medical equipment, bed mobility, and vascular signs makes it difficult to justify skilled care and provide future progress comparisons.

5. Are the objective data related to functional deficits?

Data are lacking, and the effects of edema on function are absent. A description of the patient's limitations in regard to function and pain is needed.

6. Are comparative statements and data clearly outlined?

Data are lacking in all areas, with the exception of cognition and transfers.

7. (A) Are the three components for goals present (measurable, functional, time frames)?

The goals are not functional, measurable, or time-specific. It would be helpful for a reviewer to have measurable data in order to determine the efficacy of the treatment intervention provided. A tar-get reduction such as five millimeters for edema in a time frame of two weeks would be more appropriate. In addition, stating "increase muscle activities of lower extremities" without providing baseline data for functional strength of the lower extremities is futile.

(B) Are the goals realistic for the individual case?

The goals are unrealistic for the treatment duration, which is stated as "indefinite." It is important to note that in the framework of health care today (managed care and prospective payment), a duration such as "indefinite" is not practical or clinically acceptable as a standard of practice.

8. Do you feel the proposed treatment is reasonable and necessary?

An evaluation would seem appropriate for caregiver training. Based on the limited data provided for treatment of this chronic condition, for an indefinite duration, the proposed treatment is not reasonable or necessary.

Case 2: Home Health, Progress Report

Current Baseline Data

Edema: Minimal edema.
Strength: Good control left scapular muscles.
Balance (sit and stand): Increased trunk stability.

Assessment

Reason for skilled care: No c/o. Good spirits. Cooperative. Motivated. Cont. with treatment.

Plan of Care

Specific treatment strategies: Deep massage and PROM both feet and ankles, sitting trunk exercises, electrical stimulation 100 watt/mm^2 x 30 min. both lower extremities.
Short-term goals and achievement dates:

1. Decrease edema.
2. Increase circulation.
3. Facilitate muscle activity both lower extremities.
4. Increase sitting balance.

Case 2: Home Health, Progress Report Worksheet

1. Are the "essential elements" (defined in Chapter 1) for documentation present?

Essential Element	Y, N, or N/A	Comment(s)
Attendance	N	Not addressed. The number of visits scheduled and any reasons for absence need to be documented, as attendance reflects the patient's compliance and participation in rehabilitation.
Current Baseline Data		
Cognition	N/A	Not applicable at this time, as the evaluation indicated that cognition was not impaired. It is recommended that any changes since the evaluation that may affect rehabilitation be documented.
Vision/hearing	N/A	
Vital signs	N	Not addressed in the evaluation or progress report. Based on the data, which indicate that edema is present, it is appropriate to include objective measurements such as respirations, pulse rate, and blood pressure.

Essential Element	Y, N, or N/A	Comment(s)
Vascular signs	N	Vascular signs are not addressed in the evaluation or progress report. Comparative data such as skin color and temperature would seem relevant based on the short-term goal, "Increase circulation."
Sensation/proprioception	N	Data were present in the evaluation, however, are not addressed in the progress report. Is diminished sensation a complicating factor? Comparative data are required to help the reviewer establish a need for continued skilled care.
Edema	Y	The therapist indicates "Minimal edema." The addition of a comparative statement would help a reviewer identify a change in the status. For example, *Minimal edema, previously moderate to maximal edema.* A reviewer could reasonably expect and request objective circumference measurements and the location of the edema to justify the vague description of "Minimal edema."
Posture	N	Not addressed. This appears to be an oversight by the therapist. The evaluation stated "NA" and the progress report indicates emphasis on sitting balance and trunk mobility. A description of posture would provide additional data to justify the need for skilled care.
AROM/PROM	N	Not addressed. As passive range of motion is identified as a treatment strategy, it is necessary to provide the reviewer with objective data to justify the skilled need and functional benefit of range of motion.
Strength	Y	Present information states, "Good control left scapular muscles." This description lacks comparative data and is not related to function. A reviewer would also find this information irrelevant, as the focus of care is on the lower extremities. It would be helpful to provide manual muscle test measurements of the extremities and relate the deficits to functional challenges such as in bed mobility and/or transfers.
Pain	N	Data pertaining to pain are absent in the evaluation and progress report. It is reasonable to expect that a patient with chronic edema and apparent functional limitations in mobility may be experiencing pain as a complicating factor.
Coordination	N	This area could not be assessed in the evaluation and is not addressed in the progress report. As trunk mobility, sitting balance, and scapular control are vaguely described, it would seem relevant to provide data on coordination and the impact on function (e.g., performance of activities of daily living and use of a scooter).
Bed mobility	N	This functional area was addressed as "None" in the evaluation and is missing in this report. A reviewer could reasonably expect data based on the apparent decrease in lower extremity edema, good scapular control, and increased trunk stability.
Balance (sit and stand)	Y	Balance is described as "Increased trunk stability." This description is vague, lacks comparative data, and is not related to function. As an increase of sitting balance is a short-term goal, further data such as direction of balance loss, safety concerns, and the amount of assistance to correct balance loss would be beneficial.
Transfers	N	Transfers were addressed in the evaluation, and the data are missing in this report. Has the decrease in edema improved transfer ability? Comparative data are required to assist the reviewer in establishing a need for continued skilled care.
Ambulation (level and elevated surfaces)	N/A	
Orthotic/prosthetic devices	N	Not addressed. The use of orthotics, if present, would help a reviewer in assessing the need for continued skilled care.

(continued)

Essential Element	Y, N, or N/A	Comment(s)
Wheelchair use	N	The evaluation indicated "Unable"; however, the patient was noted to be dependent on a scooter. The progress report does not address scooter use. It would seem reasonable to provide data based on the report of good scapular mobility and increased trunk control. Have these improvements influenced safety?
DME (using or required)	N	Not addressed in the evaluation or progress report. It is reasonable to expect that the patient benefits from durable medical equipment use because of the functional deficits in bed mobility and ambulation.
Activity tolerance	N	Not addressed. Data pertaining to the patient's ability to tolerate positioning for edema control or to assist with functional activities would be important to a reviewer in determining the need for continued skilled care.
Wound description, including incision status	N/A	
Special tests	N/A	
Architectural/safety considerations	N	As this patient is homebound, nonambulatory, and uses a scooter, it would seem relevant to identify architectural barriers and/or safety issues related to activities of daily living and positioning.
Treatment Diagnosis	N	Not addressed. It is important to identify the treatment diagnosis for which physical therapy services are rendered, as it may change during the course of intervention.
Assessment Reason for skilled care	Y	Although present, the statements: "No c/o. Good spirits. Cooperative. Motivated. Continue with treatment" do not justify the need for skilled care or provide expectation statements regarding future progress.
Problems	N	Not addressed. It is helpful to list the problems in order to focus treatment. A lack of focus is evident in this case.
Plan of Care Specific treatment strategies	Y	The progress report describes several modalities. The modalities are not justified because of the limited objective data. There is inadequate information regarding the application of electrical stimulation, and a reviewer would not understand why it is being used. It is also important that parameters for modalities be written clearly. The data presented are the author's interpretation of the therapist's data entry.
Frequency	N	Not addressed. The frequency helps the reviewer determine the reasonableness of the therapy services rendered in relationship to the functional progress reported. It can also help when analyzing documentation and the corresponding service billed.
Duration	N	Not addressed. The anticipated duration of service helps the reviewer determine the reasonableness of the therapy services rendered in relationship to the functional progress reported.
Patient instruction/home program	N	Not addressed. A home program is an essential element for carryover of progress made in rehabilitation. A description of the home program, program revisions, and any barriers to completion help a reviewer in determining the need for continued skilled care.
Caregiver training	N	Not addressed. The evaluation described the patient as dependent on an aide. It is important to indicate the dates and activities of teaching and training to provide evidence of skilled care.
Short-term goals and achievement dates	Y	The short-term goals are vague. All goals lack a functional, measurable, and time-specific component.

Essential Element	Y, N, or N/A	Comment(s)
Long-term goals and achievement dates	N	Not addressed. The focus of caregiver training is absent and especially evident in the omission of a long-term goal.
Rehabilitation potential	N	Not addressed. The rehabilitation potential is an essential element of documentation. It helps a reviewer determine the reasonableness of skilled care in relationship to the stated goals.

2. Is there evidence of the need for skilled intervention?

Evidence of the need for skilled intervention is lacking. The reader should note that in this particular case, the reviewer was asked to assess three months of treatment four years after the evaluation. To make an accurate decision, the reviewer analyzed all of the notes from the evaluation through the dates in question. The documentation consistently lacked measurable data, evidence of training or communication with the caregiver, and description of functional deficits. It provided repetitive, vague clinical information, as presented in this progress report.

3. Are there adequate baseline data to develop future comparisons?

No, the data provided are vague or missing. For example, "Increased trunk stability" is not measurable or related to improvements in safety or function.

4. Are the objective data related to functional deficits?

The limited available data are not related to functional deficits. A reviewer would find it helpful to understand the relationship of edema to bed mobility and transfers. The description "minimal edema" does not provide that relationship.

5. Are comparative statements and data clearly outlined?

Data are vague and there are no comparative statements.

6. (A) Are the three components for goals present (measurable, functional, time frames)?

The goals are not measurable, functional, or time-specific.

(B) Are the goals realistic for the individual case?

The goals are not realistic for this patient based on the limited data, lack of comparative statements, and omission of caregiver training for functional carryover.

7. Do you feel the treatment was reasonable and necessary?

No. In this case, the reviewer denied the dates in question and strongly advised the third-party payer to pursue further retrospective review. The reviewer stated that there was no evidence for skilled intervention and that the treatment for this chronic condition did not appear reasonable and necessary. The reviewer determined that the treatment appeared maintenance in nature and could be provided by nonskilled personnel under nursing supervision.

Case 3: Hospital, Initial Evaluation

Referral

Specific treatment requested: PT for evaluation and left leg strengthening exercises.

Data Accompanying Referral

Diagnosis/onset date: S/P femoral/popliteal bypass surgery LLE/11-18-95.

Secondary diagnoses: CABG, CAD, ASHD, diabetes, chest pain.

Medical history: Patient is a pleasant 83 year old male who underwent lower extremity femoral/popliteal bypass on 11-18-95. Patient was hospitalized 2 weeks following surgery. He relates he had continued c/o of LLE pain. Patient returned home in approximately 2 days and was readmitted to the emergency room via ambulance secondary to chest pain.

Comorbidities (complicating or precautionary information): Cardiac and pulmonary precautions.

Physical Therapy Intake/History

Date of birth: 07-05-12
Age: 83
Gender: Male
Start of care: 12-05-95
Primary complaint: Patient states attempted ambulation with walker although was unable secondary to LLE pain upon weight bearing.

Prior Therapy History: Patient denies receiving P.T. following surgery.

Baseline Evaluation Data

Vital signs: Mr. ABC presents today supine in bed with halter cardiac monitor. No I.V. or catheter. Palpable pedal pulse LLE, although weak.

Vascular signs: No discoloration noted distally. Skin in good condition other than healing incision.

Edema: Edema noted over the left distal lower extremity proximal knee extending to the toe.

AROM/PROM: BUE and RLE WFL. L knee and ankle ROM limited approximately 50% secondary to increased edema and pain.

Strength: BUE and RLE Fair +. LLE testing deferred.

Pain: Patient has consistent c/o LLE pain and edema.

Transfers: Mr. ABC requires assist for transfers and gait. Patient relates 90% independence in ADL's.

Ambulation (level and elevated surfaces): See Transfers.

Wound description, including incision status: Patient presents with healing incision approximately 15 inches in length over the medial aspect of the lower extremity approximately mid-thigh to distal knee.

Prior Level of Function

Mobility (home and community): Mr. ABC lived at home with his wife. Patient relates that prior to surgery, he was ambulating independently without assistive device.

Treatment Diagnosis: Left lower extremity edema, pain, weakness, healing incision.

Assessment

Reason for skilled care: Patient is a pleasant motivated gentleman who has had continued LLE pain and as a result has become limited in his functional mobility. Patient appears motivated to progress. Mr. ABC may benefit from daily P.T. to increase active LLE ROM to decrease pain and edema. Patient may benefit from LE strengthening, transfer and gait training safely utilizing walker.

Problems:

1. Pain and edema left distal lower extremity.
2. Decreased ROM left knee and ankle.
3. Decreased strength left lower extremity.
4. Requires assist for transfers and gait.
5. Nonambulatory secondary to left lower extremity pain with weight bearing.

Plan of Care

Specific treatment strategies: Patient to be seen for LLE ROM, strengthening, transfer, and gait training with walker. Instruction in a HEP.

Frequency: Daily.

Duration: Hospitalization.

Caregiver training: Nursing was instructed in ROM of the LLE.

Short-term goals and achievement dates:

1. Decrease pain/edema left distal lower extremity (circumferential measurements to within 5% of right).
2. Increase AROM left knee and ankle.
3. Increase right lower extremity strength to 4/5.

4. Independence in transfers.
5. (a) Ambulate 50 ft with walker, with minimal assist and contact guard assist of 1. (b). Independence in HEP.

Long-term goals and achievement dates: Patient will return to prior level of function, ambulating independently with an appropriate assistive device. Independence in HEP. Rehabilitation potential: Good.

Case 3: Hospital, Initial Evaluation Worksheet

1. Are the "essential elements" (defined in Chapter 1) for documentation present?

Essential Element	Y, N, or N/A	Comment(s)
Referral		
Reason	N	The reason for referral is not stated. However, based on the data presented in the medical history and prior level of function, a reviewer can probably determine the need for skilled therapy service.
Specific treatment requested	Y	
Data Accompanying Referral		
Diagnosis/onset date	Y	
Secondary diagnoses	Y	Secondary diagnoses are presented. However, it is recommended that abbreviations not be overutilized. For example, CABG and CAD, coronary artery bypass graft and coronary artery disease, may not be recognized by all reviewers. Remember, many reviewers may have minimal health care training.
Medical history	Y	The patient's present medical history is summarized appropriately. Because of the multiple secondary diagnoses relating to cardiac function, it would be helpful to also describe the past medical history. This would reinforce the patient's medical challenges and need for skilled care. (e.g., *Bypass surgery performed (date). History of chest pain with exertion since (date). Diabetes controlled through diet.*)
Medications	N	Not addressed. As cardiac diagnoses including arteriosclerotic heart disease, coronary artery disease, and coronary artery bypass graft are documented, it would be helpful to know what medications, if any, are being administered that may affect rehabilitation—for example, beta blockers.
Comorbidities (complicating or precautionary information)	Y	The therapist appropriately documents that cardiac and pulmonary precautions exist. A reviewer may find it helpful, in determining the need for skilled care, if the parameters are defined—for example, blood pressure/pulse rate upper and lower limits.
Physical Therapy Intake/History		
Date of birth	Y	
Age	Y	
Gender	Y	
Start of Care	Y	
Primary complaint	Y	
Referral Diagnosis		
Mechanism of injury	N/A	
Prior diagnostic imaging/testing	N	Not addressed. Considering the history of cardiac dysfunction, additional information such as previous stress testing (if available) may provide insight into the patient's functional capacity.
Prior Therapy History	Y	The therapist appropriately documents, "Patient denies receiving P.T. following surgery." It is helpful for the reviewer to know if prior therapy was provided.

(continued)

Essential Element	Y, N, or N/A	Comment(s)
Baseline Evaluation Data		
Cognition	N	Not addressed. Evaluation of cognition is important to establish the ability of a patient to participate in a rehabilitation program.
Vision/hearing	N	Not addressed. Vision and hearing deficits can affect function and are therefore important to assess.
Vital signs	Y	The therapist indicates that the pedal pulse is weak in the left lower extremity and that the patient has a cardiac monitor. Given the patient's history of cardiac and pulmonary deficits, additional data would seem relevant, such as blood pressure, pulse rate, and respirations.
Vascular signs	Y	Documentation indicates, "No discoloration noted distally. Skin in good condition other than healing incision." The site being examined is not addressed. It is helpful to provide the location to eliminate any assumptions by the reviewer.
Sensation/proprioception	N	Not addressed. Diabetes is documented as a secondary diagnosis; therefore, assessment of the lower extremities for sensation/proprioception deficits would be important in establishing the treatment plan and goals.
Edema	Y	The documentation indicates, "Edema noted over the left distal lower extremity proximal knee extending to the toe." This description may not be understood by the reviewer, as it lacks objective measurements and functional limitations. Additional information is needed, such as circumference measurements of the involved and uninvolved lower extremity, whether the edema is pitting or nonpitting, and how the edema limits functional activities.
Posture	N	Not addressed. When evaluating a patient's function, particularly ambulation, it is important to incorporate postural assessment in development of the treatment plan.
AROM/PROM	Y	Range of motion is described; however, specific range of motion measurements for the left lower extremity and the differentiation between active and passive range of motion are needed for future comparative analysis. The description "limited approximately 50% . . . " is not helpful to a reviewer. The effect of range of motion deficits on function is also lacking.
Strength	Y	Measurements are present and left lower extremity testing was deferred. A reviewer would find it helpful to know the reason why. For instance, manual muscle testing can be difficult and particularly challenging if there is pain. Documentation regarding the patient's functional strength deficits would be helpful if described in terms such as, *The patient required moderate assistance for sit to stand due to lower extremity strength deficits.*
Pain	Y	The therapist indicates, "Patient has consistent c/o LLE pain and edema." This is a vague description. A pain scale is needed to provide measurable data for future progress comparisons.
Coordination	N/A	
Bed mobility	N	Not addressed. A description of the patient's ability to reposition in bed and initiate or complete rolling are needed.
Balance (sit and stand)	N	Not addressed. A description of the patient's balance deficits would be important for developing an effective treatment plan. This is especially relevant in the area of safety because of the weight-bearing deficit and the patient's sudden onset of functional loss.

Essential Element	Y, N, or N/A	Comment(s)
Transfers	Y	The evaluation data indicates that the patient "requires assist for transfers and gait" and "Patient relates 90% independence in ADL's." These descriptions are vague and do not allow for future comparisons. A statement describing the level of assistance and the activities of daily living that are limited is needed.
Ambulation (level and elevated surfaces)	Y	Ambulation is briefly described under transfers. Information pertaining to weight-bearing status, type of assistive device, distance, level of assistance, and description of gait deficits would help the reviewer in assessing the functional limitations of the patient and the need for skilled care.
Orthotic/prosthetic devices	N/A	
Wheelchair use	N	Not addressed. With the patient's sudden decrease in function, it is likely that a wheelchair is used. A description of the patient's ability to maneuver the wheelchair would be helpful, if applicable.
DME (using or required)	N	Not addressed. This is an oversight by the therapist, as the documentation indicates use of a walker for previous ambulation attempts.
Activity tolerance	N	Not addressed. Given the cardiac and pulmonary history, a reviewer would have a more accurate picture of the patient's limitations if reference was made to functional activity tolerance. Activity tolerance could be a factor in justifying an extended duration of treatment and skilled intervention during and/or following hospitalization.
Wound description, including incision status	Y	
Special tests	N/A	
Architectural/safety considerations	N	Not addressed. Given the patient's decreased function, especially with ambulation and the current cardiac complications, it would seem that more information is necessary. For example, does the patient need to climb stairs?
Requirements to return to home, school and/or job	N	Not addressed. A description of the patient's mobility requirements to allow safe return to home would provide the reviewer with insight into the current functional limitations. Will the patient's wife be able to meet his physical assistance needs?
Prior Level of Function		
Mobility (home and community)	Y	The data indicates that prior to surgery the patient was independent in ambulation without an assistive device. This information is specific to the dysfunction being treated and helps the reviewer assess the appropriateness of the established goals and plan of care.
Employment	N/A	
School	N/A	
Treatment Diagnosis	Y	
Assessment		
Reason for skilled care	Y	A description of the patient and the need for skilled care are evident. The therapist could display more confidence by stating, *Mr. ABC is a candidate for daily PT*, rather than "Mr. ABC may benefit from daily PT."
Problems	Y	
Plan of Care		
Specific treatment strategies	Y	
Frequency	Y	

(continued)

Essential Element	Y, N, or N/A	Comment(s)
Duration	Y	The duration is listed as "hospitalization." It would be helpful to estimate the anticipated duration and indicate the number of visits.
Patient instruction/home program	N	Not addressed. Training and education are important components of treatment. They should be initiated at the time of evaluation.
Caregiver training	Y	The therapist appropriately documents that nursing was trained in range of motion activities for the left lower extremity. This is incomplete, as it is reasonable to expect that the patient would benefit from caregiver training in the areas of transfers and bed mobility as well as positioning of the left lower extremity for edema control.
Short-term goals and achievement dates	Y	Goal 1 is measurable. However, baseline data are lacking to validate circumference measurement changes in the left lower extremity. Goal 2 is not measurable and requires a specific number of degrees rather than "Increase AROM." Goals 1, 2, and 3 require a functional component. All goals lack a time frame.
Long-term goals and achievement dates	Y	
Rehabilitation potential	Y	

2. Is the overall history of the patient adequate?

No, given the multiple diagnoses regarding the cardiac and pulmonary deficits and also diabetes, further information of the patient's past medical history would enhance the reviewer's ability to assess the patient's functional limitations. In addition, the history should indicate any previous physical therapy intervention, separate from the incident involving this surgery, that may have occurred. Finally, information regarding the wife's ability to provide supportive services and the extended services available from family and/or other caregivers would be helpful.

3. Is there evidence of the need for skilled intervention?

Yes. As the patient was previously independent in ambulation at home and in a relatively short time became dependent in mobility, there is justification of the need for skilled physical therapy intervention. In addition, the patient's other comorbidities, such as diabetes and edema, further enhance the need for the skills of a physical therapist.

4. Are there adequate baseline data to develop future comparisons?

Measurable baseline data are lacking. This is particularly evident for range of motion, edema, transfers, and ambulation.

5. Are the objective data related to functional deficits?

Because of the vague descriptions such as "requires assist for transfers and gait," "Edema noted," and "ROM limited approximately 50 percent," there subsequently is no description of the patient's functional deficits. It would be helpful to know the effect of edema and range of motion deficits on transfers, bed mobility, and gait. A reviewer would also find it helpful to understand the functional limitations in activity tolerance secondary to the cardiac and pulmonary comorbidities.

6. Are comparative statements and data clearly outlined?

There are minimal baseline comparative data in the evaluation to allow for an adequate description of the patient's progress. Range of motion, circumference measurements, and levels of assistance for mobility are lacking.

7. (A) Are the three components for goals present (measurable, functional, time frames)?

No, components are frequently missed. For example, Goal 2 states, "Increase AROM left knee and ankle." This is vague and would be better stated as, *Increase active range of motion left knee extension and ankle dorsiflexion ten degrees to improve midstance weight bearing during gait training in three days.* Goal 3 describes the need for strengthening of the *right* lower extremity. This does not correlate with Problem 3, which defines a need for strengthening of the *left* lower extremity.

(B) Are the goals realistic for the individual case?

A reviewer would have difficulty determining if the stated goals are realistic, as the goals lack the proper components and baseline data for justification.

8. Do you feel that the proposed treatment is reasonable and necessary?

Based on the patient's prior level of function, multiple diagnoses, and acute functional regression, the evaluation as well as treatment are reasonable.

Case 3: Hospital, Discharge Report

Attendance: Mr. ABC was seen daily 12-05-95 and 12-06-95 for gentle range of motion, transfer training, gait training and home exercise program instruction. Mr. ABC was evaluated 12-05-95 and was discharged 12-06-95.

Current Baseline Data

Edema: Patient exhibits minimal decrease in edema left lower extremity.

AROM/PROM: Exhibits increased AROM of the left knee and ankle.

Pain: Decreased subjective complaints of lower extremity pain.

Transfers: Mr. ABC transfers with walker with minimal assist of 1.

Ambulation (level and elevated surfaces): He ambulates 10 feet with rolling walker with minimal contact guard assist. He is apprehensive and hesitant to bear weight on the left lower extremity. Requires verbal cuing for weight bearing on left lower extremity exhibiting a heel strike and toe off during gait with walker. He requires verbal cuing regarding sequencing during ambulation.

Treatment Diagnosis: LLE edema, pain, weakness, healing incision.

Assessment

Reason for skilled care: Mr. ABC exhibits decreased edema left lower extremity. He appears to be motivated to be compliant with a home exercise program. Patient hesitant to perform daily ambulation, although, has increased confidence since recent gait training. Patient being discharged from physical therapy secondary to discharge from hospital. Will recommend continued physical therapy in the home setting.

Problems:

1. Pain and edema left distal lower extremity.
2. Decreased range of motion left knee and ankle.
3. Decreased strength left lower extremity.
4. Requires assist for transfers and gait.
5. Nonambulatory secondary to left lower extremity pain with weight bearing.

Plan of Care

Specific treatment strategies: Patient discharged from physical therapy secondary to discharge from facility.

Patient instruction/home program: He is independent in a home exercise program involving left lower extremity range of motion, stretching and strengthening. Patient was encouraged to continue ambulation several times daily and with continuation of his home exercise program.

Caregiver training: Patient and wife were instructed in safe proper transfers, ambulation, negotiation of stairs and safety during functional mobility around the home and in activities of daily living.

Short-term goals and achievement dates:

1. Independence in home exercise program.
2. Safe transfers and ambulation with walker utilizing assist as needed.

Long-term goals and achievement dates: Patient will return to prior level of function, ambulating independently with an appropriate assistive device. Independent in home exercise program.

Discharge prognosis: Good.

Case 3: Hospital, Discharge Report Worksheet

1. Are the "essential elements" (defined in Chapter 1) for documentation present?

Essential Element	Y, N, or N/A	Comment(s)
Attendance	Y	
Current Baseline Data		
Cognition	N	Not addressed in the evaluation or discharge report. It would be helpful to have a description of the patient's ability to follow directions. This would help in assessing safety at home and the ability to participate in rehabilitation and in justifying continued skilled intervention outside the inpatient hospital setting.

(continued)

Essential Element	Y, N, or N/A	Comment(s)
Vision/hearing	N	Not addressed. It is helpful to know that this was assessed and that the patient has no deficits that may affect function and safety.
Vital signs	N	Vital signs were briefly addressed in the evaluation and the data are omitted in this report. Based on the cardiac and pulmonary precautions in the evaluation, it would be helpful if discharge data were provided to justify skilled care and the need for continued outpatient intervention.
Vascular signs	N	Although the duration of physical therapy intervention was limited to two days, the status should be documented, as this area was addressed in the evaluation.
Sensation/proprioception	N	This area is not addressed in the evaluation or discharge report. Any existing deficits need to be documented, as they help justify the need for skilled care.
Edema	Y	The data indicate, "Patient exhibits minimal decrease in edema left lower extremity." Comparative data are not provided to justify this conclusion. It would also be helpful to describe the functional activities that are limited.
Posture	N	Posture is not described in the evaluation or discharge report. As deficits are present in transfers and ambulation, a final assessment of posture and the impact on functional mobility are relevant.
AROM/PROM	Y	As in the evaluation, data are present. However, objective measurements such as the differentiation between active and passive range of motion and how improvements affected function are needed. For example, has the increase in knee and ankle range of motion improved heel strike and safety during gait training?
Strength	N	Not addressed. Since left lower extremity testing was deferred, it would be important to assess at the time of discharge and to relate any strength deficits to functional activities such as ambulation or transfers.
Pain	Y	As in the evaluation, the pain description in the discharge report also lacks a pain scale to provide measurable data. The effect of pain on functional activities would also be of benefit to the reviewer in determining the need for skilled care.
Coordination	N/A	
Bed mobility	N	Not addressed in the evaluation or discharge report. Since the patient's functional level is not high for ambulation, it would be helpful to know if the patient had achieved independence in bed mobility or required assistance because of lower extremity pain and strength deficits.
Balance (sit and stand)	N	Not addressed. This is an oversight in the evaluation and discharge report. As the patient was independent before the recent surgery and hospitalization, it would be reasonable to expect balance deficits.
Transfers	Y	The data indicates, "Mr. ABC transfers with walker with minimal assist of one." This brief description is helpful; however, information as to the type of transfer and level of safety is needed. For example, does the transfer include tub, shower, toilet, car, and/or wheelchair? Does the patient require a variable level of assistance based on the type of transfer performed?
Ambulation (level and elevated surfaces)	Y	A detailed description of ambulation is provided. The documentation would be enhanced by stating, "*Gait training* performed for 10 feet" rather than "*He ambulates* 10 feet . . ." It is important to demonstrate that the skills of a therapist are needed and that the patient is not practicing the functional activity. Information regarding performance on elevated surfaces such as stairs would also be helpful.

Essential Element	Y, N, or N/A	Comment(s)
Orthotic/prosthetic devices	N/A	
Wheelchair use	N	Not addressed. Since the patient did not return to total independence in ambulation, it seems likely that he would be using a wheelchair for long distances. Description about whether the patient was independent or not in its use would be helpful.
DME (using or required)	N	Not addressed. This is an oversight by the therapist, as documentation indicates use of a rolling walker.
Activity tolerance	N	Not addressed in the evaluation or discharge report. Data pertaining to the patient's activity tolerance, such as the need to pace activities, would be helpful to a reviewer in assessing functional limitations.
Wound description, including incision status	N	Not addressed. It is important to document the status of the incision, especially if there are soft tissue restrictions, pain, or challenges to healing that may affect functional progress.
Special tests	N/A	
Architectural/safety considerations	N	Not addressed. Data suggest that the patient is limited in mobility (i.e., transfers require minimal assist and ambulation distance is ten feet). It is reasonable to expect that the patient uses a wheelchair for longer distances; therefore, data pertaining to architectural barriers and safety considerations are needed.
Treatment Diagnosis	Y	
Assessment		
Reason for skilled care	Y	The assessment summarizes in vague terms the patient's functional status and describes the patient's involvement in a home program. The therapist also recommends continued skilled physical therapy; however, why therapy will be necessary is not described. An explanation of the goals that were not achieved and/or complications that remain (i.e., pain, lower extremity strength deficits, safety concerns) would help define the need for continued skilled care. The therapist's assessment of the impact of the cardiac diagnoses on functional mobility would also be helpful.
Problems	Y	
Plan of Care		
Specific treatment strategies	Y	The plan of care indicates the present treatment strategy as, "Discharged from physical therapy secondary to discharge from facility." A summary of the treatment strategies, as described in the Attendance area, is needed. The summary of modalities used helps the reviewer determine the reasonableness of the plan of care in relationship to functional progress. It can also help when analyzing documentation and the corresponding services billed.
Frequency	N	Not addressed. A summary of the frequency and duration is needed. For example, documenting that the patient *Was seen daily for two days* helps the reviewer determine the reasonableness of the frequency and duration in relationship to the functional progress reported. It can also help when analyzing documentation and the corresponding services billed.
Duration	N	See Frequency.
Patient instruction/home program	Y	
Caregiver training	Y	
Short-term goals and achievement dates	Y	The evaluation addressed five problems and goals. The discharge report does not reflect goal status. It is important to restate all goals and their status, such as achieved or not achieved.

(continued)

Essential Element	Y, N, or N/A	Comment(s)
Long-term goals and achievement dates	Y	The status of the long-term goal is not defined.
Discharge prognosis	Y	

2. Is there evidence of the need for skilled intervention?

Yes, the patient had gait deficits that required the skills of a physical therapist. Training of the patient and caregivers was also documented and helps justify the need for skilled care.

3. Are there adequate baseline data to develop future comparisons?

Baseline and comparative data are lacking in the evaluation and discharge report. More information regarding pain, edema, range of motion, strength, and balance would assist in justifying the skills of a therapist.

4. Are the objective data related to functional deficits?

The relationship between objective data and functional deficits is lacking, except for ambulation.

5. Are comparative statements and data clearly outlined?

Comparative statements do not exist in this report, as limited baseline data were provided in the evaluation.

6. (A) Are the three components for goals present (measurable, functional, time frames)?

Goal 1 is measurable; however, it is not related to function. Goal 2 is not measurable. All goals lack time frames. Five problems are given and only two goals are listed. Each problem should have a related goal or the problem should be listed as resolved. The status of the goals at the time of discharge is needed.

(B) Are the goals realistic for the individual case?

Yes. However, it would be easier for a reviewer to view them as realistic if measurable data, time frames, and the functional outcomes were identified. It appears that the goals were revised without justification.

7. Do you feel that the treatment was reasonable and necessary?

Yes, based on the fact the patient was independent in ambulation prior to surgery and exhibited deficits in transfers and ambulation. Skilled care is also evident, as a home program was established and caregiver training is documented.

Case 4: Hospital, Initial Evaluation

Referral

Specific treatment requested: Physical therapy assessment, needs strengthening exercises of extremities, ambulation with walker.

Data Accompanying Referral

Diagnosis/onset date: Dehydration, possible aspiration pneumonia/12-11-95.
Secondary diagnoses: Weakness.
Medical history: Patient is a pleasant 75-year-old female who was hospitalized in October 1995. Patient was admitted to ABC Hospital on 12-11-95 secondary to family concerns regarding patient's increased weakness, dehydration, and possible aspiration pneumonia. Past medical history involves IDDM.

Physical Therapy Intake/History

Date of birth: 01-23-20
Age: 75
Gender: Female
Start of care: 12-12-95

Prior Therapy History:
In October 1995, the patient received P.T. consult regarding education for husband regarding transfers. Patient receiving P.T. in the home for strengthening and gait training.

Baseline Evaluation Data

Cognition: Patient is noncommunicative, although, does communicate nodding yes/no.
Vascular signs: Skin appears in good condition. Circulation appears intact.
Edema: No edema noted.
AROM/PROM: BU/LE P/AAROM limited approx. 10% Minimal AROM.
Strength: BU/LE strength fair (−).
Pain: She indicates she is not in pain, but is tired and extreme ROM is uncomfortable.
Bed mobility: Requires assist for bed mobility.

Prior Level of Function

Mobility (home and community): Patient currently lives at home with husband. Family relates the patient was nonambulatory at the time of admission and requires full assistance regarding transfers.

Treatment Diagnosis: Weakness.

Assessment

Reason for skilled care: Patient appears weak and fatigued. Patient is pleasant although indicates reluctance for AROM possibly secondary to weakness. Does not indicate pain at this time.

Problems:

1. Decreased BU/LE strength and AROM.
2. Requires assist for transfers.
3. Nonambulatory, requires assist for gait.
4. Dec'd functional mobility and participation in ADL's.

Plan of Care

Specific treatment strategies: Pt. seen on a daily basis for ROM, strengthening, transfers, gait and HEP involving strengthening and AROM.
Frequency: Daily.
Duration: Hospitalization.
Caregiver training: Patient positioning in bed and chair will be discussed with nursing.
Short-term goals and achievement dates:

1. Inc. BU/LE strength and AROM.
2. (a) Transfer supine-to-sit with mod assist of one. (b) Transfer sit-to-stand mod assist of one.
3. Ambulate 5 ft. with walker mod assist of two.
4. Participate in BU/LE ROM and exercise program with verbal cuing and min assist of one.

Long-term goals and achievement dates:

1. Patient will increase general BU/LE strength to increase AROM. 2. Independent in HEP involving strengthening and AROM.

Rehabilitation potential: Good.

Case 4: Hospital, Initial Evaluation Worksheet

1. Are the "essential elements" (defined in Chapter 1) for documentation present?

Essential Element	Y, N, or N/A	Comment(s)
Referral		
Reason	N	Not addressed. A statement regarding the reason for referral is needed to help justify the need for skilled therapy intervention. For example, *Patient referred by Dr. ABC for physical therapy to improve functional strength for transfers and short distance ambulation to facilitate safe return to home with husband.*
Specific treatment requested	Y	
Data Accompanying Referral		
Diagnosis/onset date	Y	
Secondary diagnoses	Y	The secondary diagnosis is listed as "weakness." This secondary diagnosis would be more appropriate as a treatment diagnosis. If it is used as a treatment diagnosis, a functional phrase alternative such as *functional strength deficit* is suggested. Further, it would be helpful for the reviewer to have further detail as to the patient's comorbidities, such as insulin-dependent diabetes mellitus (IDDM), which is described in the medical history.
Medical history	Y	The medical history indicates a prior hospitalization, the presence of diabetes, and the multiple reasons for admission, which include possible aspiration pneumonia, dehydration, and weakness. Further detail regarding the functional deficits and their relationship to the diagnoses would be helpful. For example, has the patient had frequent bouts of pneumonia and dehydration? Is there a history of falls secondary to weakness?
Medications	N	Not addressed. As diabetes and pneumonia are indicated in the evaluation, it would be helpful to know what medications, if any, are being administered that may affect rehabilitation, such as insulin, and/or the need for oxygen.
Comorbidities (complicating or precautionary information)	N	Not addressed. It is important to include any complicating or precautionary information that may affect the patient during rehabilitation. For example, does this patient require monitoring of blood glucose levels during exercise? Does the patient require oxygen during exercise?
Physical Therapy Intake/History		
Date of birth	Y	Patient identifying information is important, as many physician offices and third-party payers file or trigger data retrieval based on date of birth.
Age	Y	
Gender	Y	
Start of Care	Y	
Primary complaint	N	The primary complaint is not identified. Is it decreased safety with transfers, decreased ambulation, and/or inability to perform activities of daily living such as dressing?
Referral Diagnosis		
Mechanism of injury	N/A	
Prior diagnostic imaging/testing	N	Not addressed. Based on the diagnosis of aspiration pneumonia, it would be helpful for the reviewer to know whether the therapist has addressed this area when determining the need for skilled care. For example, were oxygen saturation rates monitored or chest X-rays performed? This information may be relevant to the case at this time.

Essential Element	Y, N, or N/A	Comment(s)
Prior Therapy History	Y	
Baseline Evaluation Data		
Cognition	Y	Data indicates, "Patient is noncommunicative, although, does communicate nodding yes/no." This data would be better stated as, *Patient is nonverbal and communication is limited to yes/no responses.* It is also reasonable to expect further data. For example, why is the patient nonverbal? Are there residual deficits from a cerebrovascular accident or a transient ischemic attack? Also, based on the diagnosis of dehydration, it would be helpful to know if confusion is evident and whether it will affect participation in rehabilitation.
Vision/hearing	N	Not addressed. It would be helpful to know if the patient has vision or hearing deficits that may affect safety.
Vital signs	N	Not addressed. Based on the diagnosis of pneumonia and dehydration, it is reasonable to expect baseline data regarding cardiopulmonary status. Evidence of any deficits would demonstrate another need for skilled intervention.
Vascular signs	Y	The data indicate, "Skin appears in good condition. Circulation appears intact." The term "appears" does not provide a clear description. For example, how was circulation assessed?
Sensation/proprioception	N	Not addressed. Based on the patient's limited communication ability, data may be difficult to obtain. If deficits exist, it would be helpful to explain their clinical relevance.
Edema	Y	
Posture	N	Not addressed. Postural deficits have a direct effect on cardiopulmonary status, as well as on the patient's ability to perform bed mobility, transfers, and ambulation. It is important to address this area of potential concern.
AROM/PROM	Y	The evaluation indicates that upper and lower extremity passive and active assistive range of motion is limited 10 percent. Also "minimal AROM" is reported. How does a 10 percent limitation affect bed mobility, transfers, ambulation, and activities of daily living? Additional descriptive information would help the reviewer understand the patient's functional abilities and disabilities.
Strength	Y	Data indicates strength is fair minus for the upper and lower extremities. Again, as with range of motion, the description lacks a relationship to functional activities. A reviewer may also question the accuracy of fair minus strength through all extremities based on the fact "minimal AROM" was reported.
Pain	Y	Despite the patient's apparent limited communication ability, the data includes, "She indicates she is not in pain, but is tired and extreme ROM is uncomfortable." This description is vague and the source of discomfort is not described. Is the discomfort present in all extremities, and what is it due to?
Coordination	N/A	Not applicable at this time.
Bed mobility	Y	The therapist documents, "Requires assist for bed mobility." Further description is needed as to the amount of assistance for future progress comparisons. For example, a better description, such as *Rolling requires moderate assistance of one. Sit to and from supine requires maximal assistance of one*, would be helpful.
Balance (sit and stand)	N	Not addressed. Sitting and standing balance deficits are relevant to the patient's rehabilitation potential for improvement of transfers and ambulation.

(continued)

Essential Element	Y, N, or N/A	Comment(s)
Transfers	N	Not addressed. This appears to be an oversight by the therapist, as the documentation indicates that transfers are a problem. Therefore, baseline data are needed for future progress comparisons.
Ambulation (level and elevated surfaces)	N	Not addressed. Again, this is an apparent oversight by the therapist. Ambulation is listed as a problem and goal; therefore, baseline data are required for future progress comparison.
Orthotic/prosthetic devices	N/A	
Wheelchair use	N	Not addressed. As the patient appears nonambulatory, it would be important for a reviewer to know if the patient can safely maneuver a wheelchair.
DME (using or required)	N	Not addressed. Based on the patient's limited functional mobility, it is reasonable to expect that durable medical equipment such as a wheelchair, bedside commode, and/or grab bars is used at home.
Activity tolerance	N	As this patient has apparent weakness (functional strength deficit) and pneumonia, this area needs to be addressed.
Wound description, including incision status	N/A	
Special tests	N/A	
Architectural/safety considerations	N	Not addressed. Discussion with the family regarding architectural barriers and safety issues would be relevant if return to home is a goal.
Requirements to return to home, school and/or job	N	Not addressed. As the husband appears to be the primary caregiver, any requirements to return home based on his physical limitations should be defined.
Prior Level of Function		
Mobility (home and community)	Y	The data indicate that the patient lives at home with her husband, was nonambulatory at the time of admission, and required "full assistance" with transfers. Further details are required for a reviewer to determine the appropriateness of the plan of care and the need for skilled intervention. It would be helpful to define "full assistance" for transfers and to indicate the ambulatory status prior to admission. Does the patient use a walker or wheelchair?
Employment	N/A	
School	N/A	
Treatment Diagnosis	Y	"Weakness" is described as the treatment diagnosis. This term may imply to a reviewer that skilled intervention may not be required and the patient's ability to resume activities of daily living will resolve this diagnosis. It is recommended that a functional phrase alternative such as *functional strength deficit* be used.
Assessment		
Reason for skilled care	Y	The assessment stresses weakness and fatigue. A statement justifying skilled intervention is needed, as well as what the focus for treatment will be to achieve a clear functional outcome—for example, *Patient requires skilled physical therapy service to establish an individualized strengthening and range of motion program to allow progression of transfer and gait training for safe return home with husband.*
Problems	Y	The problems are listed. However, baseline data are lacking to establish that deficits exist in the areas of transfers, ambulation, and activities of daily living.
Plan of Care		
Specific treatment strategies	Y	
Frequency	Y	

Essential Element	Y, N, or N/A	Comment(s)
Duration	Y	The duration is listed as "hospitalization." It would be helpful to estimate the anticipated duration and indicate a number of visits.
Patient instruction/home program	N	Not addressed. Because of the trend for short hospital stays, an indication of a home program, initiated from the start of care, is an effective approach when justifying skilled physical therapy intervention.
Caregiver training	Y	Although present, an indication of an actual inservice to both nursing and family would justify the need for physical therapy intervention. A general statement such as "will be discussed with nursing" does not reflect that training was performed.
Short-term goals and achievement dates	Y	The goals lack time frames. Goal 1 is not related to function. Also, the short-term goals do not incorporate home programming.
Long-term goals and achievement dates	Y	The long-term goal is extremely vague. It would be better stated if a functional component and measurable component were provided for strength and range of motion. For example, *Strength will increase to good and range of motion to within normal limits to allow transfers and gait with moderate assistance of one.*
Rehabilitation potential	Y	It is the opinion of the authors that the data presented do not justify a rating of good. The patient would be better assessed at a fair level.

2. Is the overall history of the patient adequate?

No, the history lacks baseline data of the patient's prior functional deficits. For instance, what was the cause of the aspiration pneumonia? Was posture or positioning inadequate for a safe swallow? What specifically was the patient's prior level of function?

The patient's diagnoses appear incomplete. What was the cause of the October 1995 hospitalization? Are the patient's mobility and communication deficits a result of a previous neurological condition?

Although it would seem redundant to reiterate data such as the medical history in a hospital physical therapy evaluation, it is important to summarize pertinent data. Remember that a reviewer may not receive the entire medical record; therefore, the therapist needs to paint a clear picture of the patient.

3. Is there evidence of the need for skilled intervention?

No, evidence of the need for skilled intervention is lacking. Baseline data are undefined in all functional areas. It would appear this patient is debilitated only as a result of illness and that by resuming activities with the husband, who was trained during a previous admission, the patient would regain previous functional activity levels.

4. Are there adequate baseline data to develop future comparisons?

There are minimal baseline data provided in the evaluation to allow for future comparisons to justify treatment. Even basic information regarding transfers was lacking, making it difficult

for the reviewer to assess the actual limitations of this patient. In this evaluation only strength is measurable.

5. Are the objective data related to functional deficits?

The objective data, which are only measurable for strength, are not related to function. This evaluation is incomplete.

6. Are comparative statements and data clearly outlined?

Data are not outlined, except for strength.

7. (A) Are the three components for goals present (measurable, functional, time frames)?

Time frames are lacking for all goals. Goal 1 is not related to function and would be better stated as *Increase bilateral upper and lower extremity strength to fair to allow transfers with assist of one in two days.* All goals are measurable, except the first short- and long-term goals.

(B) Are the goals realistic for the individual case?

It would be difficult for the reviewer to determine if the goals are realistic secondary to the lack of baseline data.

8. Do you feel the proposed treatment is reasonable and necessary?

It would be reasonable for a reviewer to request more information regarding the patient's status and functional deficits before approving treatment in order to determine if the treatment was reasonable and necessary.

Case 4: Hospital, Progress Report

Attendance: Patient seen on a daily basis for P/AAROM BU/LE's. 10 visits.

Current Baseline Data

AROM/PROM: Patient exhibits increased resistance to PROM LUE and LE which is decreased with rotational movement. Bilateral shoulder ROM limited greater than 100 degrees secondary to muscular tightness. Patient participation in ROM is minimal. Decreased spontaneous AROM is noted.

Strength: BU/LE strength poor.

Bed mobility: Requires max assist for bed mobility and positioning.

Transfers: Pt. transfers were attempted but were unsafe secondary to patient flaccidity and decreased safety.

Treatment Diagnosis: Weakness.

Assessment

Reason for skilled care: Patient exhibits increased BU/LE weakness, decreased AROM and increased muscle tone LU/LE. Unable to maintain upright position when seated.

Problems:

1. Decreased PROM/AROM BU/LE's.
2. Decreased strength BU/LE's.
3. Increased muscle tone LU/LE.
4. Max assist for bed mobility and ADL's.
(Problems revised 12-12-95)

Plan of Care

Specific treatment strategies: Pt. seen on a daily basis for ROM, positioning and progression to strengthening if indicated.

Frequency: Daily.

Duration: Hospitalization.

Patient instruction/home program: See Caregiver training.

Caregiver training: Nursing has been instructed to continue ROM of BU/LE's, proper positioning to decrease muscle tone and proper positioning to prevent skin breakdown.

Short-term goals and achievement dates:

1. Maintain ROM BU/LE's.
2. Inc. strength BU/LE's.
3. Prevent joint contractures.
4. Educate nursing staff in ROM techniques.
(Goals revised 12-26-95.)

Long-term goals and achievement dates: Maintain ROM and prevent joint contractures secondary to muscle tightness.

Rehabilitation potential or discharge prognosis: Fair+ to good.

Case 4: Hospital, Progress Report Worksheet

1. Are the "essential elements" (defined in Chapter 1) for documentation present?

Essential Element	Y, N, or N/A	Comment(s)
Attendance	Y	The data indicate that the patient was seen daily for ten visits. In the evaluation the start of care date was 12-12-95 and the goals in the progress report were revised 12-26-95. The fourteen-day length of care and ten-visit attendance do not reflect daily intervention. It is recommended that the number of visits scheduled and any reasons for absence be identified.
Current Baseline Data Cognition	N	Not addressed. Data regarding communication were provided in the evaluation. Any cognitive deficits should be documented to help in determining the patient's ability to participate in a rehabilitation program.

Essential Element	Y, N, or N/A	Comment(s)
Vision/hearing	N	Not addressed in the evaluation or progress report. Given the minimal amount of data and the vague treatment diagnosis (weakness), the reviewer needs as much information as possible regarding additional deficits. It would be helpful to know if the patient has deficits in this area that may affect the ability to return home.
Vital signs	N	Not addressed in the evaluation or progress report. Given the primary diagnosis of possible aspiration pneumonia, data related to respiration would provide a complete picture of the patient's functional challenges that may affect participation in rehabilitation.
Vascular signs	N/A	Not applicable at this time. This area was addressed in the evaluation, and no deficits were noted. Documentation is only required if a change in status affects participation in rehabilitation.
Sensation/proprioception	N	Not addressed. Based on the patient's limited communication ability, data may be difficult to obtain. If deficits exist, it would be helpful to explain their clinical relevance.
Edema	N/A	Not applicable at this time. This area was addressed in the evaluation and no deficits were noted. Documentation is only required if a change in status affects participation in rehabilitation.
Posture	N	This area is not addressed in the evaluation or progress report. Information regarding posture is relevant in terms of this patient's ability to perform basic functional tasks such as rolling, sitting, and transfers.
AROM/PROM	Y	The data lack specific objective measurements for comparison, a description of functional deficits, and where the range limitations exist. Specific range of motion measurements would be helpful. The phrase "decreased with rotational movement" would also be difficult for a reviewer, who may have a limited rehabilitation background, to understand.
Strength	Y	Data indicate, "BU/LE strength poor." The validity of one strength grade for all extremities may be questioned. Furthermore, the data are inconsistent with data in Transfers, and a description of strength would be enhanced if a progress comparison and the relationship to function were provided—for example, *Strength of the upper and lower extremities per manual muscle testing is Poor (previously Fair minus). Patient is now unable to initiate safe standing for transfer training.*
Pain	N	Because of the data describing resistance to range of motion activities and muscle tightness, it is reasonable to expect that pain may affect participation in therapy. A description comparing data from the evaluation to present would be helpful.
Coordination	N/A	
Bed mobility	Y	The amount of assistance is described as "max." A reviewer would be unable to determine if this is a regression, as the evaluation did not provide adequate baseline data and described bed mobility as "requires assist."
Balance (sit and stand)	N	Balance is not addressed in the evaluation or progress report. This is an oversight, as the assessment describes the patient as "unable to maintain upright position when seated." It is important to describe the direction of balance loss, the amount of assistance to maintain balance, and the impact of balance deficits on functional activities.

(continued)

Essential Element	Y, N, or N/A	Comment(s)
Transfers	Y	Baseline data are not described in the evaluation. However, in the progress report transfers are described as unsafe. It would be helpful to know what safety deficits exist and how much assistance is required. For example, if maximal assistance of two is required and knee buckling occurs during standing attempts, is an alternative method of transfers recommended? Determining a safe method of transfers and training caregivers in, for example, the use of a Hoyer™ lift or sliding board transfer would require the skills of a therapist.
Ambulation (level and elevated surfaces)	N/A	Not applicable at this time.
Orthotic/prosthetic devices	N/A	
Wheelchair use	N	Wheelchair use is not addressed in the evaluation or progress report. As the patient is nonambulatory and the assessment indicates difficulty maintaining an upright position when seated, it is reasonable for a reviewer to expect that wheelchair positioning and propulsion need to be described.
DME (using or required)	N	This area is not described in the evaluation or progress report. As the patient is nonambulatory, it is reasonable to expect that a wheelchair is used.
Activity tolerance	N	Data pertaining to the patient's activity tolerance, such as the ability to tolerate range of motion activities, would be helpful to a reviewer in assessing functional limitations and the ability to tolerate a rehabilitation program.
Wound description, including incision status	N/A	
Special tests	N/A	
Architectural/safety considerations	N	Not addressed. If return to home with the husband as the primary caregiver is a long-term goal, then it would be appropriate to address architectural and safety issues. Also, a reviewer might expect information at this point regarding discharge plans and/or potential obstacles to discharge planning.
Treatment Diagnosis	Y	"Weakness" is the treatment diagnosis. This term may imply that skilled intervention is not required and that the patient's ability to resume activities of daily living will resolve this problem. It is recommended that a functional phrase alternative such as *functional strength deficit* be used.
Assessment		
Reason for skilled care	Y	The assessment provides generalized data such as "increased BU/LE weakness, decreased AROM, increased muscle tone LU/LE." It would be helpful for a reviewer if the relationship between the generalized data and functional deficits was provided. An explanation of the origin of the disabilities and why physical therapy intervention is needed would be helpful, as well as the rationale for problem and goal revision.
Problems	Y	The therapist provides data that indicates that the problem list has been revised. The reason for revision is not explained in the progress report, but would help the reviewer when determining the reasonableness of continued skilled care.
Plan of Care		
Specific treatment strategies	Y	The treatment strategies are described; however, they are lacking for bed mobility, transfer training, balance activities, and caregiver training.

Essential Element	Y, N, or N/A	Comment(s)
Frequency	Y	
Duration	Y	The duration is listed as "hospitalization." It would be helpful to estimate an anticipated duration and indicate a number of visits.
Patient instruction/home program	Y	See Caregiver training.
Caregiver training	Y	Documentation indicates nursing instruction in various activities. This demonstrates skilled intervention. It is suggested that the dates of training also be included.
Short-term goals and achievement dates	Y	The revised short-term goals lack all goal components (i.e., measurable, functional, time frames). The goals do not reinforce the need for skilled care. For example, "Maintain ROM BU/LE's" and "Prevent joint contractures" would be appropriate goals for nursing. The goal "Educate nursing staff in ROM techniques" appears to have already been achieved based on the data presented.
Long-term goals and achievement dates	Y	The goal "Maintain ROM and prevent joint contractures secondary to muscle tightness" does not relate to function and is maintenance. Is return to home a long-term goal?
Rehabilitation potential	Y	The evaluation indicates rehabilitation potential as "good," and the progress report describes it as "fair+/good." Based on the limited data presented and apparent regression, this data would not appear realistic to a reviewer without further explanation.

2. Is there evidence of the need for skilled intervention?

There is no evidence of the need for skilled intervention, except for nursing training. It would be helpful if additional data were provided for pain, strength, vital signs, balance, and activity tolerance.

3. Are there adequate baseline data to develop future comparisons?

Data for future comparisons are lacking in all areas except for bed mobility and strength, which are respectively described briefly as "max assist" and "poor."

4. Are the objective data related to functional deficits?

No, data are not related to functional deficits.

5. Are comparative statements and data clearly outlined?

There are no comparative statements in this sample of documentation.

6. (A) Are the three components for goals present (measurable, functional, time frames)?

The goals do not provide measurable data, functional outcomes, or time frames. Goal 1, "Maintain ROM BU/LE's," would be better stated as *Increase range of motion ten degrees in shoulder flexion to improve reaching during rolling in five visits*, and Goal 2, "Inc. strength BU/LE's," could be restated as *Increase strength in the left lower extremity to fair to allow standing with moderate assist of one during transfers in two weeks*.

(B) Are the goals realistic for the individual case?

No, because the goals are vaguely stated. It would be difficult for a reviewer to judge how realistic the goals are for this patient.

7. Do you feel that the treatment was reasonable and necessary?

The authors feel that the patient has multiple deficits and is in obvious need of rehabilitation intervention. However, the documentation poorly reflects this need through minimal baseline and comparative data. The one exception is the explanation of nursing training. For approval of therapy intervention, the reviewer would need and expect further information.

Case 5: Industrial Health—Workers' Compensation, Initial Evaluation

Referral

Specific treatment requested: PT eval and treat.

Data Accompanying Referral

Diagnosis/onset date: Right shoulder and chest pain, Right pectoral strain, and Right rotator cuff bursitis/09-08-96. Medications: Advil™.

Physical Therapy Intake/History

Start of care: 09-14-96

Referral Diagnosis

Mechanism of injury: Gradual onset.
Prior diagnostic imaging/testing: None.

Prior Therapy History: Had PT one and a half years ago.

Baseline Evaluation Data

AROM/PROM: WNL.
Strength: 3/5 for mid-traps on left and 2/5 for mid-traps on right.
Pain: 10 on a 0 to 10 scale. Activities that increase pain include upper extremity activities, work, repetitive lifting, and reaching. Pain decreases after patient rests for 15 minutes. Pain more severe during work and after activity.
Requirements to return to home, school and/or job: Does lots of lifting/reaching.

Prior Level of Function

Employment: ABC Electronics. Off of work.

Problems:

1. Pain in thoracic area and anterior chest.
2. Tender to palpation interscapular area.
3. Decreased upper extremity strength.

Plan of Care

Specific treatment strategies: Ultrasound, hot pack, electrical stimulation and soft tissue mobilization.
Frequency: 3x/week.
Duration: 3 weeks.
Patient instruction/home program: Instructed in towel roll.
Short-term goals and achievement dates:

1. Decrease pain 50% in two weeks.
2. Decrease tenderness 50% in two weeks.
3. Increase strength to 3+/5 in two weeks.

Long-term goals and achievement dates:

1. Independent HEP to control symptoms.

Case 5: Industrial Health—Workers' Compensation, Initial Evaluation Worksheet

1. Are the "essential elements" (defined in Chapter 1) for documentation present?

Essential Element	Y, N, or N/A	Comment(s)
Referral		
Reason	N	The reason for referral is not stated. A reviewer would find it helpful to understand the need for skilled intervention in relationship to the functional deficits. For example the statement *Patient referred for physical therapy by Dr. ABC to decrease right shoulder pain and improve right shoulder mobility to allow return to work* would demonstrate this relationship.
Specific treatment requested	Y	

Essential Element	Y, N, or N/A	Comment(s)
Data Accompanying Referral		
Diagnosis/onset date	Y	The therapist indicates the following diagnoses: "Right shoulder and chest pain," "Right pectoral strain," and "Right rotator cuff bursitis." Shoulder and chest pain may be more appropriately identified as treatment diagnoses. It is also recommended that "chest pain" be clarified. Does "chest pain" refer to pain in the shoulder region or from a cardiac condition?
Secondary diagnoses	N/A	
Medical history	N	Not addressed. It is reasonable for a reviewer to expect documentation pertaining to medical history. In this case, the multiple diagnoses presented pertaining to the right shoulder and the notation of prior therapy one and a half years previously imply that a medical history exists. Information specific to prior medical interventions, such as cortisone injections or immobilization of the right shoulder (e.g., use of a sling), would provide clinical insight to the reviewer in determining the need for skilled physical therapy intervention.
Medications	Y	The evaluation indicates that Advil™ is used. Further description of why this medication is being used and how long it has been administered would help in determining the acute or chronic nature of the diagnoses.
Comorbidities (complicating or pre-cautionary information)	N	Not addressed. Based on the multiple diagnoses presented and the report that the patient is "Off of work," it is reasonable to expect that restrictions exist that limit job responsibilities such as lifting.
Physical Therapy Intake/History		
Date of birth	N	Not addressed. This is important information, as many physician offices and third-party payers file and/or identify patients based on the date of birth.
Age	N	It may be helpful for a reviewer to know the age in the overall assessment of the patient's rehabilitation potential and for identification purposes.
Gender	N	Not addressed. Demographic information such as gender is helpful for patient identification.
Start of care	Y	
Primary complaint	N	Not addressed. As pain and limitations in job performance exist, it would be helpful to document the patient's primary complaint. Identifying this information assists in the development of the short-term and long-term goals.
Referral Diagnosis		
Mechanism of injury	Y	The mechanism of injury is documented as "Gradual onset." This is a vague description, as it does not define a specific time frame. Is the gradual onset over a time frame of days, weeks, months, or years? Based on the onset date of 09-08-96 and the start of care date of 09-14-96, a reviewer may question the accuracy of the mechanism of injury and/or the onset date because of the diagnoses presented.
Prior diagnostic imaging/testing	Y	The therapist's documentation indicates "None." It would seem reasonable based on the multiple diagnoses listed that diagnostic imaging, such as an x-ray, was performed.

(continued)

Essential Element	Y, N, or N/A	Comment(s)
Prior Therapy History	Y	The documentation indicates that the patient "Had PT one and a half years ago." A reviewer would find it helpful in assessing the need for skilled care and in determining the patient's rehabilitation potential if further details were provided. For instance, was the prior therapy intervention for a similar diagnosis? If yes, then what modalities were provided, at what frequency and duration? Were the patient's goals achieved? What additional teaching/training could be rendered to prevent another recurrence of this injury?
Baseline Evaluation Data		
Cognition	N/A	
Vision/hearing	N/A	
Vital signs	N/A	
Vascular signs	N	Not addressed. Based on the diagnoses of right shoulder and chest pain, right pectoral strain, and right rotator cuff bursitis, it would seem reasonable that girth measurements are needed for future progress comparison.
Sensation/proprioception	N	Not addressed. It is reasonable for a reviewer to expect this area to be addressed based on the diagnoses presented. Any deficits would help in justifying the need for skilled care.
Edema	N/A	See Vascular signs.
Posture	N	Not addressed. It would seem, based on the job responsibilities of lifting and reaching, that a description of postural deficits is relevant. A reviewer may seek additional information on posture as well as overall body mechanics because of their potential effect on reinjury.
AROM/PROM	Y	Range of motion is described as within normal limits. Data pertaining to what the therapist measured is needed. For example, were the trunk, neck, or upper extremities tested?
Strength	Y	The present information, "3/5 for mid-traps on left and 2/5 for mid-traps on right," provides baseline data that are helpful for the reviewer. However, the data are incomplete, and further details are required for future progress comparisons such as additional manual muscle test measurements for the left and right upper extremities and shoulder girdle musculature. Also, the impact of the strength deficits in regard to functional limitations in activities of daily living and job responsibilities would help the reviewer in determining the need for skilled intervention.
Pain	Y	The therapist documented a pain description that provides examples of activities that exacerbate and diminish pain. It would be helpful for the reviewer to know the location of the pain and what the pain rating is following the documented fifteen-minute rest. This additional information would provide the reviewer with baseline data for future progress comparisons.
Coordination	N/A	
Bed mobility	N/A	
Balance (sit and stand)	N/A	
Transfers	N/A	
Ambulation (level and elevated surfaces)	N/A	
Orthotic/prosthetic devices	N/A	
Wheelchair use	N/A	
DME (using or required)	N/A	

Essential Element	Y, N, or N/A	Comment(s)
Activity tolerance	N	Not addressed. The evaluation indicates that pain decreases following fifteen minutes of rest and that pain is more severe during work and after activity. Although the activities that increase pain are not described, it is reasonable to assume that activity tolerance needs to be addressed, as it will influence the patient's ability to return to work.
Wound description, including incision status	N/A	
Special tests	N	Not addressed. Any special tests should be listed and the clinical relevance briefly explained.
Architectural/safety considerations	N	Not addressed. As this case involves workers' compensation insurance, a patient that is "Off of work," and job responsibilities such as lifting and reaching, it is reasonable to evaluate and consider architectural barriers in both the work and home settings. Identifying architectural barriers would provide the reviewer with insight into the patient's functional limitations.
Requirements to return to home, school and/or job	Y	The therapist documents that the patient "Does lots of lifting/reaching." This is a limited description for the reviewer to determine the extent of the patient's functional limitations. The documentation would be enhanced by including information such as how often lifting/reaching occurs, the average weight of the objects lifted, and the vertical height necessary to complete the task.
Prior Level of Function		
Mobility (home and community)	N	Not addressed. Prior level of function is important to the reviewer in determining the need for skilled intervention and assessing the reasonableness of the established goals. A reviewer would want to know the patient's prior functional status specifically related to the right shoulder. For instance, was the patient able to retrieve objects from a cupboard or lift objects? Was the patient pain-free?
Employment	Y	The therapist indicates the patient's place of employment and that the patient is now "Off of work." This is vague. It would be helpful for the reviewer to be provided with an accurate description of the patient's functional abilities prior to the onset of pain. For example, *The patient previously was able to stack and lift fifty-pound boxes approximately seventy-five times a day. Presently the patient reports the inability to lift due to right shoulder pain.*
School	N/A	
Treatment Diagnosis	N	As part of the evaluation process, it is important to identify the treatment diagnosis for which physical therapy services are rendered.
Assessment		
Reason for skilled care	N	Not addressed. Identifying the need for skilled care is a necessary element in documentation. The therapist's insight into the functional limitations and expectations for improvement are important to the reviewer.
Problems	Y	A reviewer may not understand the clinical relationship between the baseline data and the three problems listed by the therapist. For example, the location of pain was not defined in the baseline data; however, Problem 1 indicates "Pain in thoracic area and anterior chest." Supporting data are needed to demonstrate why the skills of a physical therapist are required.

(continued)

Essential Element	Y, N, or N/A	Comment(s)
Plan of Care		
Specific treatment strategies	Y	Modalities such as hot packs, ultrasound, electrical stimulation, and soft tissue mobilization are listed. To a reviewer, this plan of care is incomplete, as carryover into functional activities is omitted. The plan would be enhanced by including therapeutic exercise and/or home program instruction.
Frequency	Y	
Duration	Y	
Patient instruction/home program	Y	The therapist provides a brief description of home program instruction by documenting "Instructed in towel roll." It is not reasonable to expect a reviewer to understand what this exercise entails and how it will functionally benefit the patient. Further detail is suggested.
Caregiver training	N/A	
Short-term goals and achievement dates	Y	All goals have a time frame and a measurable component. However, baseline data are lacking to measure a decrease in tenderness of 50%. All three goals are vague and do not specify locations of the pain, tenderness, and strength deficits. All goals lack a functional component.
Long-term goals and achievement dates	Y	Although present, the symptoms that the home exercise program will be controlling are not defined. Also, it would seem important to include the patient's ability to return to work.
Rehabilitation potential	N	It is important to identify the rehabilitation potential of the patient, as it helps the reviewer assess the need for and duration of skilled care.

2. Is the overall history of the patient adequate?

No, there is a lack of information regarding the patient's past and present medical history, previous physical therapy for a related or unrelated condition, and mechanism in injury. This is particularly true in relationship to the patient's job requirements, thus making it difficult for the reviewer to assess the patient's overall functional deficits (i.e., if this was a gradual onset, was it related to posture, changes in responsibilities at work or the repetitive nature of the activities performed?).

3. Is there evidence of the need for skilled intervention?

There appears to be a need for skilled care based on the diagnoses (right pectoral strain and rotator cuff bursitis), the recent onset date, and the pain described. However, the need for skilled intervention would be enhanced if a description of the functional deficits and the need for instruction in postural correction as well as body mechanics were documented. Further details regarding job responsibilities would also help the reviewer in assessing the need for skilled intervention.

4. Are there adequate baseline data to develop future comparisons?

Baseline data are lacking in all areas except for active and passive range of motion. For instance, regarding strength, the only muscle assessed is the middle trapezius. There is no distinct reflection of the strength of the right upper extremity or a comparison to the left. If the patient has functional limitations, it would seem logical that deficits in strength would be present in other muscles, or if the muscle grades are normal, that should be stated.

5. Are the objective data related to functional deficits?

No, there are no functional relationships described with the baseline data provided for pain and strength or in the problem and goal areas. For example, Problem 2 states, "Tender to palpation interscapular area" and does not address the relationship to function such as lifting at work or reaching into a cupboard at home.

6. Are comparative statements and data clearly outlined?

Data are either lacking or incomplete for vascular signs, sensation/proprioception, posture, strength, pain, activity tolerance, and architectural considerations. Limited or missing data will hamper the development of future progress comparisons.

7. (A) Are the three components for goals present (measurable, functional, time frames)?

Goals are measurable and exhibit a time frame. However, they do not have a functional component for the home or work setting. For example, Goal 1 may be better stated as, *Decrease right shoulder pain by 50% (5 out of 10) in two weeks to enable patient to improve lifting ability at work.*

(B) Are the goals realistic for the individual case?

Even though data are limited, it is felt the overall goals are realistic for this patient. However, additional baseline data would make it easier for the reviewer to determine that the goals are realistic.

8. Do you feel the proposed treatment is reasonable and necessary?

It is difficult to answer this question based on the limited evaluation data presented. Because of the severe pain, diagnoses indicated, and the "Off of work" status, it is reasonable to believe that the proposed treatment is necessary. However, it would seem appropriate for a reviewer to the request additional information prior to authorizing treatment beyond one week. A reviewer may be concerned with the limited focus on return to work and absence of baseline data.

Case 5: Industrial Health—Workers' Compensation, Discharge Report

Attendance: Total of 13 visits since evaluation.

Current Baseline Data

Strength: In mid and lower trapezius is 4-/5.
Pain: Patient reports no symptoms in thoracic and anterior chest wall. Initially had soreness and cramping anteriorly. Those symptoms are gone. Does have some soreness in the right levator scapular area after work. Is no longer tender to palpation in the interscapular area and thoracic paraspinals. Did have tenderness in the first right rib and this was mobilized from a superior position to an inferior position throughout the course of therapy.
Activity tolerance: Return to full duty at ABC Electronics.

Assessment

Reason for skilled care: The short-term goals were achieved.

Plan of Care

Specific treatment strategies: Treatment utilized: Hot pack, ultrasound, soft tissue mobilization, therapeutic exercise, instruction in HEP and electrical stimulation. Discharge patient from PT this date.
Patient instruction/home program: Is very compliant with a HEP including a towel stretch in supine, prone stretch for upper back, scapular stretch, pivot prone with blue theraband and red theraband for pain of diagonals, four point with upper extremity/lower extremity lifting. Has had difficulty with this because of wrist flexor tightness.
Short-term goals and achievement dates: All goals were achieved.

1. Decrease pain 50% in two weeks.
2. Decrease tenderness 50% in two weeks.
3. Increase strength to 3+/5 in two weeks.

Discharge prognosis: Excellent.

Case 5: Industrial Health—Workers' Compensation, Discharge Report Worksheet

1. Are the "essential elements" (defined in Chapter 1) for documentation present?

Essential Element	Y, N, or N/A	Comment(s)
Attendance	Y	The therapist indicates, "Total of 13 visits since evaluation." It is recommended that the number of visits scheduled and any reasons for absence be identified. The evaluation listed a frequency of three times per week for three weeks, which totals nine visits. A reviewer may seek an explanation for the extended duration of skilled service.
Current Baseline Data		
Cognition	N/A	
Vision/hearing	N/A	
Vital signs	N/A	
Vascular signs	N	This area is not addressed in the evaluation or discharge report. Data such as girth measurements would help in justifying the need for skilled care.
Sensation/proprioception	N	Not addressed in the evaluation or discharge report. Any changes in sensation or proprioception that may affect rehabilitation need to be documented.
Edema	N/A	See Vascular signs.
Posture	N	Posture and/or body mechanics are not addressed in the evaluation or the discharge report. As this patient's job responsibilities include lifting and reaching, a reviewer could reasonably expect skilled intervention/assessment of posture and/or body mechanics.

(continued)

Essential Element	Y, N, or N/A	Comment(s)
AROM/PROM	N/A	Not applicable at this time. As range of motion was "WNL" in the evaluation, only changes that affect rehabilitation need to be documented.
Strength	Y	The documentation indicates that strength in the middle and lower trapezius is 4-/5. No comparison is presented in relationship to the evaluation findings. It is also unclear if this muscle grade pertains to the right or left trapezius. A reviewer would also find it helpful to know the functional improvement in activities of daily living and job responsibilities.
Pain	Y	Comparative statements regarding a decrease in pain are documented for the reviewer. However, the statement "Initially had soreness and cramping anteriorly" was not reported in the evaluation. The same is true in regard to the comments discussing "palpation" and "tenderness in the first right rib." It is recommended that objective data in the evaluation, such as the pain rating, be included at discharge to provide comparative information for determining progress.
Coordination	N/A	
Bed mobility	N/A	
Balance (sit and stand)	N/A	
Transfers	N/A	
Ambulation (level and elevated surfaces)	N/A	
Orthotic/prosthetic devices	N/A	
Wheelchair use	N/A	
DME (using or required)	N/A	
Activity tolerance	Y	The discharge data indicate that the patient returned to full duties. Comparative data or the progression of duties is needed. For example, since the last report, did the patient return to light duty?
Wound description, including incision status	N/A	
Special tests	N/A	
Architectural/safety considerations	N	Not addressed. As job responsibilities include lifting and reaching, it is reasonable to consider architectural barriers for both the work and home settings.
Treatment Diagnosis	N	It is important to identify the treatment diagnosis for which physical therapy services were rendered, as it may have changed during the course of treatment.
Assessment		
Reason for skilled care	Y	The relationship between the modalities rendered and a description of their effects is not provided. An expectation statement of the therapist's insight regarding successful carryover into the workplace is also lacking. A reviewer would find it helpful if these items were included along with an explanation of the need for the extended duration beyond the nine visits indicated in the evaluation.
Problems	N	Not addressed. A reviewer would find it helpful to include the problems (and dates of resolution), as they may have changed during the course of treatment.
Plan of Care		
Specific treatment strategies	Y	The therapist lists a detailed plan of care. The addition of therapeutic exercise and instruction in a home exercise program help to justify the skilled care provided for carryover of progress into functional activities.

Essential Element	Y, N, or N/A	Comment(s)
Frequency	N	Not addressed. A summary helps the reviewer determine the reasonableness of the frequency and duration in relationship to the functional progress reported. It also helps when analyzing documentation and the corresponding services billed (e.g., *Frequency: Was seen three times per week, Duration: Was seen for eight weeks.*).
Duration	N	See Frequency.
Patient instruction/home program	Y	A detailed description of the home program is provided and justifies the need for skilled care to the reviewer. It is recommended that the frequency with which the program is performed by the patient and the dates on which the therapist provided training and/or changes to the program be documented.
Caregiver training	N/A	
Short-term goals and achievement dates	Y	It appears the goals were achieved and exceeded. It is helpful for the reviewer to assess progress if goals are upgraded during the course of treatment. The goals presented in the discharge summary are the same as those listed in the evaluation. Once again, the goals lack a functional component and are vague in regard to the location of pain, tenderness, and strength deficits.
Discharge prognosis	Y	

2. Is there evidence of the need for skilled intervention?

Yes, there is evidence of the need for skilled intervention based on the description of the home exercise program and the gains in pain management. However, the modalities utilized (hot packs, ultrasound, and electrical stimulation) were not adequately justified and were only described in the plan of care. It would be difficult for a reviewer to justify coverage of all three modalities when the application and results were not described. The lack of detail regarding the patient's job requirements also detracts from justifying the need for a therapist to develop a treatment regime to return the patient to work.

3. Are there adequate baseline data to develop future comparisons?

The evaluation was lacking in baseline data, and this has continued in the discharge report. Baseline data are lacking on the discharge report, specifically in the areas of posture, pain ratings, bilateral upper extremity strength grades, architectural considerations, and activity tolerance.

4. Are the objective data related to functional deficits?

There is no description of the relationship between data and function. This is particularly true in regard to pain, reaching, and lifting.

5. Are comparative statements and data clearly outlined?

Based on the discharge report, a reviewer would have difficulty determining coverage if a copy of the evaluation was not included with the claim. Even with the evaluation, there is a lack of comparative data. For example, there is no comparison to the initial pain rating scale; instead there are several subjective statements that neither relate to the evaluation or to function.

6. (A) Are the three components for goals present (measurable, functional, time frames)?

Goals are measurable and exhibit a time frame. However, the goals do not have any functional components related to the work setting. For example, Goal 1 may be better stated as, *Decrease right shoulder pain by 80% (8 out of 10) in two weeks to allow return to work full time.*

(B) Are the goals realistic for the individual case?

Even though the overall information is limited, it is felt that the overall goals are realistic for this patient. However, as stated in the previous questions, additional baseline data regarding posture and job requirements would assist in establishing realistic goals. In addition, goals and treatment intervention regarding posture and body mechanics would be important for a long-term successful outcome for this patient.

7. Do you feel that the treatment was reasonable and necessary?

Yes, the treatment by a physical therapist was reasonable in relationship to the diagnoses. A reviewer could question the fact that the treatment did not reflect adequate assessment and goal-related treatment intervention to the work setting. Furthermore, which was the treatment focus: return to work, pain control, or the patient's ability to perform activities of daily living?

Case 6: Industrial Health—Work Hardening, Initial Evaluation

Referral

Reason: Was referred for functional capacity assessment (FCA) and work hardening by Dr. ABC, with the goal of improving work tolerances to return to modified work as a Finish Carpenter.

Data Accompanying Referral

Diagnosis/onset date: Bilateral wrist fusion/05-12-94.

Medical history: 5/94 he underwent open reduction internal fixation procedures but symptoms and dysfunction continued following surgery. In 9/94, he underwent a left wrist bone fusion and in 3/95, a right wrist bone fusion procedure. Following delayed union on the right, he underwent refusion surgery in 2/96. Patient was on a bone growth stimulator.

Medications: He uses Valium™ to assist sleep that is interrupted by pain.

Comorbidities (complicating or precautionary information): He occasionally uses alcohol, smokes about one pack of cigarettes daily and consumes 5 cups of caffeinated coffee daily.

Physical Therapy Intake/History

Date of birth: 06-05-51

Age: 44

Gender: Male.

Start of care: 05-15-96 (Note that initial contact with the facility occurred September 1995, however, placed on hold secondary to nonunion fracture and use of a bone growth stimulator).

Primary complaint: Both pain and dysfunction continues in hands bilaterally, but he states that there has been improvement since his last surgery. He stated that his goal is to return to work in a modified capacity as a Finish Carpenter.

Referral Diagnosis

Mechanism of injury: Was injured in May 1994 while working as a carpenter framing a roof when he slipped and fell sustaining fractures of the distal radius bilaterally.

Prior Therapy History:

He has participated in rehabilitation to increase flexibility and strength in hands/wrists/arms bilaterally.

Baseline Evaluation Data

Vital signs: Blood pressure (seated/resting): 134/100, Target measure: 120/80. Cardiovascular MET level: 5.4.

Posture: Demonstrated marginal body mechanics requiring cuing to correct tendencies to use excessive spinal flexion during material handling activities.

	AROM/PROM:	
Assessed Area	**Current Measure**	**Target Measure**
ROM/Wrist Right Flexion	35°	80°
ROM/Wrist Left Flexion	30°	80°
ROM/Wrist Right Extension	35°	70°
ROM/Wrist Left Extension	30°	70°
ROM/Wrist Right Ulnar Deviation	20°	30°
ROM/Wrist Left Ulnar Deviation	20°	30°
ROM/Wrist Right Radial Deviation	25°	20°
ROM/Wrist Left Radial Deviation	15°	20°

Strength: Upper extremity strength measures related to wrist and hand was consistently greater on the left (except for forearm pronation, wrist extension, and pinch): grip—21% greater left; wrist flexion—50% greater left; forearm supination—61% greater left.

Current Safe Work Capacity

The following graph represents current safe work capacity with respect to strength levels as defined by the US Department of Labor (DOL). Ratings are based on a comparison between the individual's current ability as demonstrated on ERGOS™ and the MAXIMUM strength requirements of each level. Though an individual may demonstrate ability within a strength level, they are rated at that level only if ALL MAXIMUM requirements are met.

Occasional (3 & 4)	Typical Weight Lifted & Carried in Pounds Frequent (3 & 4)	Constant (3 & 4)	Approximate Energy Expended in METS (5)	Work Day Capacity in Hours (6) 0 1 2 3 4 5 6 7 8 +	Physical Demand Level (2)
10 or less	Neglig	Neglig	1.5–2.1	8+	Sedentary
20	10 (7)	Neg. (8)	2.2–3.5	8+	Light (1)
50	25	10	3.6–6.3	8	Medium
100	50	20	6.4–7.5	0	Heavy
100 +	50 +	20 +	Over 7.5	0	Very Heavy

(1) Even though weight lifted may be negligible, a rating of light is required when significant walking and/or standing exists or when significant seated pushing and pulling with arms or legs is involved.

(2) U.S. Department of Labor; Dictionary of Occupational Titles, Fourth Edition Supplement, Appendix D, PP 101-102, 1986.

(3) Frequency defined by the Department of Labor is 0–33% for Occasional, 34–66% for Frequent, and 67–100% for Constant.

(4) Based on the works of Snook, Legg and Myles, Mital and Matheson, the following lifting rates are used to defined DOL frequencies: Occasional—1 lift every 30 minutes, Frequent—1 lift every 2 minutes, Constant—1 lift every 15 seconds.

(5) 1 MET (energy requirement unit) equals one's oxygen/energy consumption at rest; e.g., a rating of 3 METS would equal three times one's resting oxygen/energy consumption.

(6) With allowances for change of position at will.

(7) and/or Walk/Stand/Push/Pull of Arm/Leg controls.

(8) and/or Push/Pull of Arm/Leg controls while seated.

This Participant . . .

Met all maximum SEDENTARY level DOL requirements.

Met all maximum LIGHT level DOL requirements.

Did not meet these maximum MEDIUM level DOL requirements:

27 Static Push Cart Height (24).

22 Static Push Shoulder Height (19).

50 Static Lift Knuckle Height (38).

34 Static Lift Bench Height (24).

50 Dynamic Lift Bench Height Center (40).

25 Dynamic Lift Shelf Height Center (20).

50 Carrying (40).

Pain: He reported symptoms in the wrist bilaterally ranging between 3–7 on a 0–10 pain scale.

Ambulation (level and elevated surfaces): See Activity tolerance.

Activity tolerance:

1. Static strength for lift/push-pull met LIGHT PDL requirements.

2. Dynamic lifting met LIGHT PDL requirements with tolerance at 40 pounds, floor to bench height and 20 pounds, floor to shelf height. Wrist deviation required to control and place loads at upper heights was the interfering factor affecting tolerance.

3. Unrestricted tolerance was demonstrated for sit, stand/walk, stair climb.

4. FREQUENT tolerance was demonstrated for forward reach.

5. OCCASIONAL tolerance was demonstrated for stoop, kneel, overhead reach and bilateral fingering activities.

6. He did not tolerate crouch (due to knee symptoms at donor graft site) and LESS THAN OCCASIONAL tolerance was demonstrated bilaterally for handling activities.

7. Estimated sustained MET level was at 5.4 METs, consistent with LIGHT–MEDIUM PDL work level.

This person can perform the following:

Hrs/Day	Lifting, Carrying, Pushing and Pulling
8+	Sedentary Work Lifting 10 pounds maximum and occasionally lifting and/or carrying such articles as dockets, ledgers, and small tools. Although a sedentary job is defined as one which involves sitting, a certain amount of walking and standing is often necessary in carrying out job duties. Jobs are sedentary if walking and standing are required only occasionally and other sedentary criteria are met.
8+	Light Work Lifting 20 pounds maximum with frequent lifting and/or carrying of objects weighing up to 10 pounds. Even though the weight lifted may be only a negligible amount, a job is in this category when it requires walking or standing to a significant degree or when it involves sitting most of the time with a degree of pushing and pulling of arm and/or leg controls.
0	Medium Work Lifting 50 pounds maximum with frequent lifting and/or carrying of objects weighing up to 25 pounds.
0	Heavy Work Lifting 100 pounds maximum with frequent lifting and/or carrying of objects weighing up to 50 pounds.
0	Very Heavy Work Lifting 100+ pounds occasionally with frequent lifting and/or carrying of objects weighing 50+ pounds.

Activity	Hrs/Day Frequency			
	Occasionally (1%-33% of time)	Frequently (34%-66% of time)	Continuously* (67%-100% of time)	See Notes Below
Sitting	8+	8	8	
Standing/Walking	8+	8	8	
Climbing Stairs	8+			
Climbing Ladder	NT			
Balancing				
Stooping	8	6	4	
Kneeling	8	6	4	
Crouching				
Crawling				
Reaching Forward	8+	8	7	
Reaching Overhead	8	6	4	
Reaching Bended				
Other				
Other				
Handling	6	4	2	
Fingering	8	6	4	
Feeling				
Talking				
Hearing				
Seeing Near				
Seeing Far				

* Even though a worker can perform at a continuous level, less frequency should be sought as a safety precaution.

Definitions taken from *Handbook for Analyzing Jobs*, U.S. Department of Labor.

Note: A "0" in a physical demand category is possible for any one of the following reasons. Further diagnostic/clinical testing is advised.

1. Very low MTM and/or functional performance;
2. Very high subjective report of pain increase on the activity;
3. Incomplete testing or terminated before adequate data were measured;
4. The test was not performed.

Notes: Instruction and/or limitations to be considered: To be determined upon conclusion of participation in work hardening.

Special tests: Performance vs. Job Requirements

The following shows the current ability of patient compared to the Heavy job of CARPENTER, ROUGH D.O.T. #860.381-042.

Numbers in parentheses show job requirements. Numbers in bold print show deficiencies.

Activity	Occasional		Frequent		Constant	
	LBS.	HRS.	LBS.	HRS.	LBS.	HRS.
Lifting						
Static—						
Knuckle Height	**38**(100)	8+(8)	**19**(50)	8+(8)	**8**(20)	8+(8)
Bench Height	**24**(67)	8+(8)	**12**(34)	8+(8)	**5**(14)	8+(8)
Ankle Height	**30**(67)	8+(8)	**15**(34)	8+(8)	**6**(14)	8+(8)
Shoulder Height	**22**(67)	8+(8)	**11**(34)	8+(8)	**4**(14)	8+(8)
Dynamic—Floor to						
Bench Height Left	**30**(100)	8+(8)	**15**(50)	8+(8)	**6**(20)	8+(8)
Bench Height Center	**40**(100)	8+(8)	**20**(50)	8+(8)	**8**(20)	8+(8)
Bench Height Right	**30**(100)	8+(8)	**15**(50)	8+(8)	**6**(20)	8+(8)
Shelf Height Left	**20**(50)	8+(8)	**10**(25)	8+(8)	**4**(10)	8+(8)
Shelf Height Center	**20**(50)	8+(8)	**10**(25)	8+(8)	**4**(10)	8+(8)
Shelf Height Right	(50)	(8)	(25)	(8)	(10)	(8)
Carrying	**40**(100)	**6**(8)	**20**(50)	**6**(8)	**8**(20)	**6**(8)

Activity	Occasional		Frequent		Constant	
Static—						
Pushing Cart Height	**24**(53)	8+(8)	**12**(27)	8+(8)	**5**(11)	8+(8)
Pulling Cart Height	**24**(44)	8+(8)	**12**(22)	8+(8)	**5**(9)	8+(8)
Pushing Shoulder Height	**19**(44)	8+(8)	**9**(22)	8+(8)	**4**(9)	8+(8)
Pulling Shoulder Height	**22**(34)	8+(8)	**11**(17)	8+(8)	**4**(7)	8+(8)
Sitting		8+()		8()		8()
Standing/Walking		8+(8)		8(8)		8(8)
Climbing—						
Stairs		8+(8)		8()		7()
Ladders		NT(8)		()		()
Balancing		(8)		()		()
Stooping		8()		6()		4()
Kneeling		8()		6(8)		4()
Crouching		()		(8)		()
Crawling		()		()		()
Reaching—						
Forward		8+()		8(8)		7()
Overhead		8()		6(8)		4()
Bended		()		(8)		()
Other		()		(8)		()
Other		()		(8)		()
Handling		6()		4(8)		2()
Fingering		8()		6(8)		4()
Feeling		()		()		()
Talking		()		()		()
Hearing		(8)		()		()
Seeing—						
Near		()		(8)		()
Distant		()		()		()

Note: A "0" in a physical demand category is possible for any one of the following reasons. Further diagnostic/clinical testing is advised.

1. Very low MTM and/or functional performance;
2. Very high subjective report of pain increase on the activity;
3. Incomplete testing or terminated before adequate data were measured;
4. The test was not performed.

Architectural/safety considerations: See Strength, Special tests, and Activity tolerance for current safe work capacities.

Requirements to return to home, school and/or job: At time of dictation awaiting modified job description from ABC Construction. See Special tests for closest comparison of job duties.

Prior Level of Function

Employment: Finish Carpenter. ABC Construction.

Assessment

Reason for skilled care: Results of the FCA indicated that he had tolerance for LIGHT physical demand level (PDL) work. Findings are considered valid as he demonstrated excellent consistency during testing. 100% of the coefficient of variation scores were within acceptable ranges and functional cross-validation testing revealed no inconsistencies. (Note: Coefficient of variation is a statistical measure of consistency of effort based on repeated trials of multiple static strength tests.) At the time of this report, job description for modified work as a Finish Carpenter was awaited from ABC Construction to be used to define return to work rehabilitation goals. The patient demonstrated limited bilateral wrist and hand strength and flexibility and continues to experience symptoms that interfere with productivity. Participation in work hardening is recommended to improve tolerances for work as a Finish Carpenter.

Problems: Patient continues to experience decreased flexibility and strength in bilateral wrists and hand. See Short-term goals.

Plan of Care

Duration: To 06-22-96
Short-term goals and achievement dates:

1. Increase physical conditioning
   a. Increase cardiovascular condition to the MEDIUM physical demand level, 6.3 METs. (Initially at 5.4 METs)

b. Increase overall body strength on Hoist and Total Gym to maximum.

c. Increase wrist strength, flexibility and stability to maximum.

2. Increase physical tolerances for work

a. Increase lift/carry strength to the MEDIUM physical demand level, 50 pounds to bench height, 25 pounds to shelf height. (Initially at 30-40 pounds bench and 20 pounds to shelf)

b. Perform work from low level positions of stooping and bending at a FREQUENT level and kneeling and squatting at an OCCASIONAL level.

3. Incorporation of safe workstyle principles

a. Consistent use of proper body mechanics.

b. Use of pacing, stretching and position changes to manage symptoms.

4. Adequate feasibility for competitive employment

a. Adequate productivity, safety and interpersonal behavior.

Long-term goals and achievement dates: Return to work as a Finish Carpenter with defined return-to-work guidelines.

Rehabilitation potential: While he continues to experience decreased flexibility and strength in bilateral wrists and hands, he is judged to have potential to improve capacities to meet physical job demands as a Finish Carpenter. Potential to improve tolerances to usual job duties in the heavy Physical Demand Level is not considered feasible.

Case 6: Industrial Health—Work Hardening, Initial Evaluation Worksheet

1. Are the "essential elements" (defined in Chapter 1) for documentation present?

Essential Element	Y, N, or N/A	Comment(s)
Referral		
Reason	Y	The reason for referral is stated. However, it would helpful to elaborate on what "improving work tolerances" means.
Specific treatment requested	N	The physician's order is not defined. However, it is implied in the reason for referral, which states, "Was referred for functional capacity assessment (FCA) and work hardening by Dr. ABC." A reviewer may find it helpful to review the specific treatment requested to ensure that the plan of care is accurately defined.
Data Accompanying Referral		
Diagnosis/onset date	Y	
Secondary diagnoses	N/A	
Medical history	Y	The therapist provides an adequate summary of the medical history. Additional details regarding the reason for the slow healing of the wrist fusion, where the fusion is, and the location of the bone graft site would be pertinent to the rehabilitation process. For instance, if the bone graft was taken from the knee, it may limit function because of pain.
Medications	Y	The therapist's statement "He uses Valium™ to assist sleep that is interrupted by pain" clearly reflects the medication's purpose and impact on function. A statement noting that no other medications are being taken would be helpful.
Comorbidities (complicating or precautionary information)	Y	The documentation appropriately identifies smoking and the consumption of caffeinated coffee as complicating factors. These factors may influence the patient's activity tolerance and heart rate. It would also be helpful to clarify for the reviewer if weight-bearing and/or lifting restrictions exist based on the history of a delayed union of the right wrist.
Physical Therapy Intake/History		
Date of birth	Y	
Age	Y	
Gender	Y	

Essential Element	Y, N, or N/A	Comment(s)
Start of Care	Y	"Patient was initially to be seen earlier, however, was placed on hold secondary to nonunion of the fracture." This is helpful information for the reviewer.
Primary complaint	Y	
Referral Diagnosis		
Mechanism of injury	Y	
Prior diagnostic imaging/testing	N	Not addressed. It would seem reasonable, based on the wrist fusion, that diagnostic imaging, such as an X-ray, was performed.
Prior Therapy History	Y	The prior therapy history is brief and does not reflect when the rehabilitation service was received or the outcome. Also, was the service for work hardening or standard outpatient rehabilitation? Further description of why the patient was not healing would also be helpful to the reviewer. For instance, are there other conditions affecting healing, or was the fracture of such severity that healing was delayed?
Baseline Evaluation Data		
Cognition	N/A	
Vision/hearing	N/A	
Vital signs	Y	
Vascular signs	N	Not addressed. It would seem reasonable to assess vascular signs because of the medical history (i.e., past surgeries).
Sensation/proprioception	N	Not addressed. Sensory or proprioceptive deficits secondary to past surgeries would seem applicable for safety considerations in the work environment.
Edema	N	Not addressed. Because of the surgical history, objective data identifying the existence or nonexistence of edema seems relevant for the reviewer, especially because of the potential functional impact on range of motion and strength.
Posture	Y	Adequate description. However, further objective data regarding the amount and type of cuing needed for postural correction would be helpful for future comparison.
AROM/PROM	Y	Range of motion is addressed. However, the unit of measurement (degrees), the movements pronation and supination, and the differentiation of passive versus active range of motion for the upper extremities are not defined. The information listed as "current measure" and "target measure" are helpful to a reviewer when determining skilled need. Depending on the bone graft site, range measurements of the knee may also be necessary, as function could be limited if a deficit exists.
Strength	Y	Detail is provided representing safe work capacities with regard to strength. However, the objective data in terms of specific measurements and age-related norms are not described for grip, wrist flexion, forearm pronation, and forearm supination. A reviewer would expect objective and specific measurements as per manual muscle testing or use of a dynameter.
Pain	Y	A pain rating scale is defined and a range of reported pain, "3–7," is provided. A reviewer would find it helpful to understand the relationship to function. For instance, is pain a 7 during heavy work or light work? Also, where is the pain, and how long does it last after activity?

(continued)

Essential Element	Y, N, or N/A	Comment(s)
Coordination	N	Not addressed. A reviewer may consider fine motor coordination to be an important safety factor for a Finish Carpenter. Baseline evaluation data are needed in this area.
Bed mobility	N/A	
Balance (sit and stand)	N	In the area of activity tolerance, the documentation indicates the patient's inability to tolerate a crouch position "because of knee symptoms at donor graft site." If balance is affected, it needs to be documented.
Transfers	N/A	
Ambulation (level and elevated surfaces)	Y	Ambulation is described in the area of Activity tolerance. If the bone graft involved the knee, then gait deficits, if they exist, should be described for the reviewer, as they may hinder functional progress.
Orthotic/prosthetic devices	N/A	
Wheelchair use	N/A	
DME (using or required)	N/A	
Activity tolerance	Y	
Wound description, including incision status	N	Not addressed. The impact of soft tissue restrictions, if present, would be helpful, as limitations may affect job performance.
Special tests	Y	Resources and detailed measures are outlined.
Architectural/safety considerations	Y	
Requirements to return to home, school and/or job	Y	The therapist addresses this information in Special tests. The need to obtain further information from ABC Construction was also reported. A reviewer appreciates documentation of the therapist's need and plan for obtaining additional information.
Prior Level of Function		
Mobility (home and community)	N	Although the goal of this program is work-related, it would be helpful for a reviewer to also know the impact on activities of daily living such as driving, grooming, and dressing.
Employment	Y	The description "Finish Carpenter. ABC construction" does not provide the reviewer with the functional duties previously performed.
School	N/A	
Treatment Diagnosis	N	Listing the status post wrist fusion would make the treatment diagnosis clearer for the reviewer.
Assessment		
Reason for skilled care	Y	
Problems	Y	The therapist provides an overview of the problems. The problems are then positively stated in terms of the need to "increase" a defined functional area in the short-term goal section. This is acceptable documentation. It would seem reasonable that knee pain be identified as a problem because of the impact on function.
Plan of Care		
Specific treatment strategies	N	The plan of care is an essential component of any evaluation. A statement describing the treatment strategies, such as reconditioning, education, and work task simulation, would be expected by a reviewer.
Frequency	N	Not addressed. Omission of the frequency of treatment is an oversight. A reviewer would expect the frequency of participation in therapy to be included in the documentation.
Duration	Y	
Patient instruction/home program	N	Not addressed. A reviewer could expect a reference to the home program and its components.

Essential Element	Y, N, or N/A	Comment(s)
Caregiver training	N/A	Not applicable at this time as a separate category. Patient and employer training are the core elements of this program. Patient performance versus job responsibilities are defined in Activity tolerance and reinforced throughout the evaluation in areas such as Strength and Special tests.
Short-term goals and achievement dates	Y	All goals lack a defined time frame. Goals 1b, 1c, 3a, 3b, and 4a are not measurable. For example, 1c states, "Increase wrist strength, flexibility, and stability to maximum," yet a reviewer could not reasonably be expected to know what "maximum" is. The functional components are described in the headings that state "Increase physical conditioning" and "Increase physical tolerance for work." However, a reviewer may find it helpful if the goal is specified in relationship to the job, such as in terms of lifting and/or carrying objects.
Long-term goals and achievement dates	Y	
Rehabilitation potential	Y	The therapist provides adequate information. However, it is suggested that the use of "tolerance" be presented as *physical conditioning* or *physical functioning*.

2. Is the overall history of the patient adequate?

More information needs to be provided on why healing of the fracture was delayed, the prior therapy history, and how the remaining deficits affected the patient's functional abilities. For instance, are soft tissue restrictions/edema present, and/or are there sensory or proprioceptive changes that may affect safety in the work place?

3. Is there evidence of the need for skilled intervention?

Yes, there are data indicating that in order to return to work, the patient needs to progress from light- to medium-duty work. Although goals are listed, the treatment strategies are not indicated for the reviewer. Despite the missing treatment strategies, the patient appears to require the skills of a therapist to implement, supervise, and upgrade a treatment program to achieve the goal of return to work.

4. Are there adequate baseline data to develop future comparisons?

The baseline data provided exclude a number of areas, such as muscle strength of the upper extremities, range of motion measurements for pronation and supination, differentiation of active versus passive range of motion, edema, sensation/proprioception, and fine motor coordination.

5. Are the objective data related to functional deficits?

Deficits in relationship to the patient's job requirements are clearly defined. Special tests reflect these data.

6. Are comparative statements and data clearly outlined?

Areas such as Special tests and Activity tolerance provide adequate data. As discussed in Question 4, a number of areas such as muscle strength of the upper extremities, range of motion measurements for pronation and supination, differentiation of active versus passive range of motion, edema, sensation/proprioception, and fine motor coordination require additional data.

7. (A) Are the three components for goals present (measurable, functional, time frames)?

No, not all components are present. For example, "Increase wrist strength flexibility and stability to maximum," could be a more effective goal if a measurable component were clearly defined. "Use of pacing, stretching and position changes to manage symptoms" is another example of a goal lacking specific data to allow assessment of measurable changes.

(B) Are the goals realistic for the individual case?

Yes, the goals appear to be specifically related to allowing the patient to return to the work place. The goals appear realistic based on the data provided and special tests performed.

8. Do you feel that the proposed treatment is reasonable and necessary?

Based on the diagnosis and functional limitations in job performance that are identified, this patient's proposed involvement in a work hardening program is appropriate and necessary. This is appropriately addressed on the subsequent discharge report worksheet for work hardening.

Note: It is likely that a case manager (probably a registered nurse) would oversee and approve initiation in a work hardening program. A peer physical therapist reviewer might be solicited in the event that an appeal is necessary. Regardless of who reviews the case, the therapist is still required to provide clear and accurate comparative data that will justify the need for skilled intervention to achieve the goal of the patient in returning to former or modified job duties.

Case 6: Industrial Health—Work Hardening, Discharge Report

Attendance: Absent one day, thirteen full days, nine half days.

Current Baseline Data

Vital signs: Performs at 7.6 METS.

Posture: Understands and demonstrates satisfactory body mechanics/workstyle with compliant carryover.

Strength: Performs fingering/handling at a FREQUENT level. Grip strength is at the LIGHT PHYSICAL DEMAND level. Overall average strength of left and right extremities have increased 8% since May 96. (25% since start of program.)

Ambulation (level and elevated surfaces): See Activity tolerance.

Activity tolerance: Based on current performance, this person appears to be able to return to the job with the following restrictions or modifications:

1. Performs lifting to 50 lbs. bench height, 20 lbs. shelf height, OCCASIONALLY.
2. Performs fingering/handling at a FREQUENT level.

This person can perform the following:

Hrs/Day	Lifting, Carrying, Pushing and Pulling
8+	Sedentary Work Lifting 10 pounds maximum and occasionally lifting and/or carrying such articles as dockets, ledgers, and small tools. Although a sedentary job is defined as one which involves sitting, a certain amount of walking and standing is often necessary in carrying out job duties. Jobs are sedentary if walking and standing are required only occasionally and other sedentary criteria are met.
8+	Light Work Lifting 20 pounds maximum with frequent lifting and/or carrying of objects weighing up to 10 pounds. Even though the weight lifted may be only a negligible amount, a job is in this category when it requires walking or standing to a significant degree or when it involves sitting most of the time with a degree of pushing and pulling of arm and/or leg controls.
0	Medium Work Lifting 50 pounds maximum with frequent lifting and/or carrying of objects weighing up to 25 pounds.
0	Heavy Work Lifting 100 pounds maximum with frequent lifting and/or carrying of objects weighing up to 50 pounds.
0	Very Heavy Work Lifting 100+ pounds occasionally with frequent lifting and/or carrying of objects weighing 50+ pounds.

Activity	Hrs/Day Frequency			
	Occasionally (1%-33% of time)	Frequently (34%-66% of time)	Continuously* (67%-100% of time)	See Notes Below
Sitting	8	8	8	
Standing/Walking	8	8	8	
Climbing Stairs	8	8	8	
Climbing Ladder				
Balancing				
Stooping	8	8	6	
Kneeling	8	8	6	1
Crouching				1
Crawling				
Reaching Forward	8+	8	8	
Reaching Overhead	8	8	/	
Reaching Bended				
Other				
Other				
Handling	8+	8	/	
Fingering	8	8	6	
Feeling				
Talking				
Hearing				
Seeing Near				
Seeing Far				

* Even though a worker can perform at a continuous level, less frequency should be sought as a safety precaution.

Definitions taken from *Handbook for Analyzing Jobs*, U.S. Department of Labor.

Note: A "0" in a physical demand category is possible for any one of the following reasons. Further diagnostic/clinical testing is advised.

1. Very low MTM and/or functional performance;
2. Very high subjective report of pain increase on the activity;
3. Incomplete testing or terminated before adequate data were measured;
4. The test was not performed.

Note: Instructions and/or limitations to be considered: Uses half kneel for kneel and squat due to right knee pain at bone graft site.

Architectural/safety considerations: See Activity tolerance for current safe work capacity

Assessment

Reason for skilled care: Goal of work hardening met. Based on current performance this person appears to be able to return to work with the following restrictions or modifications.

1. Performs lifting to 50 lbs. bench height, 20 lbs. shelf height OCCASIONALLY.
2. Performs fingering/handling at a FREQUENT level. Worker role behaviors (productivity, safety, interpersonal): no problems noted. Client's worker behaviors would make him/her generally acceptable as a worker. Employer has indicated ability to provide work at current capacities.

Plan of Care

Specific treatment strategies: Recommend that the patient continue with home exercise program daily. Recommend continued strength training at local health club. Will see Dr. XYZ on June 11, 1996, and Dr. ABC on June 12, 1996, for return to work release and final restrictions.

Patient instruction/home program: Home exercise program updated and reviewed on date of discharge.

Caregiver (employer) training: Return to work with the following modifications:

1. Currently lifts 50# bench height, 20# shelf height, OCCASIONALLY.
2. Performs stoop, bended reach and half kneel FREQUENTLY.
3. Performs fingering/handling at a FREQUENT level.

Short-term goals and achievement dates:

OBJECTIVES (Established at evaluation 05/15/96)	Discharge Status: 06-06-96
1. Increase cardiovascular condition to the MEDIUM physical demand level, 6.3 METs. (Initially at 5.4 METs)	Performs at 7.6 METs.
2. Increase overall body strength on Hoist and Total Gym to maximum.	Performs at 30–70# on controlled resistance exercises.
3. Increase wrist strength, flexibility and stability to maximum.	Performs fingering/handling at a FREQUENT level. Grip strength is at the LIGHT physical demand level. Overall average strength of left and right extremities has increased 8% since May 21, 1996 (25% since start of program).
4. Increase lift/carry strength to the MEDIUM physical demand level, 50# to bench height, 25# to shelf height. (Initially at 30–40# bench and 20# to shelf.)	Performs lifting to 50# bench height, 20# shelf height, OCCASIONALLY.
5. Performs work from low level positions of stooping and bending at a FREQUENT level and kneeling and squatting at an OCCASIONAL level.	Performs stoop and bended reach FREQUENTLY, uses half-kneel for kneel and squat due to right knee pain at bone graft site.

Case 6: Industrial Health—Work Hardening, Discharge Report Worksheet

1. Are the "essential elements" (defined in Chapter 1) for documentation present?

Essential Element	Y, N, or N/A	Comment(s)
Attendance	Y	Although listed, a reviewer may question compliance. For instance, how many full and/or half days were scheduled?
Current Baseline Data		
Cognition	N/A	
Vision/hearing	N/A	
Vital signs	Y	The documentation indicates that the patient performs at 7.6 METS. A reviewer would find it helpful if a comparative statement was provided. For example, *Performs at 7.6 METS initially 5.4 METS.* Also the relationship to function may not be understood by the reviewer and needs to be documented. The evaluation provided a target blood pressure of 120/80; however, no data are listed in the discharge report.
Vascular signs	N	Vascular signs are not addressed in the evaluation or the discharge report. A problem in this area is important for a reviewer to be aware of when determining the need for skilled care.
Sensation/proprioception	N	This area is not addressed in the evaluation or discharge report. A reviewer may question if sensation or proprioception is diminished. Deficits in this area have the potential to affect the safety of a Finish Carpenter.
Edema	N	Not addressed at the time of evaluation or discharge. Based on the history of surgical intervention, the presence of edema could influence functional progress.
Posture	Y	Although described, the addition of comparative data would be helpful.
AROM/PROM	N	Range of motion measurements, current and target values, are listed in the evaluation. Comparative data to objectively demonstrate the discharge status would be helpful to the reviewer in determining progress.

(continued)

Essential Element	Y, N, or N/A	Comment(s)
Strength	Y	Strength is briefly addressed, and the therapist indicates a functional increase. However, objective data are lacking to substantiate this result from a reviewer's perspective.
Pain	N	Not addressed. This appears to be an oversight by the therapist, as the patient "Uses half kneeling for kneel and squat due to right knee pain at bone graft site." Because of the pain ratings provided in evaluation and the potential impact on functional progress, a reviewer would find it helpful to know the location of pain and the comparative rating(s) from evaluation to discharge. The presence of pain during active versus passive movement and the intensity during and after activity would be helpful.
Coordination	N	Coordination is not addressed in the evaluation or the discharge report. Data pertaining to the patient's fine motor coordination would seem relevant for a Finish Carpenter because of the potential impact on safety and job performance.
Bed mobility	N/A	
Balance (sit and stand)	N	Not addressed. Data pertaining to standing balance would seem important because of the right knee pain. Does the patient compensate for kneeling and squatting by performing functional activities in half kneeling because of pain or balance loss?
Transfers	N/A	
Ambulation (level and elevated surfaces)	Y	Although ambulation is addressed in the area of Activity tolerance, data pertaining to gait deficits, if they exist, would be helpful in determining skilled need.
Orthotic/prosthetic devices	N/A	
Wheelchair use	N/A	
DME (using or required)	N/A	
Activity tolerance	Y	The patient's activity tolerance and performance level are defined. A reviewer might find it helpful if data from the evaluation were listed to clearly indicate the areas of functional progress.
Wound description, including incision status	N	The potential functional impact of soft tissue restrictions on job performance is not reflected in the evaluation or the discharge report. This information is important to the reviewer when determining the reasonableness of the skilled care provided.
Special tests	N	Not addressed. A detailed table is provided at the time of evaluation; however, data are not presented at discharge. Comparative data would be helpful for the reviewer in identifying the functional progress.
Architectural/safety considerations	Y	Although this area is primarily addressed in Activity tolerance, information about the job site would be important to the reviewer and the patient by identifying potential barriers for functional carryover.
Treatment Diagnosis	N	Listing the status post wrist fusion would make the treatment diagnosis clearer for the reviewer.
Assessment		
Reason for skilled care	Y	The assessment provides a summary of the patient's discharge status and reason for discharge. However, this could be enhanced by justifying the need for skilled intervention. For example, *Patient participated in a work hardening program following a right wrist fusion. Right knee pain was also a complicating factor. Skilled service was necessary to emphasize reconditioning and job simulation.*
Problems	N	Not addressed. It is important to identify the problem areas to demonstrate the focus of skilled rehabilitation.

Essential Element	Y, N, or N/A	Comment(s)
Plan of Care		
Specific treatment strategies	Y	The therapist's plan for the patient at the time of discharge is outlined. However, a reviewer will find it helpful when assessing functional progress and the services billed if the treatment strategies provided through the date of discharge are described—for example, *Patient was seen for reconditioning and job simulation.* It is also to the provider's credit that the program was appropriately transferred to a nonskilled setting.
Frequency	N	Not addressed. A summary of the frequency and duration is needed. For example, documenting *the patient was seen 3x/wk for 8 weeks* helps the reviewer determine the reasonableness of the frequency and duration in relationship to the functional progress reported. It can also help when analyzing documentation and the corresponding services billed.
Duration	N	See Frequency.
Patient instruction/home program	Y	It is always important that the home program be documented. The therapist indicates that the home program was updated and reviewed. However, further description of the program would be helpful. For instance, does the home program emphasize wrist strengthening or general conditioning?
Caregiver training	Y	Specific parameters were given to the employer regarding the patient's work limitations. This is an important component for the therapist to document.
Short-term goals and achievement dates	Y	The goals compared do not reflect all those established at the time of evaluation. This may be confusing to a reviewer. Were prior goals achieved? The status of the goals at discharge lack a relationship to function.
Long-term goals and achievement dates	N	Information as to the long-term placement of this employee would be helpful.
Discharge prognosis	N	It would be helpful to the reviewer for assessing the success of the skilled intervention to know the therapist's discharge prognosis. If the patient and employer adhere to the recommendations, how successful will the patient be in his job responsibilities?

2. Is there evidence of the need for skilled intervention?

There is evidence that progress was made in the area of activity tolerance and job performance. However, objective data describing what skilled service was provided to address the evaluated deficits are lacking.

3. Are there adequate baseline data to develop future comparisons?

Data at the time of discharge are limited. There is a need for objective specific discharge measurements. For example, wrist pain, right knee pain, and strength limitations were not addressed.

4. Are the objective data related to functional deficits?

No, not clearly. The documentation requires further objective data and relationship to function. For instance, does strength, pain, or deconditioning affect job performance (i.e., lifting/reaching)?

5. Are comparative statements and data clearly outlined?

This is inconsistent. A percentage of increase in strength was documented. However, posture, wrist range of motion, pain rat-ings, and activity tolerance were not compared from evaluation to discharge.

6. (A) Are the three components for goals present (measurable, functional, time frames)?

No, the goals are often not related to function. For example, increasing cardiovascular conditioning to 7.6 METS allows what improvement in the workplace?

(B) Are the goals realistic for the individual case?

Yes, based on the fact that the patient has achieved the short-term goals necessary for job performance at a modified capacity as a Finish Carpenter.

7. Do you feel the treatment was reasonable and necessary?

Yes, the treatment duration was limited and the patient was appropriately referred to a nonskilled setting. The goal of return to work at a modified capacity appears to have been achieved. The patient's complicated medical history and limited job performance indicate a need for skilled care. However, additional objective data would have strengthened this case.

Case 7: Outpatient, Initial Evaluation

Referral

Specific treatment requested: Evaluate and treat (12 visits).

Data Accompanying Referral

Diagnosis/onset date: Torn medial/lateral meniscus and ACL/ 05-25-96.

Medical history: Surgery 06-23-96. Underwent arthroscopic repair to the meniscus and ACL. Right knee Hx—3 arthroscopies on right knee. '83, '84, '86. Past med Hx— nonremarkable.

Comorbidities (complicating or precautionary information): None.

Physical Therapy Intake/History

Date of birth: 05-11-56
Age: 40
Gender: Female
Start of care: 06-24-96
Primary complaint: Right pain.

Referral Diagnosis

Mechanism of injury: Jumped up.

Baseline Evaluation Data

Sensation/proprioception: Decreased sensation around knee.
Edema: Mid pat—41cm

1" prox	2" prox	3" prox
43	43	43
1" dist	2" dist	3" dist
39"	36"	36 cm

AROM/PROM: 0 degrees ext. to 40 degrees flex. with increased pain at end range.

Strength: n/tested—poor quad contraction.

Pain: 4, Quite a bit (on a 0 to 4 scale where 0 is not at all).

Ambulation (level and elevated surfaces): WBAT with 2 crutches.

Special tests: Not tested.

Prior Level of Function

Employment: RN, not working now. Off for six weeks.

Assessment

Reason for skilled care: The patient is a 30 year old female S/ P ACL reconstruction. She complains of an aching knee pain. Significant findings include decreased ROM, moderate edema and point tenderness around the patella. She should do well with physical therapy intervention.

Plan of Care

Specific treatment strategies:

1. Modalities as needed for pain and swelling.
2. NMES to right quad to increase quad contraction.
3. Therapeutic activity/exercise to increase ROM, strength.
4. HEP.

Frequency: 3x/wk.
Duration: 4 weeks.

Short-term goals and achievement dates:

1. Independent with HEP.
2. 0 degrees ext. To 100 degrees flex.
3. Edema reduction.
4. Increase quad contraction.

Long-term goals and achievement dates:

1. Full ROM (0 degrees to 135 degrees).
2. Return to work.
3. Return to normal ADL without restriction.

Rehabilitation potential: Good.

Case 7: Outpatient, Initial Evaluation Worksheet

1. Are the "essential elements" (defined in Chapter 1) for documentation present?

Essential Element	Y, N, or N/A	Comment(s)
Referral		
Reason	N	The reason for referral is not stated. A clear statement of the reason for referral, such as *Patient referred by Dr. ABC for rehabilitation to improve right knee mobility following recent arthroscopic surgery*, would help justify skilled therapy intervention.

Essential Element	Y, N, or N/A	Comment(s)
Specific treatment requested	Y	
Data Accompanying Referral		
Diagnosis/onset date	Y	The diagnosis of a torn medial/lateral meniscus and anterior cruciate ligament (ACL) is present. However, whether the diagnosis involves the right or left extremity is not indicated. This is relevant based on the patient's medical history.
Secondary diagnoses	N/A	
Medical history	Y	The therapist appropriately documents the date of surgery to repair the meniscus and ACL. The history of arthroscopy on the right knee is also noted. However, more information specific to any functional limitations in right knee range of motion or strength may help the reviewer in assessing the prior level of function.
Medications	N	Not addressed. As pain and edema are indicated in the evaluation, it would be helpful to know what medications, if any, are being administered that may affect rehabilitation—for example, narcotics.
Comorbidities (complicating or precautionary information)	Y	The therapist indicated "None." However, this is inaccurate, as the patient is weight bearing as tolerated.
Physical Therapy Intake/History		
Date of birth	Y	Patient identifying information is important, as many physician offices and third-party payers file or trigger data retrieval based on date of birth.
Age	Y	
Gender	Y	
Start of Care	Y	
Primary complaint	Y	"Right pain" lacks description. Specifically, where is the pain, and what functional deficits are experienced by the patient?
Referral Diagnosis		
Mechanism of injury	Y	The patient "Jumped up" per the therapist's documentation. Information such as where the injury occurred would be important for the reviewer to know when determining whether the injury was an accident or was work-related and whether another third-party payer is the primary source of payment.
Prior diagnostic imaging/testing	N	Not addressed. It is reasonable to expect that an x-ray or an MRI was performed. This information may be relevant to the case at this time.
Prior Therapy History	N	Not addressed. Secondary to the previous arthroscopies on the right knee in 1983, 1984, and 1986, therapy history would be pertinent to the reviewer. For example, the therapy history would provide insight into the rehabilitation potential and any prior functional limitations in range of motion or strength.
Baseline Evaluation Data		
Cognition	N/A	
Vision/hearing	N/A	
Vital signs	N/A	
Vascular signs	N	Not addressed. Tissue temperature and color need to be assessed, as this is a recent surgical repair.
Sensation/proprioception	Y	The therapist indicates "Decreased sensation around knee." This statement is vague, and information pertaining to where the sensation is diminished and the type (e.g., light touch or temperature) should be given.

(continued)

Essential Element	Y, N, or N/A	Comment(s)
Edema	Y	Measurements are present. However, they lack clinical significance to the reviewer. Additional information is needed, such as defining the extremity (right or left) that is measured, measurements of the opposite extremity for comparative data, and whether the edema is pitting or nonpitting. The term "mid pat" as abbreviated in the evaluation may be unfamiliar to a reviewer. Also, consistency in the unit of measurement, inches versus centimeters, is recommended.
Posture	N/A	
AROM/PROM	Y	Range of motion is indicated. However, information such as the extremity being measured (right or left), opposite limb measurements for comparison, and differentiation between active and passive range of motion is needed.
Strength	Y	The therapist indicates that strength was not tested, yet provides a muscle grade of "poor quad contraction." An explanation of why the limb could not be tested would assist the reviewer in assessing the functional limitations of the patient and need for skilled therapy intervention. It would also be helpful to define how the therapist obtained a "poor quad contraction" if "n/tested."
Pain	Y	The therapist provides a definition of the pain scale used. Data such as where the pain is (knee, hip), when it occurs (with range of motion, during gait), and how the pain limits function would be helpful to a reviewer in assessing the need for skilled care. Nonspecific information such as "quite a bit" does not assist a reviewer in determining the need for skilled care.
Coordination	N/A	
Bed mobility	N/A	
Balance (sit and stand)	N	Not addressed. It would seem that sitting balance is not applicable in this case. However, the patient's safety during standing and gait (with crutches on level and elevated surfaces) is important to the reviewer. If balance is not a concern then a notation of *normal* would clarify this area of potential concern.
Transfers	N	Not addressed. The evaluation indicates range of motion, pain, and strength limitations. Transfers could be a potential safety concern; therefore, data related to transfers would provide a clear picture of the patient's challenges or safety level.
Ambulation (level and elevated surfaces)	Y	The weight-bearing status and type of assistive device are defined by the therapist. Further detail of gait deficits, pain with weight bearing, and ability to negotiate stairs/uneven surfaces would be helpful to the reviewer in determining the need for skilled care.
Orthotic/prosthetic devices	N	Not addressed. A brace is often applied following a surgical repair of the ACL. If present, its use needs to be documented.
Wheelchair use	N/A	
DME (using or required)	N	Not addressed. This appears to be an oversight by the therapist, as documentation indicates that the patient is ambulating with two crutches.
Activity tolerance	N	As this is a postsurgical evaluation, this area needs to be addressed.
Wound description, including incision status	N	Not addressed. The status of the surgical site is relevant in terms of tissue repair and complications such as infection.
Special tests	N	Not addressed. Any special tests should be listed and the clinical relevance briefly explained.
Architectural/safety considerations	N	Not addressed. Data pertaining to the patient's ability to ambulate in the community would be helpful in identifying functional deficits.
Requirements to return to home, school and/or job	N	Not addressed. A description of the patient's job requirements would provide the reviewer with insight into the patient's existing functional limitations.

Essential Element	Y, N, or N/A	Comment(s)
Prior Level of Function		
Mobility (home and community)	N	Prior level of function is of great importance to the reviewer for determining the reasonableness of therapy intervention. The medical history of three arthroscopies magnifies this importance, as a reviewer would want to know if functional limitations in strength, range of motion, or gait were present.
Employment	Y	
School	N/A	
Treatment Diagnosis	N	It is important to identify the treatment diagnosis for which physical therapy services are rendered.
Assessment		
Reason for skilled care	Y	The therapist defines the physical limitations in strength and range of motion. However, the relationship to the functional gait deficit is lacking. The reviewer may find it helpful to know the therapist's viewpoint on the necessity and/or effectiveness of the skilled intervention in the past and whether a similar outcome would be expected following this recent surgery.
Problems	N	Not addressed. It is helpful to determine the problems in order to focus treatment. (e.g., *Edema right knee, decreased functional strength right quadriceps, decreased range of motion right knee.*)
Plan of Care		
Specific treatment strategies	Y	There is a relationship between the treatments selected and the physical limitations, with the exception of "Modalities as needed for pain and swelling." In this example, the specific modality or modalities used need to be described.
Frequency	Y	
Duration	Y	
Patient instruction/home program	N	Not addressed. Training and education are important components of treatment. They should be initiated at the time of evaluation.
Caregiver training	N/A	
Short-term goals and achievement dates	Y	Goals 3 and 4 are not measurable, and goals 2, 3, and 4 lack a functional component, such as to improve stair climbing or knee extension during gait. Time frames are lacking for all goals.
Long-term goals and achievement dates	Y	The long-term goals are reasonable as a whole. However, the restrictions on activities of daily living were not defined in the evaluation.
Rehabilitation potential	Y	

2. Is the overall history of the patient adequate?

History of previous arthroscopies is present. However, the outcome of references to previous functional deficits and therapy intervention is absent. The patient's complaint of "right pain" is not descriptive. It would be reasonable, as this is the fourth attempt at rehabilitation, that the prior levels of function and outcomes from previous therapies be specified. The functional impact on employment and activities of daily living is not mentioned. Are there previous range of motion deficits affecting activities of daily living and overall function? The mechanism of injury is quite brief and does not portray the where and how. Was the patient active in sports, or was this a work-related injury?

3. Is there evidence of the need for skilled intervention?

No. Other than the fact the patient has had surgery, the evaluation is vague and nonspecific. Specific skilled modalities are not listed, nor is their impact on enhancing functional progress. In addition, NMES needs to be defined, as many reviewers would not know that it refers to neuromuscular electrical stimulation.

4. Are there adequate baseline data to develop future comparisons?

There are very few adequate baseline data, with the exception of range of motion measurements. There is no description of functional deficits (e.g., strength is described as "n/tested—poor quad contraction" and is not related to sit-to-stand difficulties, initiating stairs or negotiation of uneven surfaces). Edema is addressed in the evaluation; however, the circumference of the noninvolved extremity is not present for baseline comparison and therefore does not demonstrate the severity of the edema in the involved extremity. Pain is listed as a 4, but is not related to a limitation in the patient's function—for instance as related to transfers, gait, and/or exercise.

5. Are the objective data related to functional deficits?

There is no example of a functional relationship. Particularly evident is the lack of description of gait pattern deficits and performance of activities of daily living.

6. Are comparative statements and data clearly outlined?

Data are present for range of motion, pain, and edema for the involved extremity. Objective data from the opposite limb would assist in establishing a baseline. The reviewer can only assume it is the right knee that is being treated.

7. (A) Are the three components for goals present (measurable, functional, time frames)?

The goals are generalized and not related to function. Time frames are not present on the evaluation.

(B) Are the goals realistic for the individual case?

The goals, although not appropriately written, do appear realistic.

8. Do you feel that the proposed treatment is reasonable and necessary?

Because of the acute diagnosis and the range of motion and strength deficits, it appears that treatment is reasonable and necessary. A reviewer would need further information regarding functional deficits, such as activities of daily living and gait, in order to determine the duration for skilled service.

Case 7: Outpatient, Progress Report

Attendance: Good.

Current Baseline Data

Sensation/proprioception: Intact.
AROM/PROM: 0–95 with 100 degrees is last ROM to date.
Strength: Poor quad contraction.
Ambulation (level and elevated surfaces): 1 crutch—WBAT.

Assessment

Reason for skilled care: Good increase in ROM. Good attitude in therapy. The patient is doing really well. ROM is doing fine, however, muscle contraction (quad contraction) is lacking at this time. I recommend continued therapy.

Plan of Care

Specific treatment strategies: Continue treatment with physicians consent. (Twelve additional visits requested.)
Frequency: 3x/wk.
Duration: 4 weeks.
Short-term goals and achievement dates:

1. Knee ROM 0 extension to 130 flexion.
2. Increase ambulation control.

Rehabilitation potential: Good.

Case 7: Outpatient, Progress Report Worksheet

1. Are the "essential elements" (defined in Chapter 1) for documentation present?

Essential Element	Y, N, or N/A	Comment(s)
Attendance	Y	Present information, listed as "Good," does not identify the number of visits clearly. If the patient missed one visit, is that "good" attendance? It is recommended that the number of visits scheduled and any reasons for absence be identified.
Current Baseline Data		
Cognition	N/A	
Vision/hearing	N/A	
Vital signs	N/A	

Essential Element	Y, N, or N/A	Comment(s)
Vascular signs	N	This area is not addressed in the evaluation or the progress report. As this is a surgical patient, any changes in tissue temperature or color may help in justifying the need for continued skilled care.
Sensation/proprioception	Y	The therapist indicates "Intact." The addition of a comparative statement would clearly indicate a status change. For example, *Normal, previously decreased sensation to light touch approximately 2cm x 2cm lateral to the right patella.*
Edema	N	Not addressed. Evaluation data, treatment strategies, and goals indicated that edema reduction required skilled intervention. A reviewer may question "Continue treatment . . ." without clinical data justifying the skilled need.
Posture	N/A	
AROM/PROM	Y	Present information stating "0–95 with 100 degrees is last ROM to date" does not justify the need for skilled intervention. A reviewer may find it helpful if data such as the techniques used to improve range of motion, passive versus active range of motion comparisons, evidence of complications such as pain, and the patient's functional limitations were described.
Strength	Y	Present information states, "Poor quad contraction." More detail regarding dysfunction of the quadriceps and the skilled intervention (NMES) used to facilitate strength is needed. A reviewer may question the request for continued treatment, as it appears ineffective after four weeks.
Pain	N	Not addressed. Pain was addressed in the evaluation, and the data are omitted in this report. Is pain a complicating factor? Comparative data are required to assist the reviewer in establishing a need for continued skilled care.
Coordination	N/A	
Bed mobility	N/A	
Balance (sit and stand)	N/A	
Transfers	N	This functional area is not addressed in the evaluation or the progress report. A problem in function, such as transfers, is important for a reviewer to be aware of when determining the need for skilled care.
Ambulation (level and elevated surfaces)	Y	The data indicated that the patient is WBAT with one crutch. It would be helpful to provide a comparative statement to demonstrate functional progress, as the patient previously required two crutches. To more accurately provide a skilled picture of the patient, gait deficits need to be described. For example, decreased heel strike or knee buckling during the midstance phase of gait would provide more detail into skilled need.
Orthotic/prosthetic devices	N	This area is not addressed in the evaluation or the progress report. The use of a brace, if applicable, needs to be documented. For example, has the use of the brace increased, decreased, or required adjustment by a physical therapist?
Wheelchair use	N/A	
DME (using or required)	N	Not addressed. This appears to be an oversight by the therapist, as the patient uses a crutch.
Activity tolerance	N	Data pertaining to the patient's activity tolerance, such as ambulation distance, would be helpful to a reviewer in assessing overall functional limitations.
Wound description, including incision status	N	A comment regarding the current status of the incision is appropriate.
Special tests	N/A	

(continued)

Essential Element	Y, N, or N/A	Comment(s)
Architectural/safety considerations	N	Not addressed. Data pertaining to the patient's ability to ambulate in the community would be helpful.
Treatment Diagnosis	N	It is important to identify the treatment diagnosis for which physical therapy services are rendered, as it may change during the course of intervention.
Assessment		
Reason for skilled care	Y	The assessment does not provide a clear picture of the patient. A reviewer may not embrace the need to extend treatment as "ROM is doing fine," and the present data reflect that the treatment strategies have been ineffective, particularly in regard to strength of the quadriceps. An explanation of the complications that remain (pain or edema) would help define the need for skilled care.
Problems	N	Not addressed. It is helpful to determine the problems in order to focus treatment.
Plan of Care		
Specific treatment strategies	Y	The description provided in the evaluation is not defined in the progress report. It appears, based on the lack of data, that edema and pain are resolved. Therefore, a revised plan of care would be warranted. It also appears that use of NMES has been unsuccessful for strengthening. A reviewer may question the lack of a defined or revised plan of care.
Frequency	Y	
Duration	Y	The request for four additional weeks appears excessive based on the lack of data and ineffectiveness of quadriceps strengthening.
Patient instruction/home program	N	The involvement of the patient in a home program appears lacking. Program upgrades require skilled care and are not defined. This is a glaring omission.
Caregiver training	N/A	
Short-term goals and achievement dates	Y	The status of prior goals is not defined. The listed goals lack time frames and a clearly defined functional outcome.
Long-term goals and achievement dates	N	The omission of a long-term goal demonstrates the lack of treatment focus.
Rehabilitation potential	Y	

2. Is there evidence of the need for skilled intervention?

There is minimal evidence, with the exception of a poor quadriceps contraction, of the need for skilled intervention. There is limited description of functional deficits related to gait quality or activities of daily living, comparative data, or use of skilled treatment modalities, and there is no evidence of a home program. It is also apparent the treatment strategies to enhance quadriceps strength have been ineffective, yet no change in the plan of care is noted.

3. Are there adequate baseline data to develop future comparisons?

There are minimal data presented on range of motion and strength. Gait deficits, edema, and the home program are not described.

4. Are the objective data related to functional deficits?

No, although one of the original long-term goals was return to work, there is no description of job requirements, or how these requirements relate to the patient's ability to perform them. More description of the patient's functional deficits in this area would be essential in justifying treatment intervention for both work and home/community activities.

5. Are comparative statements and data clearly outlined?

This progress note exemplifies the lack of comparative data. This makes it very difficult for the reviewer both to assess the progress of the patient to date and to justify further coverage.

6. (A) Are the three components for goals present (measurable, functional, time frames)?

There are no time frames or functional relationships. The status of the prior goals is not defined. The long-term goal is not addressed.

(B) Are the goals realistic for the individual case?

This is difficult to answer, as the goals are vague. For example, the short-term goal "Increase ambulation control" is vague, and a reviewer would not understand the functional importance. Also, the long-term goal is not described.

7. Do you feel the treatment was reasonable and necessary?

The actual reviewer of this case was prepared to deny continued coverage for a twelve-visit extension. This decision was based on the lack of overall functional deficits, inadequate data on edema, gait limitations, assessment of strength related to function, comparative data on pain, and lack of detail on home program and job responsibilities. However, at the request of the case manager a call was placed to the treating physical therapist.

The therapist described the patient as limited in all activities of daily living, unable to drive, having an unstable gait particularly on stairs and unlevel surfaces, and unable to freely extend the knee in the last 25° of extension secondary to quadriceps weakness.

In response to this increase in detail, relating specifically to various functional deficits, twelve additional visits were approved with the understanding that the treating therapist provide the following in the next discharge and/or progress report:

1. Detailed home program.

2. Descriptive detail of gait deficits, range of motion and strength deficits, comparative data on edema/pain related to function in activities of daily living/gait, and job-related expectations/requirements.

Case 8: Outpatient, Initial Evaluation

Referral

Specific treatment requested: Referred to PT for strengthening, monitoring pulse oximeter.

Data Accompanying Referral

Diagnosis/onset date: COPD exacerbation/04-07-95.

Medical history: Pt. moved from her home to retirement community apt. in 11-94. Participated in pulmonary program twice weekly for past 8 years. Admitted to ABC Hospital 03-03-95 w/COPD exacerbation, R infiltrate and density w/lung CA suspected. Pt. recently D/C home alone from rehab hospital.

Comorbidities (complicating or precautionary information): Uses oxygen at night.

Physical Therapy Intake/History

Gender: Female
Start of care: 05-01-95

Prior Therapy History:

Referred to XYZ for IP rehab for deconditioning/steroid myopathy. By D/C from IP rehab had weaned from oxygen except for night use, was ambulatory walking 250 ft behind W/C and could walk on treadmill .7 mph for 25 minutes.

Baseline Evaluation Data

Cognition: Pt. oriented.

Vital signs: SOB w/speech. See Activity tolerance and Strength.

Edema: Blt ankle edema.

Posture: Slim woman w/dorsal kyphosis, forward head, flat lumbar spine, slightly protruding abdomen.

AROM/PROM: ROM WFL throughout.

Strength: Strength grossly 3/5, manual muscle test deferred secondary to SOB. Exhibits dec. eccentric control of quadriceps for sitting, maximum of 7 straight leg raises blt, 10 reps of hip bridging. Oxygen saturation from 87 to 90.

Bed mobility: Indep, however uses momentum to move sit to stand and c/o dizziness.

Balance (sit and stand): Balance score 13/16. Stands w/wide base of support, legs become tremulous after 20 seconds.

Ambulation (level and elevated surfaces): Tremulous, using cane as new assist device. Uses cane in either hand, uses cane backwards, slow gait uses momentum for swing phase on R, Tinetti gait score 7/12. Stairs not tested.

Activity tolerance: Oxygen saturation 87, pulse 120 at rest, dec. to 85, 119 after 3 minutes 24 seconds on treadmill at .8 mph.

Prior Level of Function

Mobility (home and community): Was independent in driving, cooking, active/social outings.

Treatment Diagnosis:

Decreased functional activity.

Assessment

Reason for skilled care: Pt. presenting with less endurance than at D/C. Will benefit from skilled PT to increase endurance to IP level, adjusting for additional home activities now required and to increase strength for functional gait/ADL's to increase balance such that pt can be ambulatory w/o assist device.

Plan of Care

Specific treatment strategies: Ther Ex including treadmill, LE ergometer, breathing exercises, etc., balance activities, gait training.

Frequency: 3x/wk.

Duration: 6 wks.

Short-term goals and achievement dates:

1. Increase treadmill duration to 15 minutes w/oxygen saturation greater than or equal to 85 x 2 wks.
2. Able to go up/down 3 training steps w/2 handrails x 1 x 2 wks.
3. Able to perform 50 reps of closed chain exercises on total gym using small excursion x 2 wks.
4. Dec. veering during gait for 1/2 distance x 3 wks.

Long-term goals and achievement dates: Indep gait w/o assist device, Indep gait off curb, Able to go up/down 8 steps w/1 handrail, Indep sit to/from stand w/o using UE, Increase Tinetti score to 24/28.

Case 8: Outpatient, Initial Evaluation Worksheet

1. Are the "essential elements" (defined in Chapter 1) for documentation present?

Essential Element	Y, N, or N/A	Comment(s)
Referral		
Reason	N	Not addressed. A statement of the reason for referral, in terms of a positive functional outcome, would be helpful. For example, *Patient referred to outpatient physical therapy by Dr. ABC following a recent decline in aerobic capacity. Pt. to increase strength, balance, and mobility skills for independent functioning at home and in the community.*
Specific treatment requested	Y	
Data Accompanying Referral		
Diagnosis/onset date	Y	
Secondary diagnoses	N	Not addressed. This appears to be an oversight by the therapist, as the medical history indicates that lung cancer is suspected. Based on this information and the diagnosis of COPD exacerbation, it is reasonable to expect secondary diagnoses exist such as venous insufficiency and edema.
Medical history	Y	
Medications	N	Not addressed. It is important to indicate what medications, if any, are being administered because of the potential side effects that may influence participation in rehabilitation—for example, steroids.
Comorbidities (complicating or precautionary information)	Y	The therapist documents that the patient "Uses oxygen at night." Further detail regarding oxygen use during exertion would be helpful. It is also reasonable to expect that other precautionary information exists, such as dyspnea during activities.
Physical Therapy Intake/History		
Date of birth	N	Patient identifying information is important, as many physician offices and third-party payers file or trigger data retrieval based on date of birth.
Age	N	It may be helpful to a reviewer to know the patient's age to determine the rehabilitation potential and for identification purposes.
Gender	Y	
Start of Care	Y	
Primary complaint	N	Not addressed. Identifying the patient's primary complaint helps the reviewer in determining the need for skilled care. For example: Is activity intolerance, a history of falls, inability to complete activities of daily living, or dizziness the primary concern?
Referral Diagnosis		
Mechanism of injury	N	The mechanism of injury, including the original date of onset, needs to be described. For example, is the diagnosis associated with pollution, smoking, bronchitis, cancer, and/or a hereditary condition?
Prior diagnostic imaging/testing	N	As the medical history describes the patient's participation in a pulmonary program for eight years, it is reasonable to expect that prior diagnostic testing has occurred. This information is relevant to the patient's ability to participate in an intensive rehabilitation program.

(continued)

Essential Element	Y, N, or N/A	Comment(s)
Prior Therapy History	Y	
Baseline Evaluation Data		
Cognition	Y	Information pertaining to the patient's alertness and ability to follow directions is needed.
Vision/hearing	N	Not addressed. It is important for a reviewer to be aware of vision and/or hearing deficits, if present, when determining the patient's rehabilitation potential.
Vital signs	Y	See Activity tolerance and Strength.
Vascular signs	N	Not addressed. Data pertaining to vascular signs, if present, need to be described. For example, assessment of capillary refill time and/or skin temperature would help justify the need for skilled rehabilitation.
Sensation/proprioception	N	Not addressed. Data pertaining to sensation/proprioception would be helpful for a reviewer in assessing functional limitations. This information is relevant because of the balance deficits, particularly the tremors in the lower extremities, and the gait deficits described in the evaluation.
Edema	Y	The therapist indicates that the patient has bilateral ankle edema. The assessment of edema needs to be expanded to include circumference measurements, data describing whether the edema is pitting or non-pitting, and any relationship to functional deficits. This is especially important for future progress comparisons.
Posture	Y	A detailed description of posture is provided. This helps the reviewer in assessing the need for skilled care. However, additional documentation of how posture affects function is needed.
AROM/PROM	Y	
Strength	Y	Data reflect the patient's functional limitations, such as, "Exhibits dec. eccentric control of the quadriceps for sitting," and the need for skilled care to monitor oxygen saturation rates.
Pain	N/A	
Coordination	N	Coordination is not addressed. However, it is relevant because of the documented balance and gait deficits such as "Stands w/wide base of support," lower extremity tremors, and slow gait requiring "momentum for swing phase."
Bed mobility	Y	
Balance (sit and stand)	Y	Standing balance is described and a score of 13/16 is reported. It is reasonable for a reviewer to assume that sitting balance is independent based on the patient's high level of function. However, the test used for scoring balance and further detail regarding the effect of lower extremity tremors on function and safety would help the reviewer in determining the patient's deficits.
Transfers	N	Not addressed. Information regarding car transfers and safety deficits when negotiating in the community would help the reviewer determine the medical necessity of skilled intervention.
Ambulation (level and elevated surfaces)	Y	Ambulation data are provided. Additional detail of the gait deficit described as "uses momentum for swing phase R" would be helpful. For instance, what is the reason for the slow gait and use of momentum? How far can the patient ambulate using a cane?
Orthotic/prosthetic devices	N/A	
Wheelchair use	N	Not addressed. This appears to be an oversight by the therapist. The prior therapy history indicates that the patient was ambulatory walking behind a wheelchair at the time of discharge from inpatient rehabilitation.

Essential Element	Y, N, or N/A	Comment(s)
DME (using or required)	N	See Wheelchair use.
Activity tolerance	Y	Activity tolerance is described in terms of oxygen saturation rates and pulse rate at rest and with exertion. It is reasonable to expect additional data regarding blood pressure and respiratory rate at rest, as well as during and after activity. Monitoring these data for safe performance of a functional activity demonstrates another need for the skills of a therapist.
Wound description, including incision status	N/A	
Special tests	N/A	
Architectural/safety considerations	N	Not addressed. It would be helpful to describe how the patient negotiates in the community, especially because of the potential need for intermittent oxygen use.
Requirements to return to home, school and/or job	N/A	
Prior Level of Function		
Mobility (home and community)	Y	The prior level of function describes the patient as "Independent in driving, cooking, active/social outings." The relationship of this data to the status at the time of discharge from inpatient rehabilitation (i.e., oxygen use only at night and ambulatory behind a wheelchair) is unclear. Further information is needed regarding the patient's functional ability for ambulation on level and elevated surfaces as well as oxygen saturation rates with exertion.
Employment	N/A	
School	N/A	
Treatment Diagnosis	Y	
Assessment		
Reason for skilled care	Y	It is recommended that the functional phrase alternative, *functional activity tolerance,* be used for the common term endurance.
Problems	N	Not addressed. It is helpful to determine the problems to focus treatment (e.g., gait deficits, decreased functional activity tolerance, decreased functional strength).
Plan of Care		
Specific treatment strategies	Y	A list of treatment strategies is provided. However, use of the term "etc." is not appropriate. Treatment modalities used need to be specifically identified.
Frequency	Y	
Duration	Y	
Patient instruction/home program	N	Not addressed. A home program is an important component of therapeutic intervention and should be initiated at the time of evaluation.
Caregiver training	N	Not addressed. Patient education and training are components of skilled care. They are lacking in this evaluation and need to be described.
Short-term goals and achievement dates	Y	The short-term goals do not reinforce the need for patient and/or caregiver training. Goals 1 and 3 are not related to function.
Long-term goals and achievement dates	Y	Five long-term goals are provided. Instruction in a home program, which is an important part of self-management, is lacking. Readers are reminded that when a time frame is not provided, the reviewer will usually conclude that the duration is the achievement date.
Rehabilitation potential	N	It is important to describe the patient's rehabilitation potential, as it helps the reviewer assess the need for and duration of skilled care.

2. Is the overall history of the patient adequate?

Yes, the history is adequate, although it would be strengthened if data pertaining to the patient's date of birth and primary complaint were included.

3. Is there evidence of the need for skilled intervention?

Yes, the patient requires skilled care because of the history of chronic obstructive pulmonary disease, gait deficits, and need for assessment of aerobic capacity.

4. Are there adequate baseline data to develop future comparisons?

In some areas there are adequate baseline data, such as oxygen saturation, Tinetti gait score, and functional strength. Additional data would have been appropriate regarding gait deficits, balance deficits, ankle edema, and transfers.

5. Are the objective data related to functional deficits?

The objective data are related to functional deficits in areas such as strength, ambulation, and balance. However, edema and activity tolerance lack this relationship.

6. Are comparative statements and data clearly outlined?

No, the comparative data are not clearly outlined for the reviewer. Although oxygen saturation rates and Tinetti gait and balance scores are present, there are not enough baseline comparative data for future progress reports. The Tinetti ratings are a beginning, but there are a lack of baseline data, specifically as to what the balance deficits are. For example, except for stating that the patient's legs become tremulous and the patient walks with a large base of support, data are lacking regarding deficits exhibited on unlevel surfaces, turns, position changes, and stairs.

7. (A) Are the three components for goals present (measurable, functional, time frames)?

Yes, all goals reflect the major components except for Goals 1 and 3, which are not related to a functional outcome.

(B) Are the goals realistic for the individual case?

Yes, the goals appear realistic and specific. This includes the long-term goals. It is suggested that goals for home program instruction and driving be included.

8. Do you feel that the proposed treatment is reasonable and necessary?

Based on the documentation presented, there is enough evidence of the need for skilled therapeutic intervention. For instance, the patient has limitations in oxygen saturation, balance, and gait, and she requires improvement in function to negotiate in the community safely.

Case 8: Outpatient, Discharge Report

Attendance: 27 visits since initiation of care. Canceled 07-03-95.

Current Baseline Data

Vital signs: See Activity tolerance.

Bed mobility: Able to come to stand w/o using UE, however, does require greater effort; able to come to stand w/light UE assist easily.

Balance (sit and stand): Goal met—Inc'd Tinetti score from 19/24, moderate risk for falls to 12 (gait) plus 15 (balance), totaling 27/28 Tinetti score, low risk for falls. She is able to squat and pick up a 2# object off floor w/o loss of balance; single leg stance 19 count on R, 11 count on L w/o UE; inc'd from 3 count previously.

Ambulation (level and elevated surfaces): Exhibits dec'd veering and is able to walk w/o device, carrying a 2# weight for 40 feet. Walks to meals in her retirement building. Goal Met—Able to go up/down 8-inch steps with CGA/SBA; able to go up/down single 6-inch step 5 times w/average oxygen saturation 88, surpassed goal—She does not require contact guard for this task. Able to go up/down 8 steps w/single rail, however, activity deferred secondary to heat in the stairway; able to go up/down curb w/o using assistive device; able to walk from PT department to facility entrance in 4 min., brings cane, however, only uses it intermittently.

Activity tolerance: Shortness of breath/decreased endurance: Goal met—inc'd treadmill duration from 10–20 minutes at .8 miles per hour w/oxygen saturation 90–93 at rest, remaining at 91 by 20 minutes; maximum duration 23 minutes; resting pulse 100–119 at rest, maximum of 128 after 20 minutes; resting pulse noted to be 95 over last 2 treatments.

Treatment Diagnosis: Decreased functional activity.

Assessment

Reason for skilled care: Patient had a fall w/decline in gait ability and function last month, missed 2 weeks of treatment secondary to illness, and was away w/family in wheelchair w/oxygen. Needed P.T. to return her to previous strength for treadmill (15 minutes) and to meet previously set goal, to increase strength for stairs, to rule out future falls ascending stairs and to improve gait quality.

Plan for home program. Patient made excellent progress—meeting goals. Has inc'd activity level, able to drive, able to tolerate PT after having a previous hair appointment.

Problems:

1. Shortness of breath/dec endurance.
2. LE weakness.
3. Slow dependent gait.

Plan of Care

Specific treatment strategies: Ther Ex, breathing exercises, treadmill, LE ergometer balance activities, gait training, pulse oximeter monitoring.

Frequency: 3/wk.

Duration: 4 wks.

Patient instruction/home program: Arrangements have been made for her to continue an exercise program in the retirement community where she resides.

Caregiver training: Patient learned to take pulse accurately. Short-term goals and achievement dates:

1. Inc. treadmill duration to 20 minutes w/oxygen saturation greater than or equal to 85 by 4 weeks.
2a. Able to go up or down 3 training steps w/2 handrails 5x's by 4 weeks.
2b. Able to perform 50 reps of closed chain exercise on total gym using small excursion by 4 weeks.
2c. Able to go up/down an 8-inch step w/contact guard, up/down a single 6-inch step w/contact guard 5 times w/oxygen saturation greater than or equal to 88 (4 wks).
2d. Able to squat, get object off floor w/o loss of balance.
3. Dec. veering during gait for 1/2 of gait distance by 4 wks.

Long-term goals and achievement dates: Indep gait w/out assist device, indep gait on/off curb, able to go up/down 8 steps w/1 handrail, indep sit to/from stand w/out using UE, increase Tinetti score to 24/28.

Case 8: Outpatient, Discharge Report Worksheet

1. Are the "essential elements" (defined in Chapter 1) for documentation present?

Essential Element	Y, N, or N/A	Comment(s)
Attendance	Y	The present data, listed as "27 visits since initiation of care. Canceled 07-03-95," do not indicate the number of visits scheduled and are inaccurate regarding the reasons for absence. The assessment indicates that the patient missed two weeks of treatment secondary to illness. A reviewer may seek additional information to ensure the accuracy of the services billed.
Current Baseline Data		
Cognition	N/A	Not applicable at this time. Only a change in status that affects safety and/or participation in rehabilitation would need to be documented.
Vision/hearing	N	Not addressed in the evaluation or discharge report. If vision and/or hearing deficits exist it would be appropriate to describe them, especially because of their role in patient safety for driving in the community.
Vital signs	Y	See Activity tolerance.
Vascular signs	N	Data pertaining to vascular signs are not described in the evaluation or discharge report. Changes in vascular signs, such as improvement in capillary refill time and/or skin temperature, would provide the reviewer with comparative data of another positive outcome from skilled intervention.
Sensation/proprioception	N	Data pertaining to sensation and proprioception are not present in the evaluation or discharge report. Given the balance and gait deficits, it would be helpful to have data in this area, or at a minimum to know that an assessment was made. Any deficits could assist in justifying the duration of skilled services provided.

(continued)

Essential Element	Y, N, or N/A	Comment(s)
Edema	N	In the evaluation, bilateral edema was reported without measurable data. A comparative summary of changes in edema and the effect on function is needed.
Posture	N	Postural deficits are described in the evaluation, but are lacking in the discharge report. Since the patient had balance deficits, a description of posture would be relevant to the rehabilitation program.
AROM/PROM	N/A	As the evaluation indicated that range of motion was within functional limits, comparative data are not required unless changes occurred that affected the rehabilitation process.
Strength	N	Data were provided in the evaluation; therefore, comparative data at discharge are needed.
Pain	N/A	
Coordination	N	Coordination is not addressed in the evaluation or discharge report. It is reasonable to expect comparative data because of the balance and gait deficits described, such as "veering."
Bed mobility	Y	The evaluation indicated that the patient was independent and used momentum for sit to stand. The discharge report implies independence and describes the patient as "Able to come to stand w/o using UE, however, does require greater effort; able to come to stand w/ light UE assist easily." Comparative data are lacking in the discharge report, and also why the skills of a therapist were needed. Is safety a concern? Was teaching and/or training provided to the patient?
Balance (sit and stand)	Y	Comparative data are provided—specifically, the Tinetti scores. Balance is also related to a functional activity such as squatting. These data display functional progress to the reviewer.
Transfers	N	This functional area is not addressed in the evaluation or discharge report. Comparative data regarding car transfers and safety deficits when negotiating in the community would help the reviewer in determining if therapy services were reasonable and necessary.
Ambulation (level and elevated surfaces)	Y	The status of ambulation goals is described in detail. There is also a relationship to function, such as ability to walk to meals. Additional comparative data pertaining to lower extremity tremors and gait quality are needed.
Orthotic/prosthetic devices	N/A	
Wheelchair use	N	Although the discharge data suggest that the patient is independent without a wheelchair, it is reasonable to expect that a wheelchair is needed occasionally because of shortness of breath or extended outings with family. An indication that the patient was instructed in energy conservation techniques to avoid overexertion would demonstrate skilled care.
DME (using or required)	N	This is an oversight by the therapist, as discharge data indicate use of a cane and a wheelchair.
Activity tolerance	Y	Detailed data are provided, such as oxygen saturation rates and pulse rate at rest and with exertion. It would be helpful to provide comparative data that are related to function, as well as additional data regarding blood pressure and respiratory rate.
Wound description, including incision status	N/A	
Special tests	N/A	

Essential Element	Y, N, or N/A	Comment(s)
Architectural/safety considerations	N	Architectural and safety considerations were not addressed in the evaluation or discharge report. A statement regarding how safely the patient negotiates in the community and at home would be helpful. For example, is balance a safety concern for long-distance ambulation? Can the patient ambulate safely on unlevel surfaces such as carpeting or grass?
Treatment Diagnosis	Y	
Assessment		
Reason for skilled care	Y	The reason for skilled care is adequate. However, a reviewer would not view the ability "to return her to previous strength for treadmill (15 minutes)" as a functional goal under the developing managed care perspective that is beginning to permeate all payer sources. Also, the statement "able to tolerate PT after having a previous hair appointment" is vague and does not present a skilled assessment related to the rehabilitation provided.
Problems	Y	The problem list helps the reviewer assess the focus of treatment.
Plan of Care		
Specific treatment strategies	Y	
Frequency	Y	The summary provided for frequency and duration for the period in question helps the reviewer determine if the functional progress reported is reasonable. It can also help when analyzing documentation and the corresponding services billed.
Duration	Y	See Frequency.
Patient instruction/home program	Y	A home program is established; however, further detail regarding the specific emphasis of the program is lacking. For example, has ambulation, stair climbing, and/or an individualized strengthening program been established?
Caregiver training	Y	Data indicate that "Patient learned to take pulse accurately." This description is brief and lacks skilled terminology. Was the patient instructed in energy conservation techniques such as monitoring cardiopulmonary stresses and pacing of activities of daily living?
Short-term goals and achievement dates	Y	The short-term goals are addressed, and the goal status at discharge is provided with the baseline data. A reviewer would find it helpful if the goal status (i.e., Goal met, Goal not met) was addressed in the goal area. Also, Goals 1 and 2b lack a relationship to function such as to improve functional strength for ambulation without a cane.
Long-term goals and achievement dates	Y	Long-term goals are provided. However, the status of the goals at the time of discharge is lacking.
Discharge prognosis	N	Not addressed. The discharge prognosis provides the reviewer with the therapist's insight into the patient's ability to maintain the stated goals without skilled intervention. This helps to assess the reasonableness of skilled care.

2. Is there evidence of the need for skilled intervention?

Evidence of teaching and training is lacking. Although the patient is evaluated as being at a moderate risk for falls, data are absent to indicate that falls occurred or that safety is jeopardized. Endurance appears to be the limiting factor. Balance testing (Tinetti) required the skills of a therapist; however, the need for the testing is undefined.

3. Are there adequate baseline data to develop future comparisons?

Baseline data are provided for activity tolerance, ambulation, and balance. There is a need to reflect more accurately the gait deficits, the amount of edema, and the effect of edema on function.

4. Are the objective data related to functional deficits?

Ambulation and balance are related to function, such as the ability to walk to meals in the retirement building and to squat and pick up objects. Functional deficits are not described for activity tolerance and bed mobility.

5. Are comparative statements and data clearly outlined?

Comparative data are present for activity tolerance, ambulation, and balance. Data are lacking for edema, strength, gait deficits, vascular signs, transfers, and vision/hearing. A description of the patient's ability to ambulate safely in the community is needed. For example, can the patient safely ambulate on unlevel surfaces?

6. (A) Are the three components for goals present (measurable, functional, time frames)?

Yes, the components are present, except for short-term Goals 1 and 2B, which lack a relationship to function.

(B) Are the goals realistic for the individual case?

The goals presented focus on endurance. For example, "Inc. treadmill duration to 20 minutes" and to "perform 50 reps of closed chain exercise" may be clinical goals, but are not functionally related to mobility within the community and activities of daily living.

7. Do you feel the treatment was reasonable and necessary?

No. This patient was performing at a high functional level without a reported incident such as a fall. Endurance building was the primary focus of the goals and treatment. Teaching and training are not documented, nor are difficulties in mobility at home or the community described.

Twenty-seven visits appear excessive and not reasonable or necessary based on the long-standing diagnosis of chronic obstructive pulmonary disease. As the patient was independent in mobility, ambulated using a cane, and only required oxygen use at night, only twelve visits were approved by the reviewer of this case.

Authors' note: This case was appealed and a full reversal was received at the second level of the appeal process. Daily notes and documentation emphasizing the functional deficits in balance, strength, and gait quality were presented as additional evidence. The patient required the skills of a therapist for progression of gait without an assistive device and to resume mobility in the community.

Additional evidence was provided indicating a fall with a resultant functional regression. This helped to justify the duration of service. Please refer to Chapter 3, page 61, to review the appeal letter written for this patient.

Case 9: Outpatient—Managed Care, Initial Evaluation

(In order to best represent the information received by the reviewer, this case contains only the initial evaluation data and the corresponding worksheet.)

Data Accompanying Referral

Diagnosis/onset date: Lumbar degenerative disc disease/One month.
Secondary diagnoses: Diabetes and hypothyroidism.
Medical history: Prior hospitalization unknown.
Medications: Glucophage™, Metoprolol™, Premarin™, Synthroid™, Diclofenac™ and Imipramine™.

Physical Therapy Intake/History

Gender: Female
Start of care: 08-05-96
Primary complaint: Patient states she has had low back pain and leg pain for three weeks.

Referral Diagnosis

Mechanism of injury: This female complains of sharp increased low back pain noted after she had been working outside cutting grass and weeding.
Prior diagnostic imaging/testing: X-rays were taken which indicate lumbar degenerative disc disease.

Baseline Evaluation Data

Sensation/proprioception: Patient denies numbness and tingling at this time. Sharp/dull and light touch testing is intact.
Posture: Standing posture presents with decreased weight bearing right lower extremity and flat lumbar spine. Patient is also noted to have forward head and C-curving of spine (thoracic area). Sitting posture is remarkable for C-curving of spine and sacral sitting.
AROM/PROM: Trunk ROM is as follows: flexion 75% motion (decreased lumbar reversal of curve), extension 25% motion, side bend right 50% (increased leg pain), side bend left 50%, rotation right 50% and rotation left 50%. Bilateral lower extremity ROM is WFL except tightness noted for hamstrings bilaterally 70°. Patient had difficulty tolerating prone positioning. Hip extension testing produced increased low back pain right side.
Strength: Bilateral lower extremity strength is WNL. Trunk, abdominal and back extensor strength is graded at F-.
Pain: Patient currently complains of a constant ache in the low back radiating into the right lateral leg, right anterior thigh and right shin. Patient also complains of pain with prolonged sitting especially if her feet are up on an ottoman. Patient states that she has difficulty falling asleep secondary

to low back pain. Patient states that she cannot tolerate laying flat on her back.
Ambulation (level and elevated surfaces): Patient states she cannot tolerate walking upright and needs to walk slightly bent over for relief. Patient states she has difficulty with ADL activities, such as making dinner. Patient states she cannot tolerate reaching overhead into cupboards to make dinner. Patient also has difficulty straightening up to take a shower. Patient states she can only walk a short distance (approximately 80 feet) before she has to sit and relax. Patient states she can only grocery shop if she leans forward onto cart.
Activity tolerance: See Ambulation.

Prior Level of Function

Mobility (home and community): Activities are listed as general.
Employment: Patient is retired.

Treatment Diagnosis: Pain and instability.

Problems:

Patient is noted to have limitations in the following areas:

1. Decreased tolerance for sit to stand transfer.
2. Decreased tolerance for ambulation.
3. Decreased tolerance for ADL activities for overhead movements, such as making dinner.
4. Low back pain which leads to decreased endurance for ADL's.

Plan of Care

Specific treatment strategies: To be seen receiving ultrasound, soft tissue mobilization, ROM, strength and endurance activities.
Frequency: To be seen 3x/wk.
Duration: For three weeks.
Short-term goals and achievement dates:

1. Decrease low back pain with modalities and exercise to increase ability to stand upright.
2. Decrease low back pain with modalities and exercise to increase walking tolerance greater than one block.

Long-term goals and achievement dates:

1. Increase walking tolerance with decreased low back pain in four weeks.
2. Increase tolerance for ADL activities, such as making dinner with increased ROM and strength.
3. Increase tolerance for transfers, such as sit to stand activity.

Case 9: Outpatient—Managed Care, Initial Evaluation Worksheet

1. Are the "essential elements" (defined in Chapter 1) for documentation present?

Essential Element	Y, N, or N/A	Comment(s)
Referral		
Reason	N	Not addressed. A clear statement of the reason for referral is needed—for example, *Patient referred by Dr. ABC for rehabilitation to decrease low back pain and improve mobility for activities of daily living.*
Specific treatment requested	N	As most third-party payers require physician involvement, a statement indicating the specific treatment requested is recommended—for example, *Physical therapy three times per week for three weeks per physical therapy plan of care.*
Data Accompanying Referral		
Diagnosis/onset date	Y	For billing purposes it would be helpful to specify the onset date in terms of a month, day, and year.
Secondary diagnoses	Y	Diabetes and hypothyroidism are documented. Based on the medications described, it would appear that depression and hypertension should also be included.
Medical history	Y	Data indicate "Prior hospitalization unknown." This description is brief. It is reasonable to assume that the patient is cognitively intact and data could be obtained through the patient interview. Data pertaining to the initial course of treatment prescribed by the physician are also needed. Has the patient been on bed rest or muscle relaxants? Is there a history of back pain?
Medications	Y	Six medications are listed. It would be helpful to provide the reviewer with insight into the effects these medications may have on rehabilitation. For example, Diclofenac™ is a nonsteroidal anti-inflammatory drug, Metoprolol™ is for hypertension, and Imipramine™ is an antidepressant.
Comorbidities (complicating or precautionary information)	N	Not addressed. It would be helpful for the reviewer to know these areas were assessed. This is easily accomplished by documenting *None.*
Physical Therapy Intake/History		
Date of birth	N	Not addressed. Patient identifying information is important, as many physician offices and third-party payers file or trigger data retrieval based on date of birth.
Age	N	The patient's age may provide insight into the rehabilitation potential.
Gender	Y	
Start of Care	Y	
Primary complaint	Y	The patient's primary complaint of low back and leg pain for three weeks is described. However, the onset date of the diagnosis is "one month." It is important to ensure consistency and accuracy when documenting to avoid a potential delay in authorization.
Referral Diagnosis		
Mechanism of injury	Y	
Prior diagnostic imaging/testing	Y	Documenting the x-ray result is helpful for determining the patient's rehabilitation potential.
Prior Therapy History	N	It would be helpful for the reviewer to know that the prior therapy history was assessed. A statement such as *no prior therapy reported* would clarify whether treatment was received for a similar condition.

Essential Element	Y, N, or N/A	Comment(s)
Baseline Evaluation Data		
Cognition	N/A	
Vision/hearing	N/A	
Vital signs	N	As the patient is taking prescription hypertension medication, vital signs need to be documented.
Vascular signs	N	As the patient has a secondary diagnosis of diabetes, vascular signs such as capillary refill should be evaluated and documented.
Sensation/proprioception	Y	
Edema	N/A	
Posture	Y	Postural deficits are described; however, data pertaining to body mechanics are needed.
AROM/PROM	Y	Range of motion measurements are provided. Additional data describing functional limitations are needed.
Strength	Y	Strength grades are provided. Any observations such as muscle spasm should be described.
Pain	Y	Descriptive terminology such as the location of pain and when pain occurs are provided. However, pain is described with phrases such as "complains of a constant ache." It would be helpful to rate pain on a defined scale to allow for future comparisons.
Coordination	N/A	
Bed mobility	N/A	
Balance (sit and stand)	N/A	
Transfers	N	Not addressed. The evaluation indicates range of motion, strength, and pain limitations. Transfers could be a potential safety concern. Any challenges or safety concerns would provide insight into the need for skilled care.
Ambulation (level and elevated surfaces)	Y	Ambulation data are described in terms of functional limitations such as: making dinner, reaching overhead, taking a shower, and grocery shopping. Although the functional limitations are helpful for the reviewer, the skills of a therapist in analyzing gait are not defined, as each statement begins with, "Patient states. . . ." Objective data are needed for the patient's present gait quality, distance, and use of an assistive device.
Orthotic/prosthetic devices	N/A	
Wheelchair use	N/A	
DME (using or required)	N/A	
Activity tolerance	Y	See Ambulation.
Wound description, including incision status	N/A	
Special tests	N	Not addressed. Any special tests should be listed and the clinical relevance briefly explained.
Architectural/safety considerations	N	Not addressed. It would be helpful for a reviewer to know if the patient is at risk for falls.
Requirements to return to home, school and/or job	N/A	
Prior Level of Function		
Mobility (home and community)	Y	The present documentation, "Activities are listed as general," is not related to function. As the patient is retired (and age is unknown), it would be important to provide more detail of the prior level of function, such as *Patient was previously free of back pain and independent in functional activities.*
Employment	Y	

(continued)

Essential Element	Y, N, or N/A	Comment(s)
School	N/A	
Treatment Diagnosis	Y	Although the diagnosis is described as "Pain and instability," this is vague. A more specific treatment diagnosis such as *radicular (spinal) pain* is needed.
Assessment Reason for skilled care	N	Not addressed. It is important to describe the reason for skilled care and the expected response to skilled intervention.
Problems	Y	
Plan of Care Specific treatment strategies	Y	The treatment strategies include ultrasound, soft tissue mobilization, range of motion, strengthening, and endurance activities. A reviewer may question the need for ultrasound and soft tissue mobilization, as objective findings relating to muscle spasm are not described. It would also seem appropriate to omit "endurance activities" and focus on *instruction in a home program* to help justify the need for the skills of a therapist.
Frequency	Y	
Duration	Y	
Patient instruction/home program	N	Not addressed. Patient training and education are important to the reviewer and need to be initiated at the time of evaluation. This is particularly true for all third-party payers and especially in a managed care environment. Patient involvement in pain management and proper body mechanics is needed.
Caregiver training	N	See Patient instruction/home program.
Short-term goals and achievement dates	Y	Although four problems are identified, only two short-term goals are described. The goals are functional; however, they lack time frames. Goal 1 is not measurable.
Long-term goals and achievement dates	Y	The long-term goals are not measurable, and wording such as "Increase tolerance" is used. Also, Goal 1 has a time frame of four weeks. This is inconsistent with the duration of three weeks. It would be more appropriate to list either four short-term goals and no long-term goal, or four short-term goals and one long-term goal.
Rehabilitation potential	N	Not addressed. Rehabilitation potential is an essential element of documentation. It provides the therapist's insight into the potential success of the rehabilitation intervention for the stated goals. This helps the reviewer assess the reasonableness of care.

2. Is the overall history of the patient adequate?

No, the history is not specific except for the mechanism of injury. It would be helpful for the therapist to document any prior therapy history related to the present diagnosis of lumbar degenerative disc disease. Is the onset date listed related to a recent exacerbation of a long-standing history of back pain, or is this the first episode of discomfort? It would also be helpful for the reviewer, in determining the necessity of skilled physical therapy, to know the effects of medication on the rehabilitation process and any intervention or education provided prior to the therapy evaluation. The statement "prior hospitalization unknown" also provides an unclear picture of the patient. Is the history of hospitalization unknown because the patient is cognitively impaired?

3. Is there evidence of the need for skilled intervention?

There are pain and limitations in functional activities such as ambulation, reaching, and activities of daily living. Objectively, posture, range of motion, and strength are limited, justifying the need for skilled intervention. A reviewer may question the use of ultrasound and soft tissue mobilization, as data are absent regarding muscle spasm. This case would be strengthened if the reason for skilled care was described and the need for patient education identified.

4. Are there adequate baseline data to develop future comparisons?

There are adequate baseline data in the areas of posture, active range of motion, strength, and ambulation. However, data are lacking in the areas of transfers and pain.

5. Are the objective data related to functional deficits?

Functional limitations in daily activities are outlined. These include reaching, ambulation, making dinner, and showering. Instructing the patient in a home program and education pertaining to back care and posture are lacking.

6. Are comparative statements and data clearly outlined?

Data are present for range of motion, strength, and posture. Additional objective data for pain and ambulation are needed.

7. (A) Are the three components for goals present (measurable, functional, time frames)?

The goals presented are not measurable. All goals are related to function. Time frames are absent with the exception of long-term Goal 1. Goal 1 lists a time frame of four weeks; however, the duration listed in the evaluation is three weeks. A reviewer may seek clarification of this information.

(B) Are the goals realistic for the individual case?

The goals appear realistic for this patient. The only goal that may be unrealistic is long-term Goal 3, as objective data are lacking regarding transfers. It is also important to note that the therapist identified four problems, and yet only two short-term goals are identified. A more consistent approach is needed.

8. Do you feel that the proposed treatment is reasonable and necessary?

Treatment appears reasonable and necessary. However, further data are needed to justify the need for nine visits. In this case, the peer reviewer recommended a modified authorization. Six visits were approved, and the nurse reviewer was advised to request evidence of a home program to include postural correction/exercises and self-management of pain (i.e., positioning, posture, and specific exercise program).

Case 10: Outpatient—Managed Care, Progress Report

(In order to best represent the information received by the reviewer, this case contains only progress report data and the corresponding worksheet. Importantly, the initial evaluation is not contained here.)

Attendance: Treatment dates 07-25-96 thru 09-15-96. Attended 7 treatments. Treatments missed 0.

Current Baseline Data

AROM/PROM: PROM—Flex 95°, Ab 90°, ER 35°, IR 60°.

Treatment Diagnosis: Rotator cuff repair/July 1996.

Assessment

Reason for skilled care: Fair progress. Improved use of arm. Decreased pain. Increased function. Slow improvement. Progress limited by the number of PT visits.

Plan of Care

Specific treatment strategies: HP, PROM, AROM, UBE, Airdyne™. Continue PT as insurance allows.

Case 10: Outpatient—Managed Care, Progress Report Worksheet

1. Are the "essential elements" (defined in Chapter 1) for documentation present?

Essential Element	Y, N, or N/A	Comment(s)
Attendance	Y	
Current Baseline Data		
Cognition	N/A	
Vision/hearing	N/A	
Vital signs	N/A	
Vascular signs	N	Vascular signs, if present, should be documented, as they demonstrate a need for skilled care.
Sensation/proprioception	N	Deficits in this area, if present, need to be addressed to justify skilled care.
Edema	N	Deficits in this area, if present, need to be addressed to justify skilled care.
Posture	N	Deficits in this area, if present, need to be addressed to justify skilled care.
AROM/PROM	Y	Passive range of motion measurements are indicated in the progress report. The reason for skilled care also states "Improved use of arm." Additional data are needed to demonstrate the skilled intervention provided, specific functional improvement, and the resultant range of motion changes. There is a need for comparative range of motion measurements and a specific functional relationship. For example, *Following joint mobilization left shoulder flexion increased by 10 degrees to 95 degrees allowing patient to comb hair* would be helpful to the reviewer.
Strength	N	Not addressed. Although the assessment implies an increase in function and "Improved use of arm," no objective measurements or specific functional tasks are documented to support this conclusion.
Pain	N	Not addressed. The assessment states, "Decreased pain"; however, data are lacking to support this conclusion. Data such as the location of the pain, when it occurs, and how it limits functional activities are needed.
Coordination	N	Deficits in this area, if present, need to be addressed to justify skilled care.
Bed mobility	N/A	
Balance (sit and stand)	N/A	
Transfers	N/A	

Essential Element	Y, N, or N/A	Comment(s)
Ambulation (level and elevated surfaces)	N/A	
Orthotic/prosthetic devices	N/A	
Wheelchair use	N/A	
DME (using or required)	N/A	
Activity tolerance	N	Because of the surgical intervention, activity tolerance would be relevant in this case, especially if the patient is off of work.
Wound description, including incision status	N	As the rotator cuff has been repaired, any soft tissue restrictions need to be described.
Special tests	N/A	
Architectural/safety considerations	N/A	
Treatment Diagnosis	Y	
Assessment		
Reason for skilled care	Y	The vague descriptions used, such as "improved use of arm" and "increased function," are unfortunately a common finding for reviewers of documentation. Data are needed to substantiate these statements. It is important to define why the skills of a therapist are needed and why the patient's goals cannot be achieved with a home program.
Problems	N	Not addressed. It is helpful to determine the problems in order to focus treatment (e.g., decreased functional left upper extremity shoulder strength, decreased left shoulder range of motion).
Plan of Care		
Specific treatment strategies	Y	The evaluation lists the following treatment strategies: "HP, PROM, AROM, UBE, Airdyne™." A reviewer may question the need for the hot pack and use of an Airdyne™, as these modalities could be incorporated into a home exercise program. As a reviewer may be unfamiliar with a device such as an Airdyne™, it would be helpful to explain what the device is and its purpose.
Frequency	N	Not addressed. Although the therapist implies that progress is limited by the patient's insurance coverage, a proactive statement of the needed therapy frequency and duration to achieve a successful outcome is needed.
Duration	N	See Frequency.
Patient instruction/home program	N	Not addressed. Especially in the managed care environment, the patient's involvement in a home program is important and an expectation of the third-party payer. Evidence of training and education helps justify the need for skilled care.
Caregiver training	N	See Patient instruction/home program.
Short-term goals and achievement dates	N	Not addressed. It is reasonable to expect goals to be established as a standard of practice. Goals provide the reviewer with insight into the patient's functional limitations and needs. This is a serious oversight in documentation.
Long-term goals and achievement dates	N	Not addressed. A statement such as *Patient's range of motion and strength will increase to within functional limits to allow return to work and pain-free activities of daily living* is needed.
Rehabilitation potential	N	Not addressed. Rehabilitation potential is an essential element of documentation. It provides the therapist's insight into the potential success of the rehabilitation intervention for the stated goals. This helps the reviewer assess the reasonableness of care.

2. Is there evidence of the need for skilled intervention?

Based on the diagnosis of a recent rotator cuff repair and passive range of motion limitations, the need for skilled care is evident despite the lack of data in this report.

3. Are there adequate baseline data to develop future comparisons?

No, data are lacking in all functional areas except for passive range of motion. (Unfortunately, reviewers often find limited data, as demonstrated in this case.)

4. Are the objective data related to functional deficits?

No, data are brief and not related to any functional deficits such as grooming, dressing, or job responsibilities.

5. Are comparative statements and data clearly outlined?

No, data are lacking in all areas except for passive range of motion. Comparative range of motion measurements are absent, and a reviewer is unable to determine the positive effect of skilled intervention.

6. (A) Are the three components for goals present (measurable, functional, time frames)?

No, goals are not listed. This is not acceptable.

(B) Are the goals realistic for the individual case?

As goals are not listed, a reviewer would not be able to determine this.

7. Do you feel the treatment was reasonable and necessary?

Based solely on the limitations in passive shoulder range of motion (i.e., flexion 95 degrees, abduction 90 degrees, external rotation 35 degrees, internal rotation 60 degrees) and the notation acknowledging a surgical repair, a limited number of visits (nine) were approved by the peer reviewer. The third-party payer was advised not to provide further authorizations without markedly improved documentation. The peer reviewer, in this particular case, advised that additional documentation must include objective data on active range of motion, strength, passive range of motion, and pain. Also requested were functional limitations of the patient for activities of daily living and work secondary to pain, as well as details of a home program with evidence of upgrading.

Case 11: Pediatric, Initial Evaluation

Referral

Reason: There is no summer physical therapy offered in his school program.

Data Accompanying Referral

Diagnosis/onset date: Developmental delay/09-14-90.
Secondary diagnoses: Spastic triplegia.
Medical history: Spastic triplegic since birth.

Physical Therapy Intake/History

Date of birth: 09-14-90
Age: 6
Gender: Male
Start of care: 06-04-96

Referral Diagnosis

Mechanism of injury: Since birth.

Prior Therapy History: Received therapy in school focusing on crawling, standing, increasing strength and balance.

Baseline Evaluation Data

Cognition: Child was evaluated using a neurodevelopmental assessment. This measures only physical developmental abilities and does not reflect cognitive functions.

AROM/PROM: Shoulder ROM is WNL on the right side and is limited by about 40% in flexion, abduction and extension on the left. He also lacks about 20 degrees of elbow and wrist supination on the left side.

Coordination: Fine motor skills are better when he is in the "W" position or on a chair. He has a gross grasp on his L and is able to pick up hand-sized objects with his left only with difficulty and only with large amounts of prodding by the therapist. He has pincer grasp with his right hand.

Balance (sit and stand): Child continues to "W-sit" for stability, although tailor sitting is possible. He gets into and out of both sitting positions independently. He continues to have protective reactions with his R arm to the right, front and back and little or no reaction with his L arm because of muscle tightness and decreased L arm abilities. As he did again, child began to "bunny hop" when he came into the clinic, but with reminders he began to use a modified 4-point. Child can balance in high kneeling. He is able to weight shift on the balance disc in this position and likes the movement. He is unable to come into or maintain a half-knee position, even following facilitation and with assistance.

Transfers: Requires moderate assist to come to stand.

Ambulation (level and elevated surfaces): He does not come to stand independently, but requires moderate assistance with this movement. He attempts to use his right UE for major weight bearing assistance when in the upright position. Can stand independently for brief periods by using his right hand on the parallel bars. The major impediment to standing is knee flexion contracture of about 60 degrees bilaterally.

Treatment Diagnosis: Decreased functional abilities, joint contractures, muscle tightness, loss of ROM and synergistic movement patterns.

Assessment

Reason for skilled care: Child would benefit from twice weekly physical therapy sessions. Has made progress since initiating therapy. This includes:

1. Ability to 4-point crawl, where he would previously only bunny-hop.
2. Child previously required maximal assistance to come to stand and now requires only moderate assistance.
3. Child previously was able to stand only with moderate assistance and is now able to stand independently for brief periods.

Plan of Care

Frequency: 2x/wk.
Short-term goals and achievement dates:

1. Child will increase his knee extension by 5 degrees when long sitting with an erect pelvis in order to allow for better balance when sitting and better ability to stand.
2. Child will crawl 100% of the time in the clinic without reminders in order to enhance his ability to move his legs and weight shift when standing.
3. Child will be able to come up to stand and maintain standing for 1 minute in order to increase his standing strength in preparation for walking.

Case 11: Pediatric, Initial Evaluation Worksheet

1. Are the "essential elements" (defined in Chapter 1) for documentation present?

Essential Element	Y, N, or N/A	Comment(s)
Referral		
Reason	Y	"There is no summer physical therapy offered in his school program," per the therapist's documentation. This is an important consideration for reimbursement, as most third-party payers assess the need for skilled care outside the school program. The reason for referral should also include information related to function and/or medical necessity. Will the child regress without skilled care? What complicating conditions exist that require skilled intervention? Also, who initiated the referral (i.e., parents, school therapists, physicians)?
Specific treatment requested	N	Most third-party payers require a physician's order prior to initiation of an evaluation and treatment. A statement reflecting this order would demonstrate the physician's involvement.
Data Accompanying Referral		
Diagnosis/onset date	Y	Developmental delay is the diagnosis provided. This is a global diagnosis. Most third-party payers will request a specific medical diagnosis, such as cerebral palsy, to justify skilled rehabilitation.
Secondary diagnoses	Y	
Medical history	Y	The medical history restates the secondary diagnosis and onset. It would be beneficial to provide more information such as pertinent birth history, developmental history, surgical history, and/or barriers to progress.
Medications	N	Not addressed. As spasticity and contractures are indicated in the evaluation, it would seem helpful to know what medications, if any, are being administered that may affect rehabilitation—for example, antispasmodics.
Comorbidities (complicating or precautionary information)	N	Not addressed. It would be helpful to know if comorbidities exist. This information is especially important if spasms or seizures are present. If absent, a notation indicating *none* is recommended.
Physical Therapy Intake/History		
Date of birth	Y	Date of birth is documented. This is helpful information, as many physician offices and third-party payers file and/or retrieve data based on date of birth.
Age	Y	
Gender	Y	
Start of Care	Y	
Primary complaint	N	Not addressed. A description of the functional deficits and the challenges reported by a parent would help in identifying the need for skilled care. For example, *The father reports difficulty with dressing because of spasming and tightness of the lower extremities.*
Referral Diagnosis		
Mechanism of injury	Y	"Since birth" lacks detail pertaining to the mechanism of injury. Is the diagnosis a result of the mother's health (i.e., drug use during pregnancy) or a complication at birth (e.g., anoxia)?
Prior diagnostic imaging/testing	N	It is reasonable to expect that prior testing has occurred to make the initial diagnosis.

Essential Element	Y, N, or N/A	Comment(s)
Prior Therapy History	Y	The data provided indicate that the patient received therapy in school that focused on crawling, standing, and increasing strength and balance. It would be helpful for a reviewer to know the frequency, duration, and prior functional limitations to provide insight into the patient's rehabilitation potential.
Baseline Evaluation Data		
Cognition	Y	Although the data describe the evaluation tool used and indicate that it does not measure cognitive function, a reviewer would find it helpful to know the patient's cognitive level. For example, can the patient follow simple or complex commands? Data relating to cognition provide the reviewer with insight into the patient's ability to participate in a skilled rehabilitation program.
Vision/hearing	N	Not addressed. The prior therapy history indicates that balance was a focus area in the school therapy program. As visual deficits may affect balance, documentation in this area would be important to a reviewer.
Vital signs	N/A	
Vascular signs	N/A	
Sensation/proprioception	N	Not addressed. It would seem reasonable that any deficits in sensation and/or proprioception should be described. Their impact on functional progress would be important to the reviewer in determining the reasonableness of care.
Edema	N/A	
Posture	N	Assessment of posture in sitting and standing needs to be addressed.
AROM/PROM	Y	Data are limited. The documentation addresses upper extremity range of motion; however, only the approximate percentage of loss is provided. The absence of lower extremity range of motion measurements is an oversight, as "knee flexion contractures of about 60 degrees bilaterally" are described in the section on ambulation. It is reasonable for a reviewer to expect specific measurements bilaterally and the differentiation of passive versus active range of motion for all extremities. Consistency in the unit of measurement, percentage of loss versus degrees, is also recommended.
Strength	N	Not addressed. This appears to be an oversight by the therapist, as "increasing strength" was one of the documented focus areas during intervention in the school program.
Pain	N	Not addressed. It would seem reasonable for a reviewer to expect that discomfort exists during stretching/range of motion activities. A description of this discomfort would help justify the need for the skills of a physical therapist to safely achieve the maximum available range.
Coordination	Y	Fine motor coordination and grasp are described. Further functional detail may be helpful to the reviewer. For example, "Fine motor skills are better when he is in the 'W' position or on a chair" could be expanded to describe how the movements "are better" and during what functional activity. The activity may be writing, manipulation of buttons while dressing, or use of utensils during feeding. Further description of how the patient is positioned, such as in what type of chair/seating system, would be helpful, as poor postural support can directly affect fine motor coordination.
Bed mobility	N	Not addressed. A reviewer would find it helpful to know if the patient is independent or if there are activities that require assistance, such as rolling.

(continued)

Essential Element	Y, N, or N/A	Comment(s)
Balance (sit and stand)	Y	Balance is described. However, additional follow through on the relationship to function would be helpful (i.e., how does the patient negotiate in home, school, and community? How is sitting balance affected by various seating available in the patient's home and school?). Also, further discussion of trunk righting skills is needed.
Transfers	Y	The therapist indicates that moderate assistance is required to come to a standing position. However, further detail regarding transitioning skills such as toileting, on/off the floor, and car/bus transfers would be helpful to the reviewer for determining functional limitations. Also, from what position is standing initiated (i.e., chair, floor or bed/mat)?
Ambulation (level and elevated surfaces)	Y	Data pertaining to ambulation are described. However, it is recommended that the amount of time the patient can stand be specified in seconds or minutes to allow for future comparison. "Can stand independently for brief periods" is not a measurable description of standing time.
Orthotic/prosthetic devices	N	It is unclear why this area is not addressed. It would seem reasonable, based on the secondary diagnosis of spastic triplegia and the treatment diagnoses of muscle tightness, loss of range of motion, joint contractures, and synergistic movement patterns, that orthotic support or referral to an orthopedist may be necessary.
Wheelchair use	N	This appears to be an oversight by the therapist, as documentation indicates the patient attends school and has limited standing ability. A reviewer could reasonably expect documentation pertaining to how the patient negotiates in his home, school, and community.
DME (using or required)	N	See Wheelchair use.
Activity tolerance	N	Not addressed. A reviewer would find it helpful to know the patient's functional activity tolerance. For example, if the patient has a wheelchair, can he propel it distances that allow independent interaction in the environment, such as during recess, at school or to seek assistance of a caregiver for toileting?
Wound description, including incision status	N/A	
Special tests	N/A	A neurodevelopmental assessment is described in the area on cognition. This type of neurodevelopmental test may provide limited clinical information to the reviewer. A functional independence test may be more appropriate for providing insight into how this patient functions at home, at school, and in the community.
Architectural/safety considerations	N	Not addressed. A reviewer would find it helpful to know how the patient is negotiating and functioning at home, at school, and in the community.
Requirements to return to home, school and/or job	N/A	
Prior Level of Function		
Mobility (home and community)	N	It would be helpful to have an overall assessment of the patient's functional ability in the home, school, and community. This is implied in the functional statements listed in the assessment area; however, it is not clearly stated.
Employment	N/A	
School	N	See Prior Level of Function: Mobility (home and community).
Treatment Diagnosis	Y	

Essential Element	Y, N, or N/A	Comment(s)
Assessment		
Reason for skilled care	Y	Although addressed, the assessment is confusing. It provides a comparison of progress that demonstrates to the reviewer that the patient has not plateaued. However, this is an evaluation, and the documentation reflects that the patient "Has made progress since initiating therapy." An explanation of when and where the progress was made may be helpful. Did the progress occur during the school therapy sessions, or since treatment in an outpatient setting last summer?
Problems	N	The documentation does not provide a list of problems that correspond to the three goals indicated. It is helpful to determine the problems in order to focus treatment.
Plan of Care		
Specific treatment strategies	N	Not addressed. It is important to describe the treatment strategies that will be used to achieve the stated goals. The treatment strategies provide the reviewer with information to help determine the appropriateness of treatment intervention. It is an expectation of third-party payers that the modalities rendered are described and correspond to the services billed.
Frequency	Y	
Duration	N	Not addressed. It is reasonable for a reviewer to expect a duration of treatment to be indicated in an evaluation. Although the documentation implies that therapy intervention is for the summer, specific time frames are recommended.
Patient instruction/home program	N	Not addressed. Training and education are important components of treatment. They should be initiated at the time of evaluation. A reviewer may question why there is not an orthopedic referral because of the severity of contractures in the lower extremities.
Caregiver training	N	No information is given as to the role of the family/caregivers in a home program. A reviewer would need to request this information from the billing provider to facilitate the ability to make a coverage decision. Justifying the need for summer therapy versus carryover by family through a home program is needed.
Short-term goals and achievement dates	Y	The goals meet the essential components of measurability and function. However, they lack a specific time frame related to the length of summer outpatient therapy. A goal to include parent involvement would also be beneficial in demonstrating carryover to home.
Long-term goals and achievement dates	N	It would be helpful to know the long-term expectations (i.e.; patient's level of ambulation). Parent involvement needs to be reflected. Specifically, is gait training meant to help improve other areas, such as transfers? Is the patient a realistic ambulator in the future? Is crawling the most appropriate long-term goal?
Rehabilitation potential	N	Not addressed. The rehabilitation potential is an essential component of documentation. It helps a reviewer assess the reasonableness of skilled care in relationship to the stated goals.

2. Is the overall history of the patient adequate?

No, especially regarding the patient's past, present, and future functional goals in the home, school, and community regarding functional transfers and ambulation. The documentation lacks information relating to birth history, developmental history, surgical history, and/or barriers to progress.

3. Is there evidence of the need for skilled intervention?

Yes, based on the age, developmental motor delays and range of motion deficits identified. However, a description of the plan of care as well as training for and details of a home program is lacking. The long-term goals of the patient are unclear, and it is questionable whether walking is a realistic goal.

4. Are there adequate baseline data to develop future comparisons?

No, measurable baseline data are lacking for future comparison. Range of motion measurements are not provided except for an approximation of the percentage of loss. Levels of assistance are not defined regarding balance. Vague terms such as "are better" (Coordination area) and "has difficulty" (Balance area) are used. Data are also omitted in such areas as passive range of motion, strength, pain, transfers, wheelchair use, and activity tolerance. Limitations related to muscle tone are not described.

5. Are the objective data related to functional deficits?

The objective data provided in the ambulation and balance areas relate to functional deficits. However, the documentation leaves a reviewer unclear as to the present functional status of the patient and the future direction of treatment intervention. This is particularly evident in limited data regarding activities of daily living, transfers (transitioning skills), and wheelchair use.

6. Are comparative statements and data clearly outlined?

Comparative statements are present regarding past functional progress in the Assessment area. However, it is unclear to the reviewer where and when the patient's progress occurred.

7. (A) Are the three components for goals present (measurable, functional, time frames)?

Yes, with the exception of time frames.

(B) Are the goals realistic for the individual case?

Yes, possibly, but because of the lack of previous and present data regarding the functional level of the patient it is difficult to predict. A reviewer may question whether "preparation for walking" is realistic because of the sixty-degree knee flexion contractures.

8. Do you feel that the proposed treatment is reasonable and necessary?

Because of the functional deficits in standing and the multiple treatment diagnoses listed, it appears treatment is reasonable and necessary. However, the reason for skilled care in an outpatient setting is not clearly stated. The reviewer needs to conclude that the patient's complicating conditions of spasticity, contractures, and progress warrants physical therapy during the summer. Realistically, a reviewer may need additional information that includes a clearly stated reason for outpatient service, objective data regarding range of motion and strength deficits, and the functional limitations at home, school, and in the community.

Case 11: Pediatric, Progress Report

Attendance: Patient was seen 2x/wk.

Current Baseline Data

AROM/PROM: Were able to get him to long sit for only brief periods of time in order to stretch his hamstrings. He did not like this position and would not assume it independently. He has not increased his knee extension, but he has begun to tolerate the stretch to a greater degree so that the degree of extension can be maintained.

Strength: He has increased his lower extremity strength so he is able to stand for longer periods of time.

Balance (sit and stand): Child began this summer by reverting to bunny hopping as his primary means of movement through the environment. Through verbal and physical reminders, he quickly began to use 4-point more frequently and was no longer bunny hopping during the last three weeks. Child is using the 4-point crawl 100% of the time now and was not doing so previously. Child comes up to a kneel standing position independently and is able to use this position for play. He cannot assume or maintain a half-kneel position without at least moderate assistance for balance and to get into this position. Child is able to maintain ball sitting for brief periods of time, but he loses his balance in all directions if the ball is moving too far in any direction. Protective reactions are present in his right upper extremity in all directions, but not in his left because of contractures and lack of movement abilities. Child relies heavily on upper extremity use in order to get up to a standing position.

Transfers: He requires moderate assistance of one for both balance and weight bearing to get to and maintain standing.

Ambulation (level and elevated surfaces): Child has hip and knee flexion contractures bilaterally which interfere with his ability to stand and bear weight. He has progressed to using the parallel bars for walking and is able to walk 8 feet more than 6 times with no difficulty. He requires assistance on his left side for upper extremity weight bearing as he has a poor grasp on the left and is unable to grip the bars effectively. With proper balancing, he is able to bear full weight on his legs for up to 1 minute depending on his mood or motivation level. This is an increase of 50 seconds from his first session this summer.

Assessment

Reason for skilled care: He has always been happy and cooperative with requested tasks and a little impetuous. Child has done very well in meeting his goals. He should continue to receive physical therapy in order to progress to goals for independence in coming to stand and in ambulation abilities.

Plan of Care

Frequency: 2x/wk.
Duration: Through the summer.

Case 11: Pediatric, Progress Report Worksheet

1. Are the "essential elements" (defined in Chapter 1) for documentation present?

Essential Element	Y, N, or N/A	Comment(s)
Attendance	Y	The therapist indicates "Patient was seen 2x/wk." A reviewer would find it helpful to know the total number of visits scheduled and any reasons for absence.
Current Baseline Data		
Cognition	N	Not addressed in the evaluation or the progress report. Documentation regarding the patient's cognitive level provides the reviewer with insight into the patient's ability to participate in a rehabilitation program and the potential to achieve established goals.
Vision/hearing	N	This area is not addressed in the evaluation or progress report. As balance can be affected by visual deficits, it is important for a reviewer to be aware of such deficits when determining the need for skilled care.
Vital signs	N/A	
Vascular signs	N/A	
Sensation/proprioception	N	Sensation and proprioception are not addressed in the evaluation or progress report. Data, if it exists, would provide the reviewer with insight into the potential challenges for gait training.
Edema	N/A	
Posture	N	This appears to be an oversight and is not addressed in the evaluation or progress report. Assessments of posture in sitting and standing need to be provided.
AROM/PROM	Y	The data indicate the patient's ability to "long sit for only brief periods of time" and that knee extension has not increased, but the patient "has begun to tolerate the stretch to a greater degree." Descriptions such as these are vague and do not provide the reviewer with objective measurable data. Upper extremity range of motion deficits are also not listed; however, they were measured in the evaluation. It is important to provide consistent measurable data to the reviewer for progress comparisons.
Strength	Y	The therapist relates an increase in strength to improvement in standing. This is a positive relationship; however, the measurable component is vaguely stated as "longer periods of time." It would be helpful to provide the number of seconds or minutes. In this case, the reviewer must read all baseline data to determine the standing time. It is also noted that strength measurements were not mentioned in the evaluation. Therefore, no data for comparison are present.
Pain	N	The data provided under AROM/PROM describe the patient as not liking the position of long sitting for stretching. The reason for the limited tolerance is not defined; however, it would seem helpful to know if pain was the factor limiting the hamstring stretch.
Coordination	N	Not addressed. Fine motor skills were briefly described in the evaluation, and data are omitted in this report except for ambulation, which describes difficulty with grasping of the parallel bars. A reviewer would find fine motor skills important when assessing the need for skilled care.
Bed mobility	N	Not addressed. It is difficult to ascertain if the patient is independent in bed mobility, as it is not described in the evaluation or progress report.

(continued)

Essential Element	Y, N, or N/A	Comment(s)
Balance (sit and stand)	Y	Balance is described; however, further description pertaining to righting reactions and various sitting postures would be helpful.
Transfers	Y	The therapist indicates that transfers required moderate assistance. As in the evaluation, data are limited and a reviewer would find it helpful if other transitional skills were described (e.g., toilet transfers, car and/ or bus transfers).
Ambulation (level and elevated surfaces)	Y	Data are provided regarding ambulation. It is suggested that use of skilled terminology, such as _Gait training has progressed to using the parallel bars_, would emphasize the skilled nature of the service delivered. Also, describing the amount of assistance for safe left grasp on the parallel bars would be helpful. A reviewer may question if ambulation is a realistic goal based on the knee and newly stated hip flexion contractures.
Orthotic/prosthetic devices	N	Not addressed in the evaluation or progress report. If orthotics are being used, it would be important for a reviewer to know when determining the need for skilled care.
Wheelchair use	N	Not addressed. This appears to be an oversight by the therapist. A reviewer would be concerned regarding this patient's ability to negotiate at home, at school, and in the community.
DME (using or required)	N	See Wheelchair use.
Activity tolerance	N	Activity tolerance is not separately described in the evaluation or progress report; it is implied only in the ambulation section. A reviewer would find it helpful to know if the patient has a wheelchair and can propel it far enough to interact during recess or to seek caregiver assistance.
Wound description, including incision status	N/A	
Special tests	N/A	
Architectural/safety considerations	N	Not addressed in the evaluation or progress report. A reviewer would find it helpful, in determining the need for skilled care, if architectural/safety considerations were described—for example, _The patient has two steps between the kitchen and living room that require daily negotiation._
Treatment Diagnosis	N	It is important to identify the treatment diagnosis for which physical therapy services are rendered, as it may change during the course of intervention.
Assessment Reason for skilled care	Y	Expectation statements are present and demonstrate the need for continued rehabilitation; however, where further care should be received is not defined (i.e., outpatient, school, or home setting).
Problems	N	Not addressed. It is helpful to determine the problem list in order to focus treatment.
Plan of Care Specific treatment strategies	N	Not addressed in the evaluation or progress report. It is important to describe the treatment strategies that will be used to achieve the stated goals. The treatment strategies provide the reviewer with information to help determine the appropriateness of treatment intervention. It is an expectation of third-party payers that the modalities rendered be described and correspond to the services billed.
Frequency	Y	

Essential Element	Y, N, or N/A	Comment(s)
Duration	Y	"Through the summer" is a vague description. A specific number of weeks or a date of discharge would be helpful.
Patient instruction/home program	N	Not addressed. Carryover of functional gains and establishment of a home program are necessary and skilled components of rehabilitation. Based on the patient's limitations in range of motion, it is reasonable to expect that a home program is necessary to prevent further contractures.
Caregiver training	N	See Patient instruction/home program.
Short-term goals and achievement dates	N	Not addressed. Goals are an essential component of physical therapy documentation. There are statements relating to the goals in the current baseline data. However, specific identification of what the goals for treatment are and the goal status are not described.
Long-term goals and achievement dates	N	The long-term goal is not addressed in the evaluation or progress report. An expectation statement is present in the reason for skilled care section that implies a long-term goal of independence in coming to stand and ambulation. A separate section identifying the long-term goal is needed.
Rehabilitation potential	N	Not addressed. The rehabilitation potential is an essential component of documentation. It helps a reviewer assess the reasonableness of skilled care in relationship to the stated goals.

2. Is there evidence of the need for skilled intervention?

Yes, based on the description of balance and ambulation. However, it would be more complete if the treatment strategies, goals, and evidence of family training were provided. There does not appear to be enough justification for skilled therapeutic intervention in the summer rather than the family providing therapy through a home program. For example, if the patient has severe muscle tone that is affecting functional progress and the skills of a therapist are required, this would enhance the justification for skilled coverage.

3. Are there adequate baseline data to develop future comparisons?

Minimal baseline data are given in this progress report. It is important to remember for continuity of care that the treating therapist in the school system would benefit greatly from a more accurate display of baseline data. Especially helpful would be the areas of range of motion, time spent in long sitting, and the amount of assistance needed for left grasp on the parallel bars.

4. Are the objective data related to functional deficits?

In part, as the data relate to the inability to stand, however, an overview of the patient's functional deficits in terms of negotiating in the home, community, and school is absent. For example the data indicates that the patient improved in ability to stand from ten seconds to one minute. This improvement is not related to transitioning skills such as a toilet transfer or activities of daily living. In light of the knee and apparent hip flexion contractures, focusing the program on increasing standing time seems inappropriate when a referral to an orthopedist is needed.

5. Are comparative statements and data clearly outlined?

No, the items measured initially, such as range of motion measurements of the shoulders and knees, are not addressed in the progress report. Hip flexion contractures are now reported; however, data are lacking. Continuity of objective data enhances the identification of the need to provide ongoing therapeutic intervention.

6. (A) Are the three components for goals present (measurable, functional, time frames)?

No, there are no short-term or long-term goals listed. Baseline data are lacking regarding the goals established in the evaluation. This places the reviewer at a disadvantage in attempting to assess the overall progress achieved.

(B) Are the goals realistic for the individual case?

This is impossible to answer as goals are not listed.

7. Do you feel that the treatment was reasonable and necessary?

As a reviewer, it would be appropriate to request more information on this case before making a coverage determination. Information requested would be: Was a home program designed for family training? Was there communication with the school therapist to coordinate treatment plans and goals? What were the specific improvements in the patient's transitional skills? What are the long-term goals for ambulation? Why is ambulation realistic? Lastly, what complicating factors exist that require the skills of a physical therapist during the summer?

Case 12: Pediatric, Initial Evaluation

Referral

Reason: Mother reports that her concerns with him are that he does not crawl and he seems to be lagging behind the other twin.

Specific treatment requested: PT for evaluation and treatment.

Data Accompanying Referral

Diagnosis/onset date: Cerebral Palsy/02-10-93.

Secondary diagnoses: Prematurity.

Medical history: He is the product of a premature delivery. He was born a twin at 28 weeks gestation with a birth weight of 2 lbs., 1 oz. He spent three months in the neonatal nursery, two of those months on a ventilator. The mother describes that he had a very small bleed while in the nursery, has had no seizures. He did have a patent ductus surgery when he was one week old. He was on an apnea monitor at home from June through October. Other than that, he has been fairly healthy.

Physical Therapy Intake/History

Date of birth: 02-10-93

Age: 17 months

Gender: Male

Start of care: 07-14-94

Primary complaint: Mom describes his primary issues as problems moving around. She claims that he feels very strong to her but seems frustrated at his inability to move or maintain a sitting position.

Referral Diagnosis

Mechanism of injury: Premature birth.

Prior Therapy History: Mother reports no previous therapy.

Baseline Evaluation Data

Vision/hearing: He currently has normal vision and hearing although he wears glasses to correct his strabismus problem on the left eye.

Posture: His spine is fairly symmetrical, although he currently demonstrates a long C-curve in upright positioning and has difficulty with extension or lordosis of the lower spine. Child presents with a moderate increase in muscle tone through his trunk and extremities. He demonstrates fairly symmetrical posturing but does have spasticity in his LE's which is primarily extensor adductor in nature and UE's which present with mild to moderate flexor tone.

AROM/PROM: Child's UE ROM is grossly WNL although he does have tightness at end range of forearm supination and shoulder flexion/abduction. His LE's show normal flexion/extension ROM but lack abduction beyond 35 degrees bilaterally and lack straight leg raise beyond 50 degrees bilaterally. Knees, ankles and feet have ROM which is grossly WNL following inhibition.

Bed mobility: He can roll from supine to sidelying and prone to supine although this is not segmental.

Ambulation (level and elevated surfaces): In a standing alignment he can bear weight, although not in a flatfoot alignment.

Orthotic/prosthetic devices: None.

Wheelchair use: He currently has no adaptive equipment.

DME (using or required): See Wheelchair use.

Special tests: Child scores a 3.5 to 4 month on the Peabody Gross Motor Scale for Development. He does demonstrate fairly good head alignment and can turn his head to observe toys. He does bear some weight after facilitation, can maintain a prone on elbows and extended arms for short periods of time. He has some skills in the 5 month range but these are scattered. In a prone position he maintains LE extension with adduction and plantar flexion of both feet. It is difficult for him to bear weight through his LE's even if properly aligned under his body. In a supine position, he is able to perform some alternate kicking but has difficulty overcoming gravity for UE play or hand/feet activities. In a propped 4-point alignment he can assume weight over UE's and LE's but has difficulty with full UE extension in this position. Sitting is a difficult position for him.

Prior Level of Function

Mobility (home and community): He is a fairly happy child. He sleeps well, has regular naps, laughs easily, will bat at toys and spin rolling objects. He is beginning to roll from prone to supine and supine to his side. He is on secondary foods.

Treatment Diagnosis: Developmental delay.

Assessment

Reason for skilled care: Child is a little boy who demonstrates moderate CP and developmental delay. His mom is eager to work with him and is very good at stimulating him as well as observing his movements and postures. Child seems motivated to move and play with toys, is very interested in a variety of toys and quickly picks up adaptations of how to activate toys. He has difficulties primarily with increase in muscle tone that makes it difficult for him to weight shift and demonstrate mobility of the UE's and LE's. He would benefit form formal PT as well as in the future, OT and speech and language therapy. Currently we are initiating a 1x/wk PT program to establish rapport and home programs with the family and will enhance formal intervention as family and physician seem to support.

Problems:

1. Decreased ROM LE's.
2. Decreased strength and control of UE's.
3. Decreased gross motor skills.

Plan of Care

Specific treatment strategies: PT for therapeutic exercise.
Frequency: 1x/wk.
Duration: Anticipate approximately one year.
Short-term goals and achievement dates:

1. Enhance ROM increase SLR to 75 degrees bilaterally.
2. Enhance weight bearing alignment in POE, 4-point, and sitting leaning on a bench surface so he can use UE's to maintain these positions with SBA for 30 seconds.
3. Facilitate gross motor development including commando crawling with facilitation, upright sitting, prone on extended arms play and standing with support.

Long-term goals and achievement dates:

1. Facilitate better tissue length and muscle strength to enhance development.

Case 12: Pediatric, Initial Evaluation Worksheet

1. Are the "essential elements" (defined in Chapter 1) for documentation present?

Essential Element	Y, N, or N/A	Comment(s)
Referral		
Reason	Y	
Specific treatment requested	Y	
Data Accompanying Referral		
Diagnosis/onset date	Y	A diagnosis of cerebral palsy is provided and the onset date is the same as the patient's date of birth. It is questionable if the onset date is accurate, as cerebral palsy is generally diagnosed after the patient has demonstrated delayed development. See Mechanism of injury.
Secondary diagnoses	Y	
Medical history	Y	This is a thorough and complete history. The patient's birth history as well as past and present medical conditions pertaining to rehabilitation are described.
Medications	N	Not addressed. It would be helpful to know what medications, if any, are being administered that may affect rehabilitation, such as Dilantin.
Comorbidities (complicating or precautionary information)	N	Not addressed. It is helpful to document *none* if precautionary information is not present to demonstrate that the area was addressed in the evaluation.
Physical Therapy Intake/History		
Date of birth	Y	Date of birth is documented. This is helpful information as many physician offices and third-party payers file and/or retrieve data based on the date of birth.
Age	Y	
Gender	Y	
Start of Care	Y	

(continued)

Essential Element	Y, N, or N/A	Comment(s)
Primary complaint	Y	The therapist documents the mother's insight into the patient's motor delays. This information helps in goal development and in determining the need for skilled care.
Referral Diagnosis		
Mechanism of injury	Y	Prematurity is indicated as the mechanism of injury. This would seem inappropriate. A reviewer may find it helpful to know the actual cause of the cerebral palsy, such as an intracranial hemorrhage or malformation of the brain.
Prior diagnostic imaging/testing	N	Not addressed. Documentation of the prior diagnostic testing that was completed to determine the diagnosis of cerebral palsy is needed.
Prior Therapy History	Y	The data indicate no prior therapy history. This helps the reviewer determine the present need for rehabilitation.
Baseline Evaluation Data		
Cognition	N	Not addressed. Data describing the patient's ability to follow simple commands or provide name recognition may be helpful in assessing cognition and the ability to participate in rehabilitation.
Vision/hearing	Y	Data indicate normal vision and hearing, although glasses are used to correct strabismus. It would be helpful to identify the source of this baseline data such as from a parent or an interdisciplinary team member's report.
Vital signs	N/A	
Vascular signs	N/A	
Sensation/proprioception	N	Not addressed. Data in this area may be important. For example, does the patient demonstrate tactile defensiveness? Abnormal responses in sensation may help to identify another need for skilled care.
Edema	N/A	
Posture	Y	Data are adequately described. However, details regarding the curvature of the spine are needed, such as the direction of the curve. A reviewer may also seek further information to explain the high trunk tone described, as it is an unusual presentation for a cerebral palsy patient.
AROM/PROM	Y	The evaluation indicates that range of motion is within normal limits with the exception of bilateral lower extremity abduction and straight leg raises. Differentiation between active and passive range of motion is needed, as well as a description of the resulting functional limitations.
Strength	N/A	Manual muscle testing at this age is not appropriate. However, data regarding use of extremities and purposeful movements would be helpful—for example, *When supported in sitting with a neutral pelvis can bring hands to midline.*
Pain	N	Pain with stretching/range of motion activities, if present, needs to be described.
Coordination	N	Not addressed as a separate area; however, data are provided in Special tests.
Bed mobility	Y	
Balance (sit and stand)	N	Not addressed as a separate area; however, data are provided in Special tests.
Transfers	N/A	Not applicable at this time.
Ambulation (level and elevated surfaces)	Y	The therapist documents that "In a standing alignment he can bear weight, although not in a flatfoot alignment." A description of the alignment would be helpful for future progress comparisons. For example, is the patient on his toes or in a supinated position? Where is the therapist providing support (i.e., under the upper extremities or with an assistive device)?
Orthotic/prosthetic devices	Y	

Essential Element	Y, N, or N/A	Comment(s)
Wheelchair use	Y	The therapist indicates that the patient does not use adaptive equipment. This would seem incomplete, as the patient has difficulty sitting. Data such as how the patient is positioned for feeding and bathing need to be described.
DME (using or required)	Y	
Activity tolerance	N	This area needs to be addressed, as the mother reports that the patient "feels very strong to her but seems frustrated at his inability to move or maintain a sitting position." Data describing how the patient moves in the home environment are needed. For example, are movements dominated by a primitive reflex? Is head righting present in a supported position? Does the patient stay where placed or roll to manipulate toys? When rolling, do the trunk and neck hyperextend?
Wound description, including incision status	N/A	
Special tests	Y	The Peabody Gross Motor Scale for Development is utilized, and although a detailed summary is documented, further objective data would be helpful for future comparison. For example, the statement "He has some skills in the 5 month range but these are scattered" could be improved by adding *these skills include rolling and prone with extended arms*. Details pertaining to how much assistance is required to obtain four-point and description of head control would be helpful. Also, what type of sitting is difficult? Functionally, is positioning in a car seat or a high chair challenging?
Architectural/safety considerations	N/A	Not applicable at this time.
Requirements to return to home, school, and/or job	N/A	
Prior Level of Function		
Mobility (home and community)	Y	The data indicating the patient's sleeping patterns and present mobility status are adequate. Additional information regarding use of a stroller and assistance for transfers and self care would be helpful.
Employment	N/A	
School	N/A	
Treatment Diagnosis	Y	
Assessment		
Reason for skilled care	Y	This description provides the reviewer with insight into the therapist's expectations for treatment and the patient's rehabilitation potential.
Problems	Y	Three problems are identified; however, a fourth problem, *Increased tone with abnormal posturing*, is needed. Also, Problem 2, "Decreased strength and control of upper extremities," needs to be expanded to include the lower extremities and trunk.
Plan of Care		
Specific treatment strategies	Y	Therapeutic exercise is the documented treatment strategy. This is vague, as the data indicate that more than one treatment strategy is needed. For example, adaptive positioning, initiation of crawling and rolling, and instruction in a home program, as well as assessment of seating/adaptive equipment needs for bathing, sitting, and feeding, would provide insight into the delivery of skilled rehabilitation.
Frequency	Y	
Duration	Y	In many such cases, third-party payers will approve a one-year duration.

(continued)

Essential Element	Y, N, or N/A	Comment(s)
Patient instruction/home program	N	Initiation of a home program is important. However, it can be overwhelming for both the parent and the patient at the time of evaluation. Data reflecting parent education that may have occurred during the evaluation are needed.
Caregiver training	N	See Patient instruction/home program.
Short-term goals and achievement dates	Y	The goals include a functional component except for Goal 1. Goal 1 may be better stated as, *Increase straight leg raise bilaterally to seventy-five degrees to improve sitting and standing posture in six weeks.* Goal 2 includes prone on elbows alignment problems; however, objective baseline data are lacking. Goal 3 would be enhanced if emphasis was placed on facilitating transitional movements. The goals are measurable except for Goal 3. All goals lack time frames.
Long-term goals and achievement dates	Y	The goal "Facilitate better tissue length and muscle strength to enhance development" is vague and lacks all three goal components. Age-appropriate skills are not identified. This goal would be better stated as *Facilitate motor development to allow independent mobility skills and age-appropriate play.*
Rehabilitation potential	N	Not addressed. Rehabilitation potential is an essential element of documentation. It provides the therapist's insight into the potential success of the rehabilitation intervention for the stated goals. This helps the reviewer assess the reasonableness of skilled care.

2. Is the overall history of the patient adequate?

Yes, a summary of the patient's past medical history and present functional level are provided. The mother appears to be an active player, and this reflects positively on potential for carryover in the home.

3. Is there evidence of the need for skilled intervention?

An adequate profile of the patient's functional deficits is presented. The therapeutic interventions described reflect that a level of skilled intervention is required. This is especially evident in the Special tests area, which indicates the patient's developmental age as scored using the Peabody Gross Motor Scale for Development.

4. Are there adequate baseline data to develop future comparisons?

Objective data are given in the areas of posture, range of motion, and bed mobility. However, there is a need to provide further detail for range of motion measurements (active versus passive); specific lengths of time for maintaining prone on elbows, upright sitting, and standing; distance for the commando crawl; and data regarding sensation.

5. Are the objective data related to functional deficits?

Yes, references to functional activities such as sitting, prone on elbows, standing, and crawling are described.

6. Are comparative statements and data clearly outlined?

Data reflect a delay in gross motor skills as defined by the Peabody Gross Motor Scale of Development. Description of standing deficits, head control, and bed mobility are provided.

However, further detailed objective data are needed regarding range of motion measurements (active versus passive), specific length of time for maintaining prone on elbows, upright sitting and standing, distance for the commando crawl, and data regarding sensation.

7. (A) Are the three components for goals present (measurable, functional, time frames)?

The goals are lacking in time frames and the third goal is not measurable. In addition, Goal 1 begins with "Enhance ROM," which is vague and requires specific range of motion measurements. Also, Goal 3 requires additional measurable information. How much and where should facilitation be applied for the commando crawl? Is the patient supported or independent in terms of positioning for upright sitting? How much assistance is required for standing? Is upper extremity support necessary, and what length of time is standing tolerated? Finally, the long-term goal "Facilitate better tissue length and muscle strength to enhance development" needs to relate to the development of independent mobility and age-appropriate play.

(B) Are the goals realistic for the individual case?

Yes, based on the data presented, it appears realistic to achieve the listed goals. It may prove difficult to achieve short-term Goal 3 (Facilitate gross motor development including commando crawling with facilitation, upright sitting, prone on extended arms play and standing with support) because of its limited measurability and the multiple components listed. The long-term goal is also vague and may be difficult to achieve, as the components for function and measurability are lacking.

8. Do you feel that the proposed treatment is reasonable and necessary?

Judging from this evaluation, treatment appears reasonable and necessary based on the diagnoses presented and evidence of a developmental delay. It may be a concern for the reviewer that, except for a notation in the assessment, there are no other data for establishing a home program and/or training of the family/caregiver. Education and home programming are expected to begin at the evaluation and need to be addressed in a short-term goal, as they are ongoing processes that require revisions and upgrades.

Case 12: Pediatric, Progress Report

Attendance: He attended 7 of 8, 2x/wk scheduled sessions.

Current Baseline Data

AROM/PROM: Child is showing increased tightness in his hamstrings as well as his adductors. Currently SLR can be achieved to 70 degrees and abduction can be achieved to 25 degrees. He has been slightly resistant to ROM activities, therefore, mom has been carrying out a program at home.

Bed mobility: He is now transitioning well prone to and from supine and moving into a slightly higher sidelying position. However, he lacks stability in his shoulder girdle showing excessive elevation in a high sidelying position and poor activity against the surface with his lower extremities.

Balance (sit and stand): Child is able to assume 4-point with minimal assistance and maintain for 30 seconds at this time. He is tolerating tall kneeling with UE support for up to 3 minutes without difficulty. Sitting continues to be a challenge for him as adduction continues to dominate in the sitting position secondary to weak trunk musculature. Side sitting is more effective and he can side sit for approximately 60 seconds with 1 UE support but is not able to actively maintain this position without external support for more than 1 minute period.

Transfers: Child is using symmetrical UE pulling with LE hip flexion and adduction. In treatment, it has been attempted to move to a more reciprocal type movement. However, this is quite a difficult pattern to break for him.

Ambulation (level and elevated surfaces): In standing, he is improving with his UE weight bearing and he will tolerate standing without back support and the support in his LE's for 30 seconds.

Orthotic/prosthetic devices: Child attended an orthopedic appointment on 6/15/95. At that time, Dr. ABC suggested Tone Reducing Ankle Foot Orthosis (TRAFO's) for him. However, the prescription has not been received by the clinic even though 3 contacts have been made to Dr. ABC. We will await prescription and then go ahead with fabricating TRAFO's.

Treatment Diagnosis: Developmental delay.

Assessment

Reason for skilled care: Child has resumed PT treatment in the clinic as the winter is now over. Initially this month he displayed crying and some other behaviors secondary to changing treatment to the clinic. However, his behavior seems to be modified and we can complete full sessions at this time. Mom continues to report that she is happy with the child's improved mobility as he is commando crawling across the floor at home.

Problems:

1. Decreased ROM.
2. Decreased strength and control of trunk and LE's.
3. Delayed gross motor skills.

Plan of Care

Specific treatment strategies: PT for therapeutic exercise, ROM, standing activities and gait.

Frequency: 2x/wk.

Patient instruction/home program: Mom is carrying out a ROM program at home.

Short-term goals and achievement dates:

1. (a) Increase straight leg raise bilaterally to 75 degrees. (b) Child will demonstrate 35 degrees bilaterally of hip abduction.
2. (a) Child will stand with minimal assistance and 1 UE support while playing for 2 minutes; Goal modified. (b) Child will assume and maintain high side lying while reaching x 5. (c) Child will tolerate tall kneeling with minimal assist for 3 minutes. Goal met. NEW GOAL: Child will maintain a 4-point position for 1 minute independently.
3. Child will commando crawl for 5 ft.
4. Child will maintain independent sitting with one UE support for 3 minutes.

Long-term goals and achievement dates:

1. Facilitate better ROM, muscle strength to enhance overall development.

Case 12: Pediatric, Progress Report Worksheet

1. Are the "essential elements" (defined in Chapter 1) for documentation present?

Essential Element	Y, N, or N/A	Comment(s)
Attendance	Y	Present information indicated, "He attended 7 of 8, 2x/wk scheduled sessions." The reason for absence needs to be described such as illness or canceled.
Current Baseline Data		
Cognition	N	Not addressed in the evaluation or progress report. Data describing the patient's cognitive status would be helpful to the reviewer for determining the potential challenges to rehabilitation and the need for skilled occupational therapy or speech–language pathology services.
Vision/hearing	N	The evaluation reported the use of glasses to correct the patient's strabismus. If visual deficits are affecting function, then a statement regarding this complicating factor is needed.
Vital signs	N/A	
Vascular signs	N/A	
Sensation/proprioception	N	Not addressed in the evaluation or progress report. If tactile defensiveness or hypersensitivity to touch exists, then the effect on function needs to be documented.
Edema	N/A	
Posture	N	Posture was addressed in the evaluation and is missing in this report. Are pregait activities challenged by postural imbalance? Is posture adversely affected by abnormal tone? Comparative data regarding posture will assist a reviewer in establishing the need for skilled care.
AROM/PROM	Y	Range of motion measurements are present for lower extremity abduction and straight leg raise. However, comparative data from the evaluation or a previous progress report are lacking. As reviewers do not always have prior information, it is helpful to provide comparisons. For example, *Hip abduction is 25 degrees, previously 35 degrees.* Also it would be helpful for active and passive range of motion to be differentiated, as well as how the range deficits affect function.
Strength	N/A	Specific manual muscle test grades are appropriately not listed based on the tonal influences affecting this patient and the patient's age. However, functional outcomes in the sections on bed mobility, balance, and ambulation reflect information on strength limitations.
Pain	N	A description of pain during stretching/range of motion is needed. Is pain the reason that the patient " has been slightly resistant to ROM activities"? The factors of pain along with the decrease in range of motion would provide the reviewer with data justifying the need for skilled care.
Coordination	N	The evaluation provided information in the Special tests area on coordination, specifically described as "alternate kicking." Comparative data would help demonstrate progress or lack of progress to the reviewer.
Bed mobility	Y	The descriptions "moving into a slightly higher sidelying position" and "poor activity against the surface with his lower extremities" may be confusing to a reviewer. This is especially true when rolling was the only activity documented in the evaluation.
Balance (sit and stand)	Y	Descriptions of sitting balance, four-point, and tall kneeling are provided. A reviewer may find it helpful to know where the patient is performing the skill, such as on tile or carpet. A description of short sitting balance would also be helpful.

Essential Element	Y, N, or N/A	Comment(s)
Transfers	Y	At the time of the evaluation this area was not appropriate for testing; however, is addressed in the progress report. Comparative data since the last progress report would be helpful for the reviewer, as well as the amount of assistance and type of transfers performed (e.g., ground to chair or ground to standing).
Ambulation (level and elevated surfaces)	Y	The data presented inform the reviewer that standing "is improving" and can be tolerated "without back support and the support in his LE's for 30 seconds." This description is vague, as comparative data are lacking. What was the prior level? Previously, the patient could not achieve a flatfoot alignment; can he do so now? There is also documentation indicating that "In standing, he is improving with his UE weight bearing." It would be helpful to know if the weight bearing is on a walker, parallel bars, or a table, and if the patient is placed in standing or can transition independently to standing.
Orthotic/prosthetic devices	Y	The patient's visit to the physician and the subsequent recommendation for TRAFO's is documented. It is suggested that the negative language stating, "However, the prescription has not been received by the clinic although 3 contacts have been made to Dr. ABC," be stated in a positive objective manner such as, *Awaiting physicians' order for TRAFO's. Calls placed to the physicians' office on (Date), (Date), and (Date).* By rephrasing the comment the therapist will avoid negative connotations about another health professional.
Wheelchair use	N	Not addressed. Data describing how the mother positions the patient for feeding and bathing are needed. Also, a description of how the mother assists the patient in mobility at home and in the community would be helpful.
DME (using or required)	N/A	Not applicable at this time.
Activity tolerance	N	Not addressed as a separate category; however, it is reflected appropriately in the balance and ambulation data.
Wound description, including incision status	N/A	
Special tests	N	Not addressed. The Peabody Gross Motor Scale for Development was scored in the evaluation. It would be reasonable to indicate the last formal testing date, scores, and the anticipated retesting date.
Architectural/safety considerations	N/A	
Treatment Diagnosis	Y	
Assessment		
Reason for skilled care	Y	The data provided do not indicate why the skills of a physical therapist are needed or contain expectation statements. An explanation of the relationship of hamstring tightness and the apparent lack of trunk control to function is needed. Is progress occurring, and if so, what further improvements can a reviewer expect? Also, the statement "Child has resumed PT treatment in the clinic as the winter is now over" may be confusing to a reviewer. What effect did winter have on the child? Was treatment canceled or were skilled services provided in the home? If provided in the home, a reviewer may assess the case to ensure that charges are reasonable and appropriately delivered within the third-party payer's guidelines.
Problems	Y	The problems are identified; however, they have been modified since evaluation. This is acceptable, provided that the changes were justified in prior progress reports. It is suggested that the addition of two problems be considered: *decreased trunk control and sitting posture* and *impaired weight shift and weight bearing in sitting and standing.*

(continued)

Essential Element	Y, N, or N/A	Comment(s)
Plan of Care		
Specific treatment strategies	Y	The evaluation listed one modality, therapeutic exercise. The progress report has described a thorough approach and has been appropriately expanded to also include range of motion, standing activities, and gait.
Frequency	Y	The progress report lists a frequency of two times per week. A reviewer may reasonably seek an explanation to justify the increase in frequency, as the evaluation indicated one time per week.
Duration	N	The evaluation anticipated a duration of one year. Duration is an essential element and needs to be addressed. A reviewer may seek clarification because of the increased frequency of service.
Patient instruction/home program	Y	The progress report appropriately indicates, "Mom is carrying out a ROM program at home." However, from a reviewer's perspective a more detailed account of the home program is needed, such as the muscle groups being emphasized.
Caregiver training	N	It is important to document dates of training, who was trained, and the demonstration of safe performance of the home program. Retraining and evidence of home program upgrades demonstrate skilled care.
Short-term goals and achievement dates	Y	The goals are measurable; however, there is a need to elaborate on function. For example, Goal 1a states, "Increase straight leg raise bilaterally to 75 degrees." Adding *to improve standing posture* provides a functional relationship. All goals lack a time frame for anticipated achievement.
Long-term goals and achievement dates	Y	The long-term goal is vague and lacks measurable and functional components. A reviewer may question what "better ROM" and "enhance overall development" entail.
Rehabilitation potential	N	Not addressed. Rehabilitation potential is an essential element of documentation. It provides the therapist's insight into the potential success of the rehabilitation intervention for the stated goals. This helps the reviewer assess the reasonableness of skilled care.

2. Is there evidence of the need for skilled intervention?

No, there is not a clear relationship describing the developmental motor delays or what skilled intervention is provided to inhibit tone or facilitate mobility. However, a home program is established and the patient appears to be functioning at a higher level in the home environment. A description of the home program upgrades would assist in justifying skilled intervention. For example, details of facilitory or inhibitory techniques used in treatment and taught to the mother for range of motion and sitting/standing activities would be helpful.

3. Are there adequate baseline data to develop future comparisons?

The data provided in the balance and range of motion areas will allow for future progress comparisons. However, measurable data are lacking for bed mobility, transfers, and ambulation.

4. Are the objective data related to functional deficits?

Yes, there is detail pertaining to functional deficits and outcomes in the areas of bed mobility, balance, and ambulation. However, data related to function are lacking for range of motion.

5. Are comparative statements and data clearly outlined?

Comparative data are implied through documentation such as "Child is showing increased tightness in his hamstrings" and "is improving with his UE weight bearing." Data and descriptions are presented but not compared to the evaluation or previous progress reports. It is important for the therapist to remember that the reviewer does not always have the evaluation or a previous progress report to reference. Therefore, before a coverage decision is rendered, these documents will often be requested by the third-party payer.

6. (A) Are the three components for goals present (measurable, functional, time frames)?

No, not consistently, particularly in regard to time frames, which are absent. Goals are measurable; however, they do not consistently relate to a functional outcome. For example, "Child will demonstrate 35 degrees bilaterally of hip abduction" lacks a functional component such as to improve standing posture.

(B) Are the goals realistic for the individual case?

Yes, however, duration is not specified, and the reviewer would want some indication of anticipated length of treatment.

7. Do you feel that the treatment was reasonable and necessary?

Yes, treatment appears reasonable and necessary based on the tonal challenges and the need for orthotic devices. Assurance of coverage could be enhanced by additional comparative data, as well as details of upgrades and training of the home program.

Case 13: Pediatric, Individualized Education Program (IEP)

Authors' note to readers: Acceptable format for IEPs varies somewhat from state to state, and new formats are often developed every few years. The following case study typifies a basic IEP format and the need for measurable functional goals that relate to the child's educational program. As the essential elements for IEP documentation are unique, a separate case study worksheet is provided. See below.

Present levels of educational performance: Gross motor skills are at the 11 to 12 month level.

Annual goal: John will increase his gross motor skills to 18 month level.

Short-term Objectives:

Short-term Objectives	Objective Criteria	Procedures	Schedule
John will develop balance reactions in standing.	70%	Clinical observation and documentation	Annually
John will ambulate 100 feet independently.	"	"	"
John will increase weight shift and transitional skills necessary for transitions from sitting to standing.	"	"	"
John will ascend and descend stairs with one railing and minimal assist.	"	"	"

Specific special education and related services which will contribute to meeting this goal: Physical Therapy

Case 13: Pediatric, Individualized Education Program Worksheet

1. Are the "essential elements" (defined in Chapter 1) for IEP documentation present?

Essential Element	Y, N, or N/A	Comment(s)
Present levels of educational performance	Y	The therapist provides the reviewer with the age equivalency for gross motor skills. However, a brief description of the functional skills observed in the school environment is needed. For example, *Gross motor skills are at the 11 to 12 month level. John sits in and transitions out of a variety of positions independently on the floor. He crawls independently and can pull up to standing on a stable object. He walks holding on to objects or with one hand held for 400–500 feet.*
Annual goal	Y	The annual goal is that the child will "Increase his gross motor skills to 18 month level." It is important to the reviewer that this goal be measurable and that it focus on functional outcomes. Documentation such as *Will increase gross motor skills to allow greater independence and safe mobility in the school environment by bringing gross motor skills to the 18 month level* would justify the need for skilled care.

(continued)

Essential Element	Y, N, or N/A	Comment(s)
Short-term objectives	Y	The following short-term objectives are listed on the IEP with the criteria to meet them 70% of the time based on clinical observation and documentation: 1. John will develop balance reactions in standing. 2. John will ambulate 100 feet independently. 3. John will increase weight shift and transitional skills necessary for transitions from sitting to standing. 4. John will ascend and descend stairs with one railing and minimal assist. These objectives are more meaningful if stated in functional terms that both parents and teachers can understand. It is important that the functional skills described relate specifically to the school environment and that the criteria developed to objectively measure each goal be specific. The following are examples of these concepts as related to the originally stated objectives: *1) John will walk from the classroom to the office and back with one hand held in five minutes. (4/5 trials)* *2) John will walk independently ten feet in the classroom from station to station. (3/5 trials)* *3) John will transition in and out of classroom chairs independently. (5/5 trials)* *4) John will walk up and down the bus steps with one hand held and one hand on the railing. (4/5 trials)*
Schedule	Y	The therapist lists the schedule (i.e., goal time frame) as "annually." Documentation regarding the extent of goal achievement needs to be more frequent than in the annual report. For instance, quarterly would seem to be a reasonable expectation.
Specific special education and related services which will contribute to meeting this goal	Y	The contributing service is listed as physical therapy. This is incomplete, and all staff who will be involved in facilitating one or more goals should be identified, such as the occupational therapist, classroom teacher, and classroom aides. The IEP is a general plan for the child and requires the specific input of each team member to be optimally effective.

Case 14: Skilled Nursing Facility, Initial Evaluation

Data Accompanying Referral

Diagnosis/onset date: L-Malleolus decubitus ulcer/12-03-96.

Secondary diagnoses: S/P CVA, progressive dementia.

Medical history: 89 year old female, long-term resident of ABC Care Center since 7-92. History of recurrent UTI's, History of R-Intraocular implant, History of TB.

Comorbidities (complicating or precautionary information): Wound Healing Risk Factors: Impaired mobility, nonambulatory, unable to achieve full-side rolling indep'ly, S/P CVA with questionable sensation on LLE, impaired circulation.

Physical Therapy Intake/History

Age: 89
Gender: Female
Start of care: 01-05-97

Prior Therapy History: Had prior PT at ABC Care Center.

Baseline Evaluation Data

Cognition: General: Alert/oriented to person; Disoriented to place/time; Able to follow commands; Slurred speech. Patient does not have knowledge of disability.

Vascular signs: See Wound description.

Sensation/proprioception: Light touch-impaired LLE but question cognition.

Posture: With unsupported sit, severely forward and to the left; Kyphotic thoracic spine; decreased lumbar extension.

AROM/PROM: RUE/RLE ROM WFLs, except R-ankle PF 0°; Tone: LUE/LLE hypotonic. LUE/LLE PROM limitations: Shld flex 130°, Shld ABD 120°, Shld external rotation 0°, Hip extension –20°, Knee extension –20°, Ankle DF 0°.

Strength: Unable to assess strength secondary to cognition and cooperation. L < R.

Pain: Denies any pain at rest.

Bed mobility: Rolling R/L, moving sideways and bridging requires Max A; Sit to/from supine requires Max A.

Transfers: Sit to/from stand, pivot and bed/chair/wheelchair transfers all require Max A.

Ambulation (level and elevated surfaces): Nonambulatory.

Wheelchair use: W/C position: Head control—forward flexion; Trunk control—leans left, but mostly forward; Has lap buddy which prevents severe forward flexion.

DME (using or required): Wheelchair.

Wound description, including incision status: Wound evaluation: L-lateral malleolus Stage IV, oblong in shape 2.6 cm inferior-superior x 1.9 cm, depth at anterior border 0.3 cm at midpoint with tunneling and green drainage; Depth at posterior border 0.1 cm, at superior border 0.2 cm, at middle of ulcer 0 depth. 25% of wound inferior aspect meaty red tissue, remaining of ulcer marbleized w/greenish yellow necrotic tissue (10% of red/pink tissue). No odor noted. Drainage on dressing noted with slightly brownish red drainage at inferior aspect and dime-size amount of greenish drainage. Inflamed pink area around periphery approximately 1 cm; Wound debrided to 50% clean; Foot purplish with decreased circulation; Appeared to be Stage IV inflammatory stage.

Prior Level of Function

Mobility (home and community): Previously ulcer-free.

Treatment Diagnosis: L-Malleolus decubitus ulcer.

Assessment

Reason for skilled care: In summary, patient appears to be a good candidate for skilled P.T. services with emphasis on closure of wound and prevention of additional skin breakdown; will continue with whirlpool to increase circulation.

Problems:

1. L-Malleolus decubitus.
2. Dec'd bed mobility.

Plan of Care

Specific treatment strategies: Ther activities, wound care, whirlpool, electrical stim or US.

Frequency: 5x/wk.

Duration: 8 weeks.

Patient instruction/home program: Restorative nursing recommendations—Reposition patient every 2 hours while in bed, and keep left-lateral malleolus in a pressure-free position utilizing pillow. Please utilize figure 8 dressing with paper tape.

Short-term goals and achievement dates:

1a. Wound will be necrotic free. (2 wks)

1b. Wound will demonstrate beefy red granulation base. (3 wks)

1c. Wound will be free of infection thru course of wound healing. (6 wks)

2. Able to initiate 1/2 side rolling to Rt., utilizing bedrail with Min A for L-side pressure relief. (4 wks)

Long-term goals and achievement dates:

1. Achieve partial thickness wound closure and prevent further skin breakdown.

Rehabilitation potential: Good

Case 14: Skilled Nursing Facility, Initial Evaluation Worksheet

1. Are the "essential elements" (defined in Chapter 1) for documentation present?

Essential Element	Y, N, or N/A	Comment(s)
Referral		
Reason	N	The reason for skilled therapy involvement versus nursing care is not defined. Is the referral due to nursing observation of wound deterioration despite attempts to promote wound closure with topical applications and/or proper positioning to alleviate pressure? A statement such as *Patient referred by Dr. ABC for physical therapy to promote wound closure as prior interventions including wet to dry dressings and positioning have been unsuccessful*, would help justify skilled intervention.
Specific treatment requested	N	As physician involvement is required by most third-party payers, it is helpful to document the specific treatment requested to ensure reimbursement. For example, *Daily whirlpool and electrical stimulation to the left malleolus—Stage IV ulcer, debridement, positioning and bed mobility training.*
Data Accompanying Referral		
Diagnosis/onset date	Y	
Secondary diagnoses	Y	Secondary diagnoses include a status post cerebrovascular accident and progressive dementia. It would be helpful for the reviewer to know whether the cerebrovascular accident involves the right or left extremities because of the potential sensation deficits and positioning challenges. In this case, the reviewer needs to study the baseline data to determine that the secondary diagnosis is a status post *right* cerebrovascular accident.
Medical history	Y	The history indicates prior medical conditions unrelated to wound care and describes the patient as a long-term resident. The history does not describe prior and/or present wound care treatments used by nursing that were/are successful, or more importantly, unsuccessful. Listing the therapeutic interventions previously performed and their effect on wound closure would help a reviewer decide that the most clinically appropriate and cost-effective treatment is being provided.
Medications	N	Not addressed. It is important to indicate present medications or recent changes in medication that may provide insight into the patient's circulatory impairment, such as anticoagulants.
Comorbidities (complicating or precautionary information)	Y	The list of wound healing risk factors is helpful for the reviewer when determining the appropriateness of the treatment duration.
Physical Therapy Intake/History		
Date of birth	N	Patient identifying information is important, as many physician offices and third-party payers file or trigger data retrieval based on date of birth.
Age	Y	
Gender	Y	
Start of Care	Y	
Primary complaint	N	Not addressed. The patient's primary complaint needs to be identified. Is pain, limited mobility, or risk of amputation a concern?
Referral Diagnosis		
Mechanism of injury	N	Not addressed. It is important to include the date of onset and course of events that have occurred or contributed to the present decubitus ulcer. For example, are positioning challenges, nutritional risk factors, and/or circulatory deficits contributing factors?

Essential Element	Y, N, or N/A	Comment(s)
Prior diagnostic imaging/testing	N	If testing of the circulatory system (e.g., Doppler) was performed, it needs to be documented.
Prior Therapy History	Y	The statement "Had prior PT at ABC Care Center" is incomplete. It would be helpful for the reviewer to know what type of intervention the patient received and the discharge status. Did the prior intervention emphasize mobility skills related to the cerebrovascular accident or wound care?
Baseline Evaluation Data		
Cognition	Y	
Vision/hearing	N	Not addressed. It is important to evaluate vision and hearing, as deficits may directly affect the patient's ability to participate in therapeutic activities, positioning changes, and nutritional intake.
Vital signs	N	Not addressed. Information regarding distal pulses is important and should be documented.
Vascular signs	Y	See Wound description.
Sensation/proprioception	Y	The data indicate that light touch appears impaired in the left lower extremity. This information helps the reviewer determine the need for the skills of a therapist to safely perform the treatment modalities prescribed for promoting wound closure.
Edema	N	Not addressed. It would be beneficial for the reviewer to know that this area was assessed by the therapist and not overlooked. Based on the location and depth (Stage IV) of the wound, baseline measurements may be indicated for future comparisons.
Posture	Y	Postural deficits are described. However, data specific to left lower extremity positioning in bed are needed.
AROM/PROM	Y	Active and passive range of motion deficits are provided. However, the relationship to functional deficits is needed. For example, is bed mobility or positioning affected?
Strength	Y	The therapist indicates the cognitive challenges to manual muscle testing. A reviewer would find it helpful to know if the patient's strength is sufficient to perform functional activities such as rolling, scooting, and/or bridging.
Pain	Y	The patient "Denies any pain at rest" per the therapist's documentation. This description is brief. It would be beneficial for the reviewer to know if movement results in pain. If yes, then the location of pain and its effect on function are needed.
Coordination	N	Not addressed. As the data indicate that the patient has a secondary diagnosis of a cerebrovascular accident and that the left extremities are hypotonic, it is reasonable to expect documentation pertaining to coordination because of the potential effect on mobility training and positioning.
Bed mobility	Y	The therapist identifies key areas that affect positioning such as bridging and rolling.
Balance (sit and stand)	N	Not addressed. Based on the postural deficits described, it is reasonable to expect that balance deficits may affect positioning of the lower extremities. Baseline data would provide the reviewer with another reason for skilled care.
Transfers	Y	
Ambulation (level and elevated surfaces)	Y	

(continued)

Essential Element	Y, N, or N/A	Comment(s)
Orthotic/prosthetic devices	N/A	It seems that data pertaining to orthotic/prosthetic devices are not applicable because of the patient's nonambulatory status. However, wound closure may be compromised, as the left extremity is hypotonic and pivot transfers are performed. It would be important to document use of a device, if applicable.
Wheelchair use	Y	A description of wheelchair positioning is given. Further data regarding the effects of lower extremity positioning on wound closure are needed.
DME (using or required)	Y	
Activity tolerance	N	This an apparent omission. The patient's ability to tolerate therapeutic exercises and proper positioning for the duration of treatment is not provided. Activity tolerance would have a direct effect on the patient's rehabilitation potential.
Wound description, including incision status	Y	The wound description is detailed and thorough. It provides data pertaining to the wound's location, size, drainage, odor, stage, and tissue description. The data also indicate that debridement was performed. If treatment such as ultrasound was performed, it needs to be documented.
Special tests	N	Not addressed. Any special tests should be listed and the clinical relevance briefly explained (e.g., doppler).
Architectural/safety considerations	N/A	
Requirements to return to home, school and/or job	N/A	
Prior Level of Function		
Mobility (home and community)	Y	Data indicate that the patient was "Previously ulcer-free." This description is helpful; however, additional information regarding the patient's functional mobility is needed, such as, *Patient performed rolling independently and transitional movements with minimal assist upon discharge from PT (date).*
Employment	N/A	
School	N/A	
Treatment Diagnosis	Y	
Assessment		
Reason for skilled care	Y	The therapist indicates that treatment emphasis will be on wound closure and that whirlpool will increase circulation. It would be helpful to provide an expectation statement that the patient will improve. For example, *In view of the multiple wound healing risk factors (impaired circulation, questionable sensation left lower extremity, and impaired mobility), this patient will benefit from skilled services to debride necrotic tissue and stimulate fibroblast mobilization. Therapeutic activities will help in positioning and facilitation of wound closure.*
Problems	Y	Two problems are identified. This demonstrates a focused treatment plan.
Plan of Care		
Specific treatment strategies	Y	The treatment strategies include therapeutic activities, wound care, whirlpool, and electrical stimulation or ultrasound. Use of multiple wound care modalities is not acceptable to most third-party payers. In this case the justification to use whirlpool to improve circulation is provided; however, the therapist needs to clarify whether electrical stimulation or ultrasound is the other modality of choice.
Frequency	Y	
Duration	Y	

Essential Element	Y, N, or N/A	Comment(s)
Patient instruction/home program	Y	Restorative nursing recommendations are documented.
Caregiver training	N	The therapist provides restorative nursing recommendations. However, documentation of an actual training session is needed to further justify the importance of skilled physical therapy intervention.
Short-term goals and achievement dates	Y	
Long-term goals and achievement dates	Y	
Rehabilitation potential	Y	

2. Is the overall history of the patient adequate?

No, the history of this patient is unclear and the prior level of function is vague. The data provided do not give the reviewer a clear picture of the patient. For instance, what was the patient's prior level of function in terms of ambulation, transfers, and, more importantly, for bed mobility/self-positioning skills and their effect on skin integrity?

A reviewer would also benefit from data related to prior and present wound treatment methods performed by nursing and/or physical therapy. It is unclear if the history of prior therapy treatment was related to mobility skills or wound care. Additional history would provide the reviewer with a better knowledge base to determine if the plan of care is reasonable and necessary.

3. Is there evidence of the need for skilled intervention?

It is apparent that skilled intervention is needed based on the severity of the wound (Stage IV), complicating factors (hypotonicity and sensation deficits), and the level of functional immobility.

4. Are there adequate baseline data to develop future comparisons?

The wound description is excellent and will lend itself well to future comparisons. However, data are lacking in areas such as edema, left extremity active range of motion, and positioning.

5. Are the objective data related to functional deficits?

The emphasis of this evaluation appears to be wound care; however, the data leave a lot to inference. For instance, was there a functional regression in bed mobility, transfers, and/or ambulation because of the wound? The prior level of function is not stated in regard to these areas. Is maximal assistance required for bed mobility because of strength, the status post

cerebrovascular accident, pain, and/or cognition? Depending on the third-party payer, these omissions may result in a shorter length of approval for treatment.

6. Are comparative statements and data clearly outlined?

Wound data are present. Data in the areas of edema, left extremity active range of motion, activity tolerance, and the amount of verbal cuing for safe performance of bed mobility activities are lacking.

7. (A) Are the three components for goals present (measurable, functional, time frames)?

All goals have time frames and are appropriate. The wound baseline data provided in the evaluation described the size/amount of drainage and listed percentages. The short-term goal would be enhanced if percentages and measurements were used. By using this strategy, the therapist would clearly define the amount of progress, and subsequent achievement of goals, for the reviewer.

Goal 1b may be difficult to understand for a reviewer who is unfamiliar with wound care terminology. A suggested revision: *Wound base will demonstrate beefy red appearance <u>consistent with new capillary formation</u> in 3 weeks.*

(B) Are the goals realistic for the individual case?

Yes, the goals appear realistic.

8. Do you feel that the proposed treatment is reasonable and necessary?

Based on the fact that this is a Stage IV wound, it appears that skilled care is reasonable and necessary.

Case 14: Skilled Nursing Facility, Discharge Report

Attendance: Ill. 01-26-97, expired 01-27-97.

Current Baseline Data

AROM/PROM: Initially, ROM R-extremities WFL's, LLE: Hip ext –20°, Knee extension –20°; Presently, R-extremities ROM WFL's; LLE –20° hip extension (S), –20° knee extension (S).

Strength: Unable to follow directions for MMT. Initially unable to assess strength secondary to cognition and cooperation, left < right.

Bed mobility: Initially Max A for R/L rolling, moving sideways and bridging; Max A for sit to/from supine. Presently, requires Max A for all mobilities.

Transfers: Sit to stand, pivot and toilet transfers with Max A. Presently, requires Max A for all transfers.

Ambulation (level and elevated surfaces): Initially nonambulatory; Presently, nonambulatory.

Wound description, including incision status: Initially, L-lateral malleolus Stage IV, 2.6 cm x 1.9 cm x .3 cm, 25% of wound meaty, red tissue remaining marbleized with greenish yellow necrotic tissue. No odor/drainage noted. Presently, wound measures as of 01-24-97, 2.1 cm x 2.0 cm x .3 cm after debridement, serous drainage, yellow eschar tunneling noted; Patient receiving whirlpool to L malleolus along with HVPC, 5x/week.

Treatment Diagnosis: L-Malleolus decubitus ulcer.

Assessment

Reason for skilled care: Whirlpool to keep infection free and HVPC to help promote fibroblast mobilization. Patient discharged from physical therapy secondary to expiring on 01-27-97.

Problems:

1. L-Malleolus decubitus.
2. Dec'd bed mobility.

Plan of Care

Specific treatment strategies: Ther Activities, Wound Care, Whirlpool, Electrical Stim or US.

Frequency: 5x/wk.

Duration: 8 wks.

Patient instruction/home program: Not applicable. Pt. expired.

Short-term goals and achievement dates:

1a. Wound will be necrotic free—Met.

1b. Wound will demonstrate beefy red granulation base. (3 wks)

1c. Wound will be free of infection thru course of wound healing. (6 wks)

2. Able to initiate 1/2 side rolling to Rt., utilizing bed rail with Min A for L-side pressure relief. (4 wks)

Long-term goals and achievement dates: Achieve partial thickness wound closure and prevent further skin breakdown.

Rehabilitation potential: Good.

Case 14: Skilled Nursing Facility, Discharge Report Worksheet

1. Are the "essential elements" (defined in Chapter 1) for documentation present?

Essential Element	Y, N, or N/A	Comment(s)
Attendance	Y	Two dates are listed with a corresponding reason for absence. It is recommended that the number of visits scheduled be identified.
Current Baseline Data		
Cognition	N	Not addressed. The evaluation described cognition. Comparative data at the time of discharge, especially changes that may have affected participation in rehabilitation, need to be documented.
Vision/hearing	N	This area is not addressed in the evaluation or discharge report. Any deficits that affect the patient's ability to participate in therapeutic activities, positioning changes, and nutritional intake would help justify the need for the skills of a therapist.
Vital signs	N	Not addressed in the evaluation or discharge report. Information regarding distal pulses is important and should be documented.
Vascular signs	N	Vascular signs were addressed in the evaluation; however, they are lacking in the discharge report. A reviewer may reasonably question if the whirlpool treatment could have been performed by nonskilled personnel.

Essential Element	Y, N, or N/A	Comment(s)
Sensation/proprioception	N	The evaluation indicated that light touch appeared impaired in the left lower extremity. However, this complicating factor is lacking in the discharge report. It is important to document sensation deficits, as they reinforce the need for the skills of a therapist to safely use treatment modalities such as electrical stimulation and whirlpool.
Edema	N	Although not addressed in the evaluation or discharge report, any deficits in edema would be important for a reviewer to be aware of when determining if the care provided was skilled.
Posture	N	Not addressed. Posture was described in the evaluation. Comparative data would help the reviewer identify challenges affecting left lower extremity positioning and wound healing.
AROM/PROM	Y	Comparative data are appropriately provided for active range of motion and indicate no change in status. A reviewer would find it helpful if the skilled approach to treatment and barriers to progress were described in terms of a functional outcome in order to determine the reasonableness of skilled care. For example, *Static stretch performed within patient's tolerance to improve hip extension for rolling. Pain monitored.* Also comparative data for passive range of motion are needed. Terminology such as "(S)" may not be familiar to a reviewer.
Strength	Y	The therapist indicates comparative data regarding the cognitive challenges to manual muscle testing. However, a reviewer would find it helpful to know if the patient's strength was sufficient to initiate functional activities such as rolling, scooting, and/or bridging.
Pain	N	Pain is not addressed in the discharge report. If the patient experienced pain during rehabilitation, it would be important for a reviewer to know that when determining the reasonableness of the skilled care provided.
Coordination	N	Not addressed in the evaluation or discharge report. If deficits exist, comparative data are needed because of the potential effects on mobility training and positioning.
Bed mobility	Y	Comparisons are provided, and no progress has occurred since the evaluation. A reviewer may question the effectiveness of therapeutic activities and retrospectively deny treatment related to mobility. This decision may be because evidence of ongoing skilled training or complicating factors such as pain and decreased strength are lacking.
Balance (sit and stand)	N	This area is not addressed in the evaluation or discharge report. It is reasonable to expect that balance deficits exist that may affect positioning and bed mobility training. Comparative data would demonstrate another need for skilled care.
Transfers	Y	Comparisons are provided, and no progress has occurred since the evaluation. A reviewer may question the effectiveness of therapeutic activities and retrospectively deny treatment related to mobility. This decision may be because evidence of ongoing skilled training or complicating factors such as pain and decreased strength are lacking.
Ambulation (level and elevated surfaces)	Y	
Orthotic/prosthetic devices	N/A	Orthotic/prosthetic use is not identified in the evaluation or discharge report and appears not applicable in this case. If a device exists, the amount of use and/or need for adaptation should be described because of the potential impact on skin integrity.

(continued)

Essential Element	Y, N, or N/A	Comment(s)
Wheelchair use	N	Wheelchair positioning is described in the evaluation. However, comparative data are lacking in the discharge report. A reviewer would find it helpful to know the skilled approach used to improve wheelchair positioning and the resultant effects, if any, on lower extremity positioning or nutritional intake.
DME (using or required)	N	Not addressed. This is an apparent oversight by the therapist, as the patient requires maximal assistance for mobility and the evaluation indicated use of a wheelchair.
Activity tolerance	N	The patient's tolerance for participation in rehabilitation is not provided. Data would be helpful for a reviewer to retrospectively assess the patient's functional limitations.
Wound description, including incision status	Y	Comparative data regarding the wound are provided. The modalities used are listed. However, data on modality parameters are not provided, such as the length of treatment and water temperature.
Special tests	N/A	
Architectural/safety considerations	N/A	
Treatment Diagnosis	Y	
Assessment		
Reason for skilled care	Y	The therapist indicates the treatment rationale for use of high-volt pulsed current and the reason for discharge. This information, although helpful, does not provide the reviewer with data supporting the effectiveness of the treatment provided before the patient expired. Also, in a retrospective review process, the whirlpool may be found to be maintenance in nature, as the discharge data provided does not support the presence of circulatory deficits.
Problems	Y	
Plan of Care		
Specific treatment strategies	Y	The treatment strategies listed include therapeutic activities, wound care, whirlpool, and electrical stimulation or ultrasound. Use of multiple wound care modalities is not acceptable to most third-party payers. In this case, the whirlpool appears maintenance in nature and electrical stimulation is the modality of choice. It is recommended that the therapist avoid the appearance of an *as needed* modality, in this case ultrasound, as it has the potential to be interpreted as unreasonable.
Frequency	Y	The summary provided for the frequency and duration for the period in question helps the reviewer determine if the functional progress reported is reasonable. It can also help when analyzing documentation and the corresponding services billed.
Duration	Y	See Frequency.
Patient instruction/home program	Y	The therapist indicates that a home program (restorative nursing recommendations) is not applicable as the patient expired. Although this is true, a summary of the recommendations in place through discharge would help emphasize that skilled care was provided.
Caregiver training	N	Although the patient expired, it is important to summarize any teaching and training previously provided to the patient and/or nursing as evidence of skilled care.
Short-term goals and achievement dates	Y	The goals for the period in question are provided, and one goal has been met. It would be helpful to describe the status of all goals at discharge.

Essential Element	Y, N, or N/A	Comment(s)
Long-term goals and achievement dates	Y	It would be helpful to list the status of the goal at discharge.
Discharge prognosis	Y	The discharge prognosis is appropriately not listed, as the patient expired. However, the therapist provided the rehabilitation potential. It would be helpful to clarify that this was the potential to meet the goals established prior to the patient's expiration.

2. Is there evidence of the need for skilled intervention?

Wound care is skilled based on the severity of the wound (Stage IV) and the progress reported (wound is free of necrotic tissue and has decreased in size). However, the need for skilled intervention for mobility is not described.

3. Are there adequate baseline data to develop future comparisons?

Baseline data were adequate, allowing comparisons of evaluation to discharge in the key treatment areas for this report, such as wound description, bed mobility, and strength. However, data in the areas of edema, range of motion, and amount of verbal cuing for bed mobility training are lacking.

4. Are the objective data related to functional deficits?

There is no direct relationship to functional deficits. This is particularly evident in the area of bed mobility skills. To justify bed mobility skills (therapeutic activities as listed in the plan of care), a reviewer would seek to identify barriers to progress such as pain or strength deficits.

5. Are comparative statements and data clearly outlined?

Comparative statements are present, particularly for the areas of wound description, transfers, range of motion (although active and passive were not clearly differentiated), and bed mobility. Comparative data are lacking for cognition, durable medical equipment, posture, and wheelchair use.

6. (A) Are the three components for goals present (measurable, functional, time frames)?

Yes, however the status of all goals at discharge is not clearly described.

(B) Are the goals realistic for the individual case?

Yes, except for Goal 2, which states "Able to initiate 1/2 side rolling to Rt., utilizing bedrail with Min A for L-side pressure relief." The data do not support the expectation that progress could occur in the area of bed mobility.

7. Do you feel the treatment was reasonable and necessary?

It was felt that the electrical stimulation provided was reasonable and necessary based on the wound description. The use of whirlpool, unless defined as a sterile technique and/or for improving circulation, presents as maintenance in nature and does not require the skills of a therapist. Improving bed mobility also is not reasonable or necessary, as it appears to be a long-standing problem and cognitive deficits may prevent the patient from benefiting from participation in a rehabilitation program. Depending on the third-party payer, additional evidence of the need for whirlpool and the patient's ability to participate in therapeutic activities may be needed.

It also seems that, in the amount of time that had passed, a restorative program could have been established for nursing to carry out all activities, except the electrical stimulation for wound care. All other modalities may be denied after two weeks, which appears to be enough time to establish a safe and effective restorative program in this particular case.

Case 15: Skilled Nursing Facility, Initial Evaluation

Data Accompanying Referral

Diagnosis/onset date: CVA/10-07-96.
Secondary diagnoses: TIAs and UTIs.
Medical history: 74 year old resident, difficult to get history.
Comorbidities (complicating or precautionary information): G-tube.

Physical Therapy Intake/History

Age: 74
Gender: Male
Start of care: 10-28-96

Baseline Evaluation Data

Cognition: General status: Alert, cooperative and able to follow commands. Oriented to person. Place/time unable to ascertain due to decrd. communication ability. Communication is aphasic.
Vision/hearing: Appears WFL.
Vital signs: Respiratory: G.
Sensation/proprioception: Not able to test secondary to speech.
Posture: Erect. Leans/falls to L.
AROM/PROM: ROM/Strength: LUE is WFL throughout, strength 0 throughout. RUE is WFL throughout, strength WFL throughout. LLE is WFL throughout, strength: Hip Ext and Knee Ext T/P; Hip Abd/Add T; IR/ER NT; all others 0. RLE is WFL throughout, strength WFL throughout. Tone: LUE/LLE flaccid. RUE/RLE normal.
Strength: See AROM/PROM.
Coordination: Gross/Fine: R = G. L = 0.
Bed mobility: Requires Max assist throughout.
Balance (sit and stand): Sitting F. Direction of loss to the L w/Mod assist to correct. Standing P. Direction of loss to the L w/Max assist to correct.
Transfers: Requires Max assist throughout. Toileting NT.
Ambulation (level and elevated surfaces): Not able to walk.
Activity tolerance: Good.
Wound description, including incision status: Skin appears intact.

Prior Level of Function

Mobility (home and community): Appears patient was independent in all mobility prior to CVA.

Treatment Diagnosis: Debility.

Assessment

Reason for skilled care: This 74 year old man was independent in mobility prior to CVA on 10-07-96. He will require skilled long-term care to regain Max independence in functional mobility.

Problems:

1. Decreased strength.
2. Max assist to perform bed mobilities.
3. Max assist to perform transfers.
4. Inability to walk.

Plan of Care

Specific treatment strategies: Eval, Ther Ex, Ther Activities and Gait Training.
Frequency: 5x/wk.
Duration: 4 wks.
Patient instruction/home program: Restorative nursing recommendations: Will need to provide Max assist w/all functional mobility, but encourage him to assist. Reposition every 2 hrs to retain skin integrity.
Short-term goals and achievement dates:

1. P strength in LLE. (4 wks)
2. Resident will perform sit to/from supine w/Mod assist. (4 wks)
3. Resident will do a stand pivot transfer w/Mod assist. (4 wks)
4. Resident will walk 1 length of parallel bars w/Mod assist. (4 wks)

Long-term goals and achievement dates:

1. Resident will perform bed mobility/transfers independently and will walk w/CGA and large base quad cane.

Rehabilitation potential: Fair.

Case 15: Skilled Nursing Facility, Initial Evaluation Worksheet

1. Are the "essential elements" (defined in Chapter 1) for documentation present?

Essential Element	Y, N, or N/A	Comment(s)
Referral		
Reason	N	The reason for referral is not stated. Documentation such as *Patient referred by Dr. ABC for rehabilitation following a recent cerebrovascular accident to regain independent mobility for return to home* would help justify the need for skilled care.
Specific treatment requested	N	Not addressed. Most third-party payers require physician involvement as a prerequisite for payment. A statement reporting the initial physician's order is needed.
Data Accompanying Referral		
Diagnosis/onset date	Y	The diagnosis/onset of a "CVA/10-07-96" is present; however, whether the diagnosis has resulted in left or right hemiparesis is not specified. A reviewer would find it helpful if this information was clearly presented.
Secondary diagnoses	Y	
Medical history	Y	The therapist documents, "74 year old resident, difficult to get history." This medical history is brief and incomplete. Additional data pertaining to the cause of the cerebrovascular accident, such as hypertension, hemorrhage, or thrombosis, and the history of hospitalization, if applicable, are needed.
Medications	N	Not addressed. Given the neurological diagnosis of a cerebrovascular accident, it would be helpful to know what medications, if any, are being administered that may affect rehabilitation, such as anticoagulants.
Comorbidities (complicating or precautionary information)	Y	
Physical Therapy Intake/History		
Date of birth	N	Not addressed. Patient identifying information is important, as many physician offices and third-party payers file or trigger data retrieval based on date of birth.
Age	Y	
Gender	Y	
Start of Care	Y	
Primary complaint	N	Not addressed. It is important to document the concerns that led the patient to seek rehabilitation.
Referral Diagnosis		
Mechanism of injury	N	Not addressed. The course of events leading to the diagnosis helps give the reviewer insight into the patient's rehabilitation potential and need to be documented.
Prior diagnostic imaging/testing	N	Not addressed. It is reasonable to expect that diagnostic testing such as an MRI was performed. This information may be relevant to the case at this time.
Prior Therapy History	N	It would seem reasonable that the patient was hospitalized and physical therapy services were initiated in the acute care setting, as the patient has a history of TIAs and a diagnosis of a cerebrovascular accident. Information about the focus of any prior treatment and the patient's functional status would be relevant for continuity of care. If no therapy history exists, then a statement such as *No therapy history noted in the medical record* would be helpful to the reviewer in assessing the present skilled therapy needs.

(continued)

Essential Element	Y, N, or N/A	Comment(s)
Baseline Evaluation Data		
Cognition	Y	
Vision/hearing	Y	
Vital signs	Y	Respiratory status is reported as "G". As no pulmonary diagnoses are documented, the relevance of this brief description is questionable. Baseline pulse rates and blood pressure measurements may be needed because of the diagnosis of a cerebrovascular accident of unknown origin.
Vascular signs	N/A	
Sensation/proprioception	Y	Sensation/proprioception was not tested "secondary to speech." This would be better stated as *Testing incomplete secondary to communication barrier as the patient appears unable to answer yes/no consistently because of expressive aphasia.*
Edema	N	Not addressed. Because of the flaccid tone reported in the left extremities, it is reasonable to expect that edema may be present and could affect positioning, range of motion, and/or mobility. Documentation of circumference measurements and the type of edema (pitting or nonpitting) would demonstrate another need for skilled care.
Posture	Y	Data indicate that posture is "Erect. Leans/falls to L." A description of whether this assessment occurred in sitting or standing and how it affects functional activities (such as safety during activities of daily living and/or wheelchair propulsion) would be helpful for future progress comparisons.
AROM/PROM	Y	Descriptions of range of motion and strength measurements are summarized. It would be helpful to differentiate between active and passive range of motion.
Strength	Y	There appears to be inconsistent information regarding the left lower extremity strength. The documentation states that active range of motion is present at the left hip and knee (strength T/P) but also describes the left lower extremity as "flaccid." This inconsistency may be confusing to a reviewer.
Pain	N	No data are present. Clinical observation regarding possible pain should be noted. Those observations should not depend on verbal responses from the patient.
Coordination	Y	
Bed mobility	Y	Bed mobility is described as "Requires Max assist throughout." Additional data would be helpful for future progress comparisons. Is the patient able to initiate movement? Are verbal cues required? Is balance a limiting factor?
Balance (sit and stand)	Y	Sitting and standing balance deficits are described in terms of direction of loss and the amount of assistance to correct. Additional detail relating the balance deficits to functional activities such as transfers, ambulation, and wheelchair propulsion would be helpful in determining the need for skilled care.
Transfers	Y	Transfers are described as "Requires Max assist throughout. Toileting NT." Additional data would be helpful for future progress comparisons. Is the patient able to initiate movement? Are verbal cues required? Is balance a limiting factor?
Ambulation (level and elevated surfaces)	Y	The evaluation indicates that the patient is "Not able to walk." Additional data would be helpful for future progress comparisons. For instance, can the patient bear weight through the lower extremities in standing? What is the patient's posture? How much assistance is needed to stand?

Essential Element	Y, N, or N/A	Comment(s)
Orthotic/prosthetic devices	N	The data indicate that the left extremities are flaccid, the patient is unable to walk, and transfers require maximal assistance. If an orthotic device is used to increase joint stability and prevent injury, it should be documented.
Wheelchair use	N	Not addressed. This is an apparent oversight by the therapist. It is reasonable to expect that the patient requires the use of a wheelchair. Data pertaining to the patient's positioning in the wheelchair and ability to propel the wheelchair safely would be helpful in identifying another need for skilled care.
DME (using or required)	N	See Wheelchair use.
Activity tolerance	Y	The patient's activity tolerance for participation in rehabilitation needs to be expanded. The patient presents with an acute cerebrovascular accident, requires maximal assistance for mobility, and has decreased functional strength. For example, *Patient tolerates thirty minutes of bed mobility training at this time.*
Wound description, including incision status	Y	
Special tests	N/A	
Architectural/safety considerations	N	If the long-term goal is to return home, then that environment needs to be assessed.
Requirements to return to home, school and/or job	N	A clear statement of the requirements to return home, if applicable, should be provided. The documentation does not provide insight into the patient's long-term goal. Is the goal return to home, or was the patient a long-term resident of a skilled nursing facility? This information is important to the reviewer for future assessment of functional progress and the duration of care.
Prior Level of Function		
Mobility (home and community)	Y	The therapist documents, "Appears patient was independent in all mobility prior to CVA." This statement is inconclusive. Was the patient independent? A reviewer may question the accuracy of this prior level, as the medical history was "difficult to get" and the patient is aphasic. It is important to accurately report the prior level of function by seeking data from the patient, other interdisciplinary team members, and/or family.
Employment	N/A	
School	N/A	
Treatment Diagnosis	Y	The therapist indicates "Debility" as the treatment diagnosis. This is a weak diagnosis for justifying the need for skilled physical therapy service. From a reviewer's perspective, debility may imply that the patient will recover mobility through the course of routine daily activities with nonskilled personnel. In this case, the treatment diagnosis may be better addressed as a *gait abnormality*.
Assessment		
Reason for skilled care	Y	The reason for skilled care restates the prior level of function and the need for "skilled long-term care to regain Max independence in functional mobility." Based on the evaluation data, the prior level of function (independent in mobility) is questionable in accuracy. A statement such as *Patient requires the skills of a therapist to improve balance and facilitate use of left extremities following a recent cerebrovascular accident to regain independent mobility.* would help justify the need for skilled care.
Problems	Y	Four problems are identified. This demonstrates a focused treatment plan.

(continued)

Essential Element	Y, N, or N/A	Comment(s)
Plan of Care		
Specific treatment strategies	Y	
Frequency	Y	
Duration	Y	A four-week duration is documented. Based on the functional deficits, a longer duration such as eight weeks is suggested.
Patient instruction/home program	Y	
Caregiver training	N	Not addressed. This area is an apparent oversight by the therapist because of the flaccid tone in the left lower extremities and potential for injury. A reviewer would expect instruction to the patient, nursing, and/or family. Documentation of actual training would demonstrate another need for skilled therapy.
Short-term goals and achievement dates	Y	The three goal components are present except for Goal 1, which does not contain a functional component. Goal 1 states, "P strength in LLE. (4 wks)." The addition of the phrase *to allow standing in parallel bars* would be helpful.
Long-term goals and achievement dates	Y	The long-term goal is stated, however, it would be helpful if the reviewer knew the number of feet the patient was expected to ambulate. It is also suggested that a functional phrase alternative be used for "walk" (e.g., *ambulate*.)
Rehabilitation potential	Y	Given that the rehabilitation potential is presented as "fair," it is recommended that this be further clarified in the assessment. A reviewer may question the rehabilitation potential, as the documentation does not provide complicating factors or comorbidities that would hinder progress.

2. Is the overall history of the patient adequate?

No, the history is inadequate. Accuracy of the prior level of function is questionable. A documented commitment by the therapist to ensure accuracy would be beneficial—for instance, *"Will contact social services to confirm prior level of function."* The patient's prior place of residence is also unclear. It would be helpful for a reviewer to know if the patient lived at home with family or was a long-term nursing home resident. It is also important to establish in the documentation information regarding hospitalization for the cerebrovascular accident or if any prior therapy was rendered for this diagnosis.

3. Is there evidence of the need for skilled intervention?

The skills of a physical therapist are needed because of the acute onset date of the cerebrovascular accident, the presence of flaccid extremities, and documented limitations in strength, balance, and mobility.

4. Are there adequate baseline data to develop future comparisons?

There are adequate baseline data for range of motion, balance, and strength. Further detail would be helpful in the areas of bed mobility, transfers, ambulation (standing), and wheelchair propulsion skills.

5. Are the objective data related to functional deficits?

A relationship between the functional deficits in bed mobility, transfers, and ambulation in regard to the patient's impaired strength, range of motion, and balance is not provided. How-ever, it seems practical that a reviewer could identify the relationship based on the data presented.

6. Are comparative statements and data clearly outlined?

The data are clearly outlined except for vital signs, posture, ambulation, activity tolerance, and wheelchair use.

7. (A) Are the three components for goals present (measurable, functional, time frames)?

The three goal components are present with the exception of Goal 1, which does not contain a functional component. Goal 1 states, "P strength in LLE. (4 wks)." The addition of the phrase, *to allow standing in parallel bars* would be helpful. The long-term goal "Resident will perform bed mobility/transfers independently and will walk w/CGA and large base quad cane," could be improved if a phrase such as *to allow return to home* or *to and from the dining room* was added. Also, replacing the term "walk" with *ambulation and specifying a distance for ambulation* is recommended to demonstrate skilled care.

(B) Are the goals realistic for the individual case?

Yes, based on the objective data provided the goals are realistic. However, it is questionable that the long-term goal can be achieved in a duration of four weeks.

8. Do you feel the proposed treatment is reasonable and necessary?

The proposed treatment is reasonable and necessary based on the acute diagnosis, abnormal tone, diminished strength, and limited mobility.

Case 15: Skilled Nursing Facility, Progress Report

Attendance: Scheduled 5x/wk, missed 12-25-97—holiday.

Current Baseline Data

Strength: In LLE is F– to F hip; P+ to F– knee; Ankle continues at 0.

Bed mobility: Rolls L independently; R w/CGA and VC. Sit to supine w/Mod assist. Supine to sit w/Min assist and VC.

Balance (sit and stand): Sitting G. Can stand for 1 min. x 8 in parallel bars, w/assist only to facilitate L-knee ext. Dynamic standing: continues to need Min+ assist, due to decrd weight shift to R and decrd consistency of L-knee ext.

Transfers: Continues to come to stand w/Min assist and pivots continue to require Min/Mod assist.

Ambulation (level and elevated surfaces): Was ambulating 50' x 2 w/large base quad cane. Needs Min assist to block L-knee 25% of the time and for balance. Places cane properly 75% of the time w/o VC.

Wheelchair use: Is in an appropriate w/c. Wheels around facility independently.

Treatment Diagnosis: Debility.

Assessment

Reason for skilled care: Resident initially made G progress, then was placed on Haldol™, due to severe agitation on the nursing unit. PT was not informed of this, but did note a regression and documented as such. As this regression continued, we discussed this w/nursing and learned of the medication change. Nursing is now in the process of decreasing the Haldol™, and we anticipate improvement as the medication decreases. Family continues to want to take resident home. Resident is regular in attendance and family is supportive. Resident remains impulsive, but less so than documented previous month. Is showing somewhat better judgement. Has begun to progress again, now that medication has been reduced.

Problems:

1. Decreased strength.
2. Max assist to perform bed mobilities.
3. Max w/ability to perform transfers.
4. Inability to walk.

Plan of Care

Specific treatment strategies: Ther Ex, Ther Activities, Gait Training.

Frequency: 5x/wk.

Duration: 4 wks.

Patient instruction/home program: Restorative nursing recommendations: Emphasis on repositioning patient in w/c when he complains of discomfort. Must sit patient all the way back in the chair so buttocks are fully supported.

Short-term goals and achievement dates:

1. F+ strength in LLE to improve LLE wt. bearing. (4 wks)
2. Resident will perform all bed mobility w/supervision. (4 wks)
3. Resident will do a stand/pivot transfer w/supervision. (4 wks)
4. Resident will walk 100' x 2 w/large base quad cane and CGA of 1. (4 wks)

Long-term goals and achievement dates: Resident will perform bed mobility/transfers w/CGA and will walk w/large base quad cane for 200' x 2 w/CGA.

Rehabilitation potential: Fair.

Case 15: Skilled Nursing Facility, Progress Report Worksheet

1. Are the "essential elements" (defined in Chapter 1) for documentation present?

Essential Element	Y, N, or N/A	Comment(s)
Attendance	Y	The data describe the scheduled frequency, a date of absence, and the reason for absence. This is helpful for the reviewer.
Current Baseline Data		
Cognition	N	This appears to be an oversight by the therapist, as the reason for skilled care indicates impaired judgement, agitation, and impulsiveness. Any changes in cognition since the evaluation need to be reported. The reviewer will seek documentation indicating that the patient is able to actively participate in the rehabilitation program.

(continued)

Essential Element	Y, N, or N/A	Comment(s)
Vision/hearing	N	As this area was addressed in the evaluation and deficits were not reported, further documentation is not required unless a functional change occurs.
Vital signs	N/A	If applicable, data pertaining to deficits that affect rehabilitation should be reported.
Vascular signs	N/A	
Sensation/proprioception	N	Following a cerebrovascular accident, it is possible that neglect of an extremity may occur. If applicable, this should be documented.
Edema	N	Not addressed in the evaluation or progress report. If present, deficits that affect function need to be described.
Posture	N	This functional area is addressed in the evaluation; however, it is absent in the progress report. Given the patient's balance deficits, it seems appropriate to provide postural data.
AROM/PROM	N/A	The evaluation data indicated that range of motion was within functional limits. As this is not a defined problem area, it is appropriately not addressed.
Strength	Y	The therapist provides left lower extremity strength grades. Comparative data for the reviewer are needed. A reviewer may also find it helpful to know the skilled approach to treatment. Does the patient participate in an individualized strengthening program? Are physical cues necessary to prevent muscle substitution? What skilled facilitation techniques are used (i.e., vibration, proprioceptive neuromuscular facilitation)?
Pain	N/A	
Coordination	N	Data pertaining to changes in coordination of the left extremities would be helpful. For example, *Patient is able to place the left lower extremity appropriately to achieve a safe base of support during gait training. Previously required moderate physical assist.*
Bed mobility	Y	Data indicates the amount of assistance for bed mobility. Further data indicating the amount of verbal cuing and comparative statements are needed. For example, data describing rolling as "R w/CGA and VC" would be better described as, *Rolling to right with contact guard assist and minimal verbal cuing to initiate reaching with left upper extremity. Previously required moderate assistance and maximal verbal cues.*
Balance (sit and stand)	Y	Balance is described; however, comparative data would help the reviewer determine functional progress.
Transfers	Y	Data pertaining to balance are provided. However, statements such as, "*Continues* to come to standing . . . " may be interpreted as maintenance. A reviewer may question the need for transfer training unless additional data are provided that indicate barriers to progress, skilled training, or safety concerns.
Ambulation (level and elevated surfaces)	Y	Ambulation is described in terms of quality, level of assistance, distance, device, and safety. Comparative data are needed to help the reviewer determine functional progress. Also, the data begin with the statement, "*Was* ambulating" This may be difficult for a reviewer to understand. Has the regression occurred since the medication change? What is the present status? A regression in functional skills due to complicating factors may help to justify an extended duration of skilled care.
Orthotic/prosthetic devices	N	Not addressed. If an orthotic device is used to increase knee or ankle stability, it needs to be documented. In this case ankle strength is zero and it would seem reasonable to assess the need for an ankle foot orthosis.

Essential Element	Y, N, or N/A	Comment(s)
Wheelchair use	Y	Although data are provided and indicate the patient's independence in wheelchair use, comparative data are lacking and a reviewer would be unable to determine if functional progress occurred.
DME (using or required)	N	Not addressed. This is an oversight by the therapist, as the patient uses a wheelchair and a cane.
Activity tolerance	N	Activity tolerance is not addressed in the progress report. Data such as tolerance for standing activities would be helpful for assessing functional limitations.
Wound description, including incision status	N/A	
Special tests	N/A	
Architectural/safety considerations	N	Architectural/safety considerations were not documented in the evaluation. Based on the patient's progress, data should be included at this time. For example, will the patient return home, and are stairs and/or curbs potential barriers? Is a home assessment required?
Treatment Diagnosis	Y	The therapist indicates "Debility" as the treatment diagnosis. This is a weak diagnosis for justifying the need for skilled physical therapy service. From a reviewer's perspective, debility may imply that the patient will recover mobility through the course of routine daily activities with nonskilled personnel. In this case, the treatment diagnosis may be better addressed as a *gait abnormality*.
Assessment		
Reason for skilled care	Y	The reason for skilled care describes the complications from a medication change that resulted in a functional regression. It also provides a statement indicating expected progress. This helps the reviewer when determining a reasonable treatment duration.
Problems	Y	Four problems are identified. This demonstrates a focused treatment plan. However, the problems as listed do not take into consideration the patient's progress and need to be rewritten to reflect that progress.
Plan of Care		
Specific treatment strategies	Y	
Frequency	Y	
Duration	Y	
Patient instruction/home program	Y	Restorative nursing recommendations are provided in the evaluation and progress report. Program upgrades are not clearly identified. It is important that carryover to nursing be indicated, as progression and/ or regression of the patient's program is another means for justifying skilled care. Objective data to guide caregivers in the amount of assistance for transfers and transitional skills are needed.
Caregiver training	N	Teaching and training of caregivers are not mentioned. The reason for skilled care notes a regression, and yet no evidence of the need for skilled training of caregivers is provided. A reviewer may be concerned about the limited attempt at carryover and limit the coverage duration.
Short-term goals and achievement dates	Y	All three goal components are present. The goals are measurable, functional, and time-specific.
Long-term goals and achievement dates	Y	The evaluation indicated a long-term goal of independent mobility. Presently this has been revised to contact guard assistance. It would be helpful to indicate the date of revision and clarify in the goal whether the patient will remain in the long-term care setting or return to home with supportive services.
Rehabilitation potential	Y	

2. Is there evidence of the need for skilled intervention?

Yes, skilled care appears necessary based on the objective data such as strength, balance deficits, challenges described in standing, and the patient's gait quality. The reason for skilled care may be strengthened with the addition of the clinical needs of the patient. For example, *Patient is an excellent candidate for continued skilled care because of the need for facilitation of strength in the left lower extremities, improvement of balance and safety to achieve contact guard assistance for transfers, bed mobility and ambulation.*

3. Are there adequate baseline data to develop future comparisons?

The data presented for standing balance, bed mobility, strength, transfers, and ambulation are adequate to allow for future progress comparisons.

4. Are the objective data related to functional deficits?

The objective data pertaining to balance deficits are linked to standing activities. The relationship of strength to functional deficits in ambulation, bed mobility, or transfers is not clearly described.

5. Are comparative statements and data clearly outlined?

Data pertaining to the defined problem list are evident. However, comparative statements are lacking throughout this report. The authors suggest that comparisons be clearly indicated. This will eliminate the potential for the reviewer to draw an erroneous conclusion regarding functional progress.

6. (A) Are the three components for goals present (measurable, functional, time frames)?

Yes.

(B) Are the goals realistic for the individual case?

No, the measurable components of short-term Goals 2 and 3 are inconsistent with the long-term goal. They indicate that supervision is required for bed mobility and transfers; however, the long-term goal indicates contact guard assistance. A reviewer may reasonably request clarification.

7. Do you feel that the treatment was reasonable and necessary?

Yes, but depending on the third-party payer, the authors would authorize a limited number of additional visits and expect improvement in transfers, bed mobility, and ambulation along with increased documentation of carryover to nursing. Clarification of the goals would also be requested.

Case 16: Subacute, Initial Evaluation

Referral

Reason: Pt. is admitted now to ABC facility because she is not ambulatory and is unable to care for herself.

Data Accompanying Referral

Diagnosis/onset date: S/P L hip fx ORIF/03-15-95.
Secondary diagnoses: Atrial fib, S/P CVA/10-94, S/P MVR, S/P CABG, adult onset DM, arthritis, ASHD, anemia, HTN, S/P THR 1990 R.
Medical history: DX: Fractured L hip, comminuted peritrochanteric fx. ORIF done 03-16-95 with Richard hip screw.
Comorbidities (complicating or precautionary information): Per order Dr. XYZ—orthosurgeon: LLE to be protected from unusual stress. To be nonwt. bearing. 1 attendant to be responsible for protecting LLE during transfers.

Referral Diagnosis

Mechanism of injury: Pt. fell at home 03-15-95 while transferring from bed to commode.

Baseline Evaluation Data

Cognition: Oriented to person, not to place or time; alert; motivation—good; directives ability—good, follows 3 step commands. Poor short-term memory.
Sensation/proprioception: Normal. Light touch intact R and L LE's.
Edema: Edema—yes. Pitting edema to knee.
Posture: Lies supine with LLE externally rotated. Standing—flexed hips and R knee—does not come to full standing.
AROM/PROM: Pt. is R handed.

Physical Therapy Intake/History

Gender: Female
Start of care: 03-28-95

	RIGHT			LEFT		
COMMENT	MMT	ROM	LOCATION	ROM	MMT	COMMENT
Tight sh abd flex beyond 90 degrees	G–/P–	WFL/WFL	Shoulder EXT/ FLX	WFL/WFL	G–/G–	
	G–/P–	WFL	ADD/ABD	WFL/WFL	G–/G–	
	NT	WFL	IR/ER	WFL	NT	
	G/G	WFL	Elbow EXT/FLX	WFL	G+/G	
	G+/G+	WFL	SUP/PRO	WFL	G+/G+	
	N/N	WFL	Wrist EXT/FLX	WFL	N/N	
	G	WFL	Grasp	WFL	G+	
			Other			
	G–/G	/90	Hip EXT/FLX	/65	Not tested due to recent FX	
	F+/F–	0/–4	ADD/ABD	0/10		
	X	WFL/WFL	IR/ER	0/WFL		Not measured—not enough hip and knee flexion
	G–/G	–22/WFL	Knee EXT/FLX	–20/WFL		
	N/cannot break contraction	–6/WFL	Ankle DF/PF	–10/WFL		

Strength: See AROM/PROM.
Pain: Pain—yes. Just distal to knee 6/10. Denies L hip pain.
Bed mobility: Max assist sit to and from supine. Mod assist rolling R and L.

Balance (sit and stand): CGA supported (bilat UE's) static and dynamic on side of bed. Patient unable to balance unsupported in sitting. Max assist to assume standing in parallel bars. Once on her feet required mod assist to maintain standing. Plus 1 person to support and align LLE and maintain.

Transfers: Max assist of 3. (2 assists for sliding board transfer plus 1 assist to support and align LLE, bed to and from w/c.)

Ambulation (level and elevated surfaces): Pt. nonambulatory. Pt. NWB LLE. Gait analysis: Sit to stand at parallel bars—1 max, 1 mod assist and 1 contact guard assist to ensure NWB LLE.

Wheelchair use: W/C mobility max assist.

Activity tolerance: Standing endurance 10 sec.

Architectural/safety considerations: Lives in 1 story home with 1 step at entrance.

Requirements to return to home, school and/or job: Daughter can assist Pt. with transfer and amb. (no lifting) post. discharge.

Prior Level of Function

Mobility (home and community): Pt. lives with 91 yr. old husband and daughter. Ambulated with walker indep. level surfaces. Negotiated steps with rail and SBA.

Treatment Diagnosis: Functional dependence, generalized weakness.

Assessment

Reason for skilled care: Pt. assets: Able to follow directions, good family support. Pt. liabilities: Decreased AROM hips, knees and ankles; R shoulder flexors and abductor muscles less than antigravity strength, pain left knee, decreased short-term memory, functional dependence, generalized weakness and NWB status LLE. Pt. is a good candidate to improve ROM, strength and thereby functional ability.

Pt.'s progress will depend somewhat on healing of the L hip fracture her wt. bearing status.

Plan of Care

Specific treatment strategies: Hot packs to L knee for pain relief, strengthening and ROM exercises trunk, UE's and RLE, AAROM ex. LLE, functional training (bed mobility, transfers, pre-gait activities progressing to ambulation as M.D. orders for wt. bearing change, safety training), caregiver instruction, w/c mobility training.

Frequency: 6x/wk, 7 as tolerated.

Duration: 3 months.

Caregiver training: Goals and plans reviewed with patient, staff, family/significant others.

Short-term goals and achievement dates:

1. Pt. will propel w/c 15 ft with verbal cues, tactile cues to get her started—on straight path.
2. Pt. will roll to either side with min assist, sit up and lie down with mod assist of 1.
3. Pt. will perform sliding board transfer with 1 mod assist and 1 to protect LLE.
4. Pt. will stand in parallel bars with mod assist and 1 assist to protect LLE for 15 sec.
5. Pt. caregivers will be knowledgeable in providing necessary assistance with bed transfers.

Long-term goals and achievement dates:

1. Pt. will be independent in bed mobility.
2. Patient will be independent in w/c management.
3. Pt. will perform stand pivot transfers w/c, chair, bed, toilet, WB LLE as ordered by physician with CGA.
4. Ambulation goals to be set when Pt. is allowed wt. bearing.

Rehabilitation potential: Good.

Case 16: Subacute, Initial Evaluation Worksheet

1. Are the "essential elements" (defined in Chapter 1) for documentation present?

Essential Element	Y, N, or N/A	Comment(s)
Referral		
Reason	Y	The reason for referral is stated. A reviewer can determine the need for skilled care as the patient is "not ambulatory and is unable to care for herself."
Specific treatment requested	N	Physician involvement is a common reimbursement requirement. Documenting the physician's initial order will help the reviewer identify that this requirement has been met.
Data Accompanying Referral		
Diagnosis/onset date	Y	

Essential Element	Y, N, or N/A	Comment(s)
Secondary diagnoses	Y	Secondary diagnoses are listed and provide the reviewer with insight into the patient's multiple deficits that may affect the frequency, duration, and/or tolerance of an extensive rehabilitation program. It is important to realize that abbreviations may not be understood by the reviewer. For example, "S/P MVR" is an unfamiliar diagnosis and needs to be clarified.
Medical history	Y	The therapist appropriately documents the date and type of hip surgery performed. More information specific to the secondary diagnoses and their effect on rehabilitation may also be helpful to the reviewer.
Medications	N	Not addressed. Based on the complexity of the diagnoses listed, it seems appropriate to indicate medications that may affect rehabilitation, such as anticoagulants or narcotics.
Comorbidities (complicating or precautionary information)	Y	Weight-bearing restrictions are described. This information is helpful to the interdisciplinary team in terms of patient safety and to the reviewer when determining the need for skilled care.
Physical Therapy Intake/History		
Date of birth	N	Not addressed. Patient identifying information is important, as many physician offices and third-party payers file or trigger data retrieval based on date of birth.
Age	N	It may be helpful for a reviewer to know the patient's age in the overall assessment of rehabilitation potential and for identification purposes.
Gender	Y	
Start of Care	Y	
Primary complaint	N	Not addressed. Information regarding the patient's primary complaint would provide the reviewer with insight into the patient's goals and/or potential barriers to functional progress.
Referral Diagnosis		
Mechanism of injury	Y	The therapist indicates that the patient fell while transferring from the bed to the commode. This is important information to a reviewer, as it identifies a functional task that will require evaluation to ensure the patient's safety.
Prior diagnostic imaging/testing	N	Not addressed. It is reasonable to expect that an x-ray was performed. This information may be relevant to the case, especially because of the patient's nonweight-bearing status.
Prior Therapy History	N	Not addressed. Secondary to the multiple secondary diagnoses, such as "S/P CVA/10-94" and "S/P THR 1990 R", it is reasonable to expect that the patient has received previous physical therapy services. If applicable, it would be helpful to know how the patient responded to the prior therapy intervention to help determine the patient's rehabilitation potential.
Baseline Evaluation Data		
Cognition	Y	Despite poor short-term memory, the documentation supports the patient's ability to follow directives. This demonstrates to the reviewer that the patient can actively participate in the rehabilitation program.
Vision/hearing	N	Not addressed. Given the age and multiple diagnoses of this patient, a reviewer would find it helpful to know if visual and/or hearing deficits exist that may affect rehabilitation.
Vital signs	N	Not addressed. It is reasonable to expect baseline vital sign data regarding pulse rate and blood pressure, as the secondary diagnoses indicate hypertension, arteriosclerotic heart disease, and a history of coronary artery bypass grafts.

(continued)

Essential Element	Y, N, or N/A	Comment(s)
Vascular signs	N	Not addressed. It is reasonable to expect baseline data, such as skin color and/or skin temperature of the lower extremities, because of the recent surgical intervention.
Sensation/proprioception	Y	
Edema	Y	"Pitting edema to knee." is documented. However, specific measurements of edema comparing the left and right lower extremities would be helpful. Further description of the pitting edema and how/if the edema limits function is needed.
Posture	Y	A description of left lower extremity positioning in supine and "flexed hips and R knee" in standing is provided. It would be helpful to include the position of the head and trunk to enhance the understanding of potential deficits in balance and ambulation.
AROM/PROM	Y	Data are provided for range of motion measurements. However, differentiation of passive and active range of motion and what functional limitations exist is needed. The data omit certain measurements such as shoulder external and internal rotation. Also, some of the range of motion data appear implausible, such as hip abduction/adduction, which is listed as "0/–4" for the right lower extremity.
Strength	Y	Numerous upper and lower extremity muscle groups are addressed and provide the potential for effective comparative data. However, because of the apparent inconsistencies in available data, it is difficult to formulate specific comparisons. A description of how strength deficits affect function is needed.
Pain	Y	A numerical score of "6/10" and the location of pain are stated. It is important when using a pain scale to define the rating. For example, is 10 maximal pain or absence of pain? Also, is the pain a chronic problem (arthritis) or acute in nature?
Coordination	N	Not addressed. Reference to the patient's ability to demonstrate coordination of the upper extremities, for use of a walker, would assist the reviewer in assessing another potential deficit area requiring the skills of a therapist.
Bed mobility	Y	Bed mobility requires "Max assist sit to and from supine. Mod assist rolling R and L," per the therapist's documentation. It might be helpful to know what limits the patient in rolling. Is it pain, decreased strength, and/or trunk/pelvic immobility?
Balance (sit and stand)	Y	Although addressed, further data pertaining to the direction of balance loss, inability to weight shift, pain, and/or strength deficits would better describe the patient's balance deficits for future comparison (e.g., *Patient exhibits sitting balance loss to the left and posteriorly when reaching for objects and requires contact guard assistance to correct*).
Transfers	Y	
Ambulation (level and elevated surfaces)	Y	A detailed description is provided in terms of the amount of assistance, device, and weight-bearing status. The therapist's use of terminology such as "gait analysis" helps demonstrate the need for the skills of a therapist.
Orthotic/prosthetic devices	N/A	
Wheelchair use	Y	The patient requires maximal assistance for wheelchair mobility in the evaluation. If the patient can initiate or assist in the propulsion of the wheelchair, this should be described.
DME (using or required)	N	Not addressed. This is an oversight by the therapist, as the patient used a walker prior to hospitalization.

Essential Element	Y, N, or N/A	Comment(s)
Activity tolerance	Y	Data indicate "Standing endurance 10 sec." Further description of where the patient is standing, how much support is required, and how the patient resumes sitting (i.e., safely or with assist) would be helpful. The use of a functional phrase alternative for "endurance" is also recommended, such as *functional activity tolerance.*
Wound description, including incision status	N	Not addressed. The status of the surgical site is relevant in regard to potential soft tissue injury.
Special tests	N/A	
Architectural/safety considerations	Y	
Requirements to return to home, school and/or job	Y	Data indicate "Daughter can assist Pt. with transfer and amb. (no lifting) post. discharge." Further detail of lifting activity restrictions and the availability of the daughter and husband for assistance would help to establish goals for safe discharge to home.
Prior Level of Function		
Mobility (home and community)	Y	
Employment	N/A	
School	N/A	
Treatment Diagnosis	Y	The treatment diagnoses are "functional dependence" and "generalized weakness." A functional phrase alternative such as *functional strength deficit* is recommended, as "generalized weakness" may imply that improvement could occur without skilled therapy intervention.
Assessment		
Reason for skilled care	Y	A detailed assessment is provided. The division of assets and liabilities provides a clear picture of the patient's functional status.
Problems	N	Not addressed. It is helpful to determine the problems in order to focus treatment. In this case the assessment describes the patient's liabilities; however, this description does not correspond to the short-term goals established.
Plan of Care		
Specific treatment strategies	Y	The detailed list of treatment strategies is helpful to a reviewer in assessing the reasonableness of the treatment plan.
Frequency	Y	The frequency is documented as "6x/wk, 7 as tolerated." A nonvariable frequency is recommended. It would be more appropriate to indicate a treatment frequency of *7x/wk* and describe the reason for absence in the Attendance section of upcoming reports.
Duration	Y	Although this patient is elderly and has complicating factors, three months could be viewed as excessive by a third-party payer. More appropriate to this case would be an eight-week duration.
Patient instruction/home program	N	Not addressed. Home program/restorative nursing recommendations should be initiated at the time of evaluation and upgraded as the patient progresses. A reviewer would want to know who was trained in what functional activities and when.
Caregiver training	Y	The data indicate that the goals and plan were reviewed with the patient, staff, and family. Although patient involvement is important, training is not identified. Information pertaining to who was trained, when, and in what is needed.
Short-term goals and achievement dates	Y	The goals are comprehensive; however, they lack time frames.
Long-term goals and achievement dates	Y	
Rehabilitation potential	Y	

2. Is the overall history of the patient adequate?

Overall the history is adequate. However, given the multiple diagnoses and cardiopulmonary deficits, the reviewer might appreciate additional information, such as how these diagnoses contribute to the functional deficits.

3. Is there evidence of the need for skilled intervention?

A clear picture of the patient is presented to justify the need for skilled intervention. The therapist presents a diverse amount of baseline data indicating the need for skilled therapy intervention in areas such as bed mobility, transfers, range of motion, and ambulation.

4. Are there adequate baseline data to develop future comparisons?

Yes. The baseline data are described and provide a clear picture of the patient's deficits. To enhance comparative data for future notes, additional description of coordination, sitting, and standing balance may be helpful. Also, the data pertaining to range of motion and strength need to be consistent.

5. Are the objective data related to functional deficits?

Most of the data are related to functional deficits; however, they could be enhanced in the areas of posture, AROM/PROM, strength, edema of the knee, and balance. It would also seem important to differentiate active and passive range of motion, particularly at key joints such as the ankle, hip, and knee.

6. Are comparative statements and data clearly outlined?

The data described are clearly outlined and will provide a springboard for comparative data in future notes.

7. (A) Are the three components for goals present (measurable, functional, time frames)?

The goals are well written; however, they do lack time frames. Goal 5, "Pt. caregivers will be knowledgeable in providing necessary assistance with bed transfers," would be more measurable if rewritten as *The patient will perform bed transfers safely with moderate assist from nursing personnel in 2 weeks*. It also would be beneficial for the reviewer to know if return to home is a long-term goal.

(B) Are the goals realistic for the individual case?

Yes, the patient has multiple comorbidities and a lengthy medical history. These factors are considered in the evaluation and the treatment plan. The goals appear realistic for this individual.

8. Do you feel that the proposed treatment is reasonable and necessary?

Based on the data provided and the justification for skilled intervention, physical therapy intervention appears reasonable and necessary. The patient appears to have good potential to improve in all functional deficit areas. However, the reviewer may monitor the patient's rehabilitation potential to return home with family because of the limited short-term memory described.

Case 16: Subacute, Discharge Report

Reader please note: The authors have prepared this example presuming the reviewer has all prior reports available.

Attendance: 71 visits.

Current Baseline Data

Posture: Posture is flexed, hips and knees, which pt. can partially correct with cues. CGA and cues for safe technique.

Pain: Patient does not c/o left hip pain—Pt. c/o L distal knee pain which limits weight bearing activities.

Bed mobility: At beginning of month: Rolling side to side required SBA and occ. cuing for technique and sequencing. Pt. inconsistently laid down with SBA and cues (or min. assist to lift LLE). Pt. sat up with SBA and no cues. At discharge: Rolling and sit to and from supine done with SBA and occasional cues for technique. If lying down to R side, pt. uses bedrail on hosp. bed, in step fashion, to lift LE's onto bed.

Transfers: At beginning of month: Sit to stand—CGA from w/c or high mat table. Min assist from low armless surfaces plus cues for sequencing. CGA and cues in stand pivot transfers WBAT LLE. Cues for safety and technique. Car transfer done with CGA and cues to car, min. assist from car (assist to stand up from low car seat). At discharge: Sit to stand—SBA from w/c and all mat tables and beds. Cues for hand placement. Care transfer done with CGA and cues, using walker. Bed, chair and toilet transfers done with SBA (and approx. 25% cuing).

Ambulation (level and elevated surfaces): At the beginning of month: WBAT LLE. Used wheeled walker. Endurance varied from 15–50 ft. level surfaces. Endurance limited by Pt. c/o L knee pain primarily, fatigue secondarily. Gait characterized by flexed hips and knees. Pt. exhibited antalgic gait on LLE. Cues required for walker placement, correct technique with sit to and from stand. Steps-min/mod assist (inconsistent) to ascend 1 step with walker, CGA to descend plus cues. At discharge: WBAT LLE. Uses std. walker. Level surfaces 25–65 ft. Endurance limited by pt. c/o knee pain. SBA (CGA if pt's knees begin to flex). Pt. has antalgic gait on L. Curbs—Pt. is able to negotiate 1 step with walker (curb) with CGA and cues for technique. Stairs—with 2 rails require CGA of 1 and cues. Stairs with 1 rail requires CGA of 2 at times mod. assist (inconsistent). However, pt's endurance does not permit a walk of more than 5 ft. to and from stairs/curb plus negotiating stairs/curbs.

Wheelchair use: At beginning of month: Indep. around P.T. gym. 130 ft. Cues to apply brakes. Cues to mod. assist to manage footrests. At discharge: Indep. around P.T. gym. 130 ft. Cues to apply brakes and manage footrests.

DME (using or required): Equipment has been ordered—hospital bed. Pt. has own walker and commode.

Activity tolerance: See Ambulation.

Treatment Diagnosis: Weakness, functional dependence.

Assessment

Reason for skilled care: Patient has made significant functional progress since WBAT LLE was initiated last month. Pt. has reached full benefit of inpatient P.T. She is being discharged home 6-20 to live with daughter (who will assist pt.) and Pt's husband. Home P.T. recommended to instruct and train pt. and family in the home environment, continue functional training, etc.

Plan of Care

Specific treatment strategies: Physical therapy for: ROM and strengthening ex. LLE and RLE, functional training (bed mobility, transfers, gait training, safety training) w/c mobility training, caregiver instruction, development of home ex. program.

Frequency: 6x/wk, 7 as tolerated.

Duration: 4 weeks.

Patient instruction/home program: See Caregiver training.

Caregiver training: Pt's daughter has been instructed to assist pt. with transfers, ambulation and a home ex. program. Pt. has had a day pass home—daughter reported transfers went well, but pt. was not able to ambulate secondary to knee pain. Nurses aides have been instructed to walk with pt. 1x each shift. Routine therapy aide has been instructed to walk with pt. and assist her with her ex. program.

Short-term goals and achievement dates:

1. Pt. will perform all bed mobility tasks with supv. (for safety).
2. Pt. will transfer bed, chair, toilet and car with SBA.
3. Pt. will ambulate 100 ft. with wheeled walker and SBA.
4. Pt. caregiver will be knowledgeable in providing necessary assistance for pt's mobility tasks.
5. Pt. will negotiate 1 single step (in/out of house) with CGA.
6. Pt and caregiver will perform indep. ex. prog. for LE.

Long-term goals and achievement dates: Pt. will be discharged home.

Case 16: Subacute, Discharge Report Worksheet

1. Are the "essential elements" (defined in Chapter 1) for documentation present?

Essential Element	Y, N, or N/A	Comment(s)
Attendance	Y	The visits from the start of care are recorded (71). The data need to describe the number of treatments scheduled and any reason for absence.
Current Baseline Data		
Cognition	N/A	Not applicable at this time. Cognition was addressed in the evaluation. It would be important to include any changes in cognition that may affect the patient's safe return to home.
Vision/hearing	N	This area was not addressed in the evaluation or discharge report. It would be important for a reviewer to know if any deficits exist when determining if skilled care was reasonable and necessary.
Vital signs	N	Vital signs, such as pulse rate and/or blood pressure, are not addressed in the evaluation or discharge report. If monitoring of vital signs is required, they would provide additional support of the need for skilled intervention.
Vascular signs	N	Vascular signs were not addressed in the evaluation or discharge report. Because of the documented surgical intervention, baseline and discharge data would be relevant.

(continued)

Essential Element	Y, N, or N/A	Comment(s)
Sensation/proprioception	N/A	Not applicable at this time. Sensation/proprioception were reported as normal in the evaluation; therefore, it would only be important to document changes in this area that affect rehabilitation.
Edema	N	As pitting edema was briefly described in the evaluation, it would be helpful for the reviewer if comparative data were provided. Documentation of any functional deficits resulting from the edema should also be included.
Posture	Y	The data for posture are helpful to the reviewer when determining the need for skilled care, as they have a direct relationship to ambulation ability. The addition of comparative data would be helpful.
AROM/PROM	N	Not addressed. Active range of motion measurements were provided in the evaluation; therefore, it is reasonable to expect discharge data. Range of motion limitations of the hips and knees have a direct effect on gait quality. It would be helpful for the reviewer to know if contractures or muscle tightness exist.
Strength	N	Strength grades were provided in the evaluation; however, comparative data are missing in the discharge report. As strengthening is identified as a treatment strategy and functional limitations in transfers and ambulation are present, it is reasonable for a reviewer to expect data.
Pain	Y	Data indicate "L distal knee pain which limits weight bearing activities" and that the left hip is pain-free. As a pain rating was provided for the knee in the evaluation, a discharge rating is needed. Also, a reviewer may find it helpful if further details were provided describing whether pain is a chronic condition and what activities increase or decrease pain. For instance, is the patient pain-free when sitting?
Coordination	N	Not addressed in the evaluation or discharge report. The data indicate that environmental barriers, such as elevated surfaces, are challenging and require cuing for technique. The patient also uses a walker for ambulation. It is therefore reasonable to expect data pertaining to coordination.
Bed mobility	Y	The therapist provides comparative data for the month in question. This is helpful to the reviewer for determining the patient's functional progress.
Balance (sit and stand)	N	As balance is addressed in the evaluation, comparative data are needed in the discharge report. Data describing the relationship of balance to safety help demonstrate another functional challenge requiring the skills of a therapist.
Transfers	Y	The therapist provides comparative data for the month in question. This is helpful in determining the patient's functional progress. However, a reviewer may not understand wording such as "and approx. 25% cuing."
Ambulation (level and elevated surfaces)	Y	A description of gait and comparative statements are present. Further data pertaining to the amount of verbal cuing required and a description of the gait pattern on unlevel surfaces, such as carpet, would further define the need for skilled therapy.
Orthotic/prosthetic devices	N/A	
Wheelchair use	Y	Comparative data are provided. This is helpful to the reviewer; however, the skilled nature of the service provided would be emphasized if the data included wording such as *Instruction in managing footrests and applying brakes provided*. Also, additional data on how the patient negotiates the wheelchair in the community and on the nursing unit would be helpful in demonstrating functional carryover.

Essential Element	Y, N, or N/A	Comment(s)
DME (using or required)	Y	Although durable medical equipment needs are addressed, the need for a wheelchair at home is not indicated. Based on the documented improvement in wheelchair skills, a reviewer may question the reasonableness of the wheelchair training provided during the last month of care.
Activity tolerance	Y	This area is addressed in the data provided for ambulation. Comparative statements are present. It is recommended that a functional phrase alternative, such as *activity tolerance*, be used for the term "endurance." This helps to reflect the skilled aspect of the care provided.
Wound description, including incision status	N	Not addressed. A comment regarding the status of the incision is appropriate, especially with respect to soft tissue mobility restrictions that may affect the patient's gait pattern.
Special tests	N/A	
Architectural/safety considerations	N	Not addressed. Evidence of a home assessment and/or discussion with the family regarding safety issues in the home is needed and would be another justification of the need for skilled care. As the fall that resulted in the hip fracture occurred during a bed-to-commode transfer, it would be helpful to ensure proper placement and height of the bed and commode. Also, are scattered rugs a safety issue?
Treatment Diagnosis	Y	The treatment diagnoses are "functional dependence" and "weakness." A functional phrase alternative such as *functional strength deficit* is recommended, as "weakness" may imply that improvement could occur without skilled therapy intervention.
Assessment		
Reason for skilled care	Y	Documentation is present and indicates the progress made, the discharge plan, and recommendations for continued physical therapy. Further description of why the patient is a candidate for continued skilled therapy is needed.
Problems	N	Not addressed. It is helpful to identify the problems that are resolved and/or remain at the time of discharge.
Plan of Care		
Specific treatment strategies	Y	The detailed list of treatment strategies describes the skilled services provided.
Frequency	Y	The frequency of service provided is "6x/wk, 7 as tolerated." A nonvariable frequency is recommended. It would be more appropriate to indicate a treatment frequency of *7x/wk* and describe the reason for absence in the Attendance section.
Duration	Y	A summary of the duration in relationship to the functional progress reported is provided. It also is helpful to the reviewer when analyzing documentation and the corresponding services billed.
Patient instruction/home program	Y	See Caregiver training.
Caregiver training	Y	The therapist indicates that instruction has occurred. It may be helpful to provide additional detail about what exercises are emphasized in the home program and what, if any, recommendations were made to the patient and family to control and/or monitor knee pain.
Short-term goals and achievement dates	Y	The short-term goals are present; however, the status of the goals at discharge is needed.

(continued)

Essential Element	Y, N, or N/A	Comment(s)
Long-term goals and achievement dates	Y	The long-term goal "Pt. will be discharged home" is not measurable or functional. Will the patient have good strength, be independent with a walker for mobility, and/or perform a home exercise program?
Discharge prognosis	N	Not addressed. It would be helpful for determining the success of skilled intervention and the need for continued skilled care to know the therapist's insight into the patient's discharge prognosis. If the patient and caregivers follow the therapy recommendations, how successful will the patient be at home?

2. Is there evidence of the need for skilled intervention?

Yes, this is a strong candidate for skilled intervention with multiple functional deficits, including transfers and ambulation.

3. Are there adequate baseline data to develop future comparisons?

There are many examples of baseline data and comparative descriptions. The reviewer is provided with a clear picture of the patient's progress in all areas of functional deficit except edema, strength, range of motion, and how pain limited the patient's gait pattern and safety, particularly on unlevel surfaces.

4. Are the objective data related to functional deficits?

Yes, the therapist relates data to functional activities; however, further details of the effects of knee pain with ambulation would be helpful. Also, the effects of edema, strength deficits, and range of motion limitations on functional activities are lacking.

5. Are comparative statements and data clearly outlined?

Comparative statements are present for bed mobility, wheelchair use, transfers, and ambulation. Comparative data are lacking in the areas of pain, edema, strength, and range of motion.

The strength of the discharge report would be enhanced if more comparisons were given between the patient's status at evaluation and that at the time of discharge. A reviewer may not have access to the original evaluation. The reviewer's job is much easier if there are data from the patient's initial evaluation.

6. (A) Are the three components for goals present (measurable, functional, time frames)?

Except for time frames, the components for goals are present. It would be helpful to indicate the goal status at discharge, such as goals met or not met.

(B) Are the goals realistic for the individual case?

Yes, they are realistic and cover all areas such as caregiver training and home program.

7. Do you feel that the treatment was reasonable and necessary?

The patient made progress in bed mobility, wheelchair use, transfers, and ambulation. The instruction of caregivers and implementation of the home program was documented. Therefore, this treatment intervention was well documented as reasonable and necessary.

Case 17: Subacute, Initial Evaluation

Referral

Reason: P.T. was initiated 03-15-96 upon healing of fracture and order from ortho physician.

Specific treatment requested: P.T. evaluation. Wt. bearing as tolerated.

Data Accompanying Referral

Diagnosis/onset date: Left femur fracture, CVA with left hemiplegia/11-03-95.

Medical history: This patient has a history of CVA with left hemiplegia and left hip fx 6-95. She was living at home until 11-95 when she was riding in a handicapped van, fell out of her w/c and fractured her left femur. This fracture was treated with closed reduction and strict nonwt. bearing (transferred with total body lift) and no physical therapy per M.D. order.

Comorbidities (complicating or precautionary information): Weight bearing as tolerated.

Physical Therapy Intake/History

Gender: Female
Start of care: 03-15-96

Referral Diagnosis

Mechanism of injury: See Medical history.

Baseline Evaluation Data

Cognition: Oriented x 3, alert, able to follow directions.

Sensation/proprioception: Intact pinprick right and left soles of feet; Light touch intact R and LLE, position sense intact R and L great toes.

AROM/PROM: WFL except left sh. abd 90°, left sh. E.R. 0°, left elbow ext. –20°, left sup. 65°, left hip flex 88°, left hip abd 10°, left knee flex 70°. Left leg length discrepancy; 5cm.

Strength: Motor control—G to N RUE. F- to G RLE; LLE demonstrated minimal flexor and extensor synergistic movement of LLE hip to ankle. LUE is dominated by min. flexor and extensor synergies at sh. and elbow and flexion at fingers.

Pain: Pt. c/o bilat. foot pain and left ant. thigh pain.

Bed mobility: Min. assist sit to and from supine.

Balance (sit and stand): Sitting balance—Independent static unsupported, supv. dynamic unsupported. Standing balance—max. assist static supported—pt. falls backward in flexed position.

Transfers: Max. assist with stand—pivot transfer. Pt. does not come to full standing.

Ambulation (level and elevated surfaces): Sit to stand—Max. assist of 2 to come to full standing. Once standing—1 mod. assist to continue to stand at parallel bar.

Orthotic/prosthetic devices: Uses left AFO.

Wheelchair use: Indep. using right extremities.

Prior Level of Function

Mobility (home and community): Prior to recent femur fracture, pt. was able to ambulate with CGA, left AFO, hemiwalker.

Treatment Diagnosis: Left femur fracture, CVA with hemiplegia/11-03-95.

Assessment

Reason for skilled care: Pt. is weak following prolonged immobility while left femur fracture healed. She will benefit from P.T. services to increase strength, endurance, ROM and function to previous levels.

Plan of Care

Specific treatment strategies: Evaluation completed. P.T. treatment to consist of therapeutic exercise (strengthening and ROM), functional training (bed mobility, balance and transfer training), aquatic therapy, safety awareness training, caregiver instruction.

Frequency: 6x/wk, 7 as tolerated.

Duration: 2 months.

Short-term goals and achievement dates:

1. Pt. will transfer sit to and from supine with SBA and cues.
2. Pt. will stand up from w/c with 1 mod assist and cues.
3. Pt. will stand–pivot transfer with 1 mod assist and cues.
4. Caregivers will be knowledgeable in assisting pt. with transfers.

Long-term goals and achievement dates:

1. Pt. will ambulate 130 ft. with hemiwalker and left AFO with CGA of 1.
2. Pt. will stand/pivot transfer w/c to and from bed, chair and toilet with CGA of 1.
3. Caregiver will be knowledgeable in assisting pt. with amb and transfer activities.

Case 17: Subacute, Initial Evaluation Worksheet

1. Are the "essential elements" (defined in Chapter 1) for documentation present?

Essential Element	Y, N, or N/A	Comment(s)
Referral		
Reason	Y	Although the information indicates that the referral was initiated "upon healing of fracture," the treatment objective is not described, such as return to home or work. Also, the location of the fracture is needed.
Specific treatment requested	Y	
Data Accompanying Referral		
Diagnosis/onset date	Y	The diagnosis and onset date are listed as "Left femur fracture, CVA with hemiplegia/11-03-95." This would suggest that the fracture and cerebrovascular accident (CVA) occurred concurrently. This may be confusing to a reviewer, as the medical history indicates that the CVA occurred in June.
Secondary diagnoses	N	Not addressed. This is an oversight as the patient has a history of a CVA and a left hip fracture.
Medical history	Y	
Medications	N	Not addressed. As pain is indicated in the evaluation, it would be helpful to know what medications, if any, are being administered that may affect rehabilitation, such as narcotics.
Comorbidities (complicating or precautionary information)	Y	The data indicate that the patient is weight bearing as tolerated. This is important treatment information. However, it would be helpful if further detail was given regarding the patient's comorbidities and complicating factors. This seems relevant because of the history of a CVA.
Physical Therapy Intake/History		
Date of birth	N	It is important to include patient identifying information, as many physician offices and third-party payers file or trigger data retrieval based on date of birth.
Age	N	The patient's age is not identified. If this is a geriatric patient, the age may suggest the potential for multiple comorbidities. As examples, does the patient have a history of multiple CVAs, arteriosclerotic heart disease, or diabetes?
Gender	Y	
Start of Care	Y	
Primary complaint	N	The patient's primary complaint is not described. Is it pain, decreased strength, and/or decreased mobility?
Referral Diagnosis		
Mechanism of injury	Y	The mechanism of injury, "fell out of her w/c," is described in the medical history. This information helps the reviewer determine primary and secondary payers.
Prior diagnostic imaging/testing	N	Not addressed. It is reasonable to expect that an x-ray and/or an assessment of bone density was performed to determine the weight-bearing status for this patient. These data may be relevant to the case at this time.
Prior Therapy History	N	Prior therapy history is not addressed. As the patient has a history of a left hip fracture, a reviewer would appreciate a summary of the patient's response to prior skilled intervention (following the CVA) to help in determining rehabilitation potential.

Essential Element	Y, N, or N/A	Comment(s)
Baseline Evaluation Data		
Cognition	Y	
Vision/hearing	N	Not addressed. Given the patient's history of a CVA, any vision and/or hearing deficits could be relevant to the patient's rehabilitation potential and therefore need to be described.
Vital signs	N	Not addressed. It would be important, if applicable, to provide baseline data regarding pulse rate and blood pressure, as the patient has a history of a CVA of unknown origin (i.e., is the patient hypertensive?).
Vascular signs	N	Not addressed. Vascular changes should be described if they exist from the left femur fracture, history of left hip fracture, and left hemiplegia.
Sensation/proprioception	Y	The therapist indicates "Intact pinprick right and left soles of feet; Light touch intact R and LLE, position sense intact R and L great toes." These data are helpful in eliminating potential challenges to rehabilitation. However, a reviewer may not understand why sensation needs to be assessed. For example, in this case to state that sensation was evaluated *for safe use of orthotics* would be helpful.
Edema	N	Not addressed. Because of the patient's limited mobility (nonweight-bearing status for approximately four months), decreased range of motion, and strength deficits, it would be important to document any edema and its effect on function.
Posture	N	Not addressed. Given the patient's medical history, including a CVA and fall from a wheelchair, it is reasonable to expect postural changes that influence function. For example, does the patient's sitting and standing posture affect balance?
AROM/PROM	Y	Range of motion measurements are provided with emphasis on the areas of deficits. However, the relationship between the left upper and lower extremity deficits and functional limitations is not described. For example, a five-centimeter leg length discrepancy could affect the patient's ability to stand and distribute weight in transfers and ambulation. It is also important to differentiate passive versus active range of motion.
Strength	Y	A description of strength is provided. However, the documentation lacks evidence of a functional relationship. For example, how does the synergistic patterning affect the patient's ability to bear weight through the left lower extremity?
Pain	Y	The therapist indicates "Pt. c/o bilat. foot pain and left ant. thigh pain." It would be helpful to rate the pain on a defined pain scale for future comparisons and describe the relationship of pain to the patient's ability to tolerate rehabilitation.
Coordination	N	Not addressed. A description of how the left extremity synergies affect function may be helpful to the reviewer in determining the need for skilled care.
Bed mobility	Y	
Balance (sit and stand)	Y	
Transfers	Y	The type of transfer and assistance level are described. The therapist also indicates "Pt. does not come to full standing." Details explaining why the patient cannot come to full standing are needed to help the reviewer assess transfer and gait potentials.
Ambulation (level and elevated surfaces)	Y	The amount of assistance to assume a standing position is documented. Further description of the factors limiting standing/ambulation need to be defined. Are muscle tone, strength, pain, and/or range of motion contributing factors?

(continued)

Essential Element	Y, N, or N/A	Comment(s)
Orthotic/prosthetic devices	Y	
Wheelchair use	Y	
DME (using or required)	N	This appears to be an oversight by the therapist, as the patient previously used a hemiwalker and a wheelchair.
Activity tolerance	N	Not addressed. It is important for the reviewer to know the patient's activity tolerance in the rehabilitation program.
Wound description, including incision status	N/A	Not applicable at this time, as therapy was initiated four months post-op. However, documentation pertaining to soft tissue restrictions should be described, if applicable.
Special tests	N/A	
Architectural/safety considerations	N	The data indicate that the patient previously lived at home and that the mechanism of injury was a fall from a wheelchair. Because of these factors, it is reasonable to anticipate the need to assess safety considerations and architectural barriers. Of course, this presumes that the patient will be returning home.
Requirements to return to home, school and/or job	N	Requirements for the patient to return home are needed, such as the availability of assistance from supportive services and/or family.
Prior Level of Function		
Mobility (home and community)	Y	The data indicate that the patient ambulated with a hemiwalker and contact guard assist. Additional data pertaining to the use of supportive services and/or how the patient negotiated transitional areas, such as unlevel surfaces within the community, would help present a clear picture of the patient's needs.
Employment	N	Not addressed. As the patient's age is unknown, it would be helpful to address the patient's prior level of function at school and/or job, if indicated.
School	N	See Employment.
Treatment Diagnosis	Y	The treatment diagnosis indicates a "Left femur fracture, CVA with left hemiplegia." The reviewer may not understand this, as the medical history indicates that the CVA occurred months before the femoral fracture. The treatment diagnosis may best be described as a *gait disturbance*.
Assessment		
Reason for skilled care	Y	The data indicate "Pt. is weak following prolonged immobility while left femur fracture healed. She will benefit from P.T. services to increase strength, endurance, ROM and function to previous levels." Further data specific to functional deficits, such as transfers and ambulation and why the skills of a therapist are needed, rather than focusing on debility from inactivity, are important. For example, it may be better to state, *The patient presents with a left femur fracture and is now able to participate in a skilled therapy program as weight-bearing restrictions are reduced.*
Problems	N	Not addressed. It is helpful to determine the problems in order to focus treatment (e.g., decreased bed mobility, decreased transfers, inability to ambulate).
Plan of Care		
Specific treatment strategies	Y	A P.T. evaluation was ordered. As most payer sources require physician involvement prior to the initiation of treatment, documentation indicating that orders will be pursued or have been received would be helpful to the reviewer. A reviewer may question the relationship of aquatic therapy to function. They may also question the omission of gait training, as ambulation is a goal.

Essential Element	Y, N, or N/A	Comment(s)
Frequency	Y	The frequency is listed as "6x/wk, 7 as tolerated." A nonvariable frequency is recommended. It would be more appropriate to indicate a treatment frequency of *7x/wk* and describe the reason for absence in the Attendance section of upcoming reports.
Duration	Y	This is an acute case, and some reviewers may prefer to see the duration stated in weeks rather than months.
Patient instruction/home program	N	Not addressed. A home program/restorative nursing recommendations should be initiated at the time of evaluation and upgraded as the patient progresses. Program upgrades require the skills of a therapist and demonstrate the effectiveness of skilled care.
Caregiver training	N	Restorative nursing recommendations are not documented, and subsequently caregiver training is not described. As the patient's weight-bearing restrictions were discontinued, it would be appropriate to provide instruction to nursing regarding changes in mobility, such as standing pivot transfers, bed mobility, and wheelchair positioning.
Short-term goals and achievement dates	Y	All goals contain a functional component. The goals are measurable, except for Goal 4, which states, "Caregivers will be knowledgeable in assisting pt. with transfers." All goals lack time frames. A goal regarding ambulation is needed.
Long-term goals and achievement dates	Y	The long-term goals are documented. The goals are functional. All goals lack a time frame, and Goal 3, which states, "The caregiver will be knowledgeable . . . ," is not measurable.
Rehabilitation potential	N	It is important to identify the rehabilitation potential of the patient, as it helps the reviewer assess the need for and duration of skilled care.

2. Is the overall history of the patient adequate?

Although a fair amount of detail is given in the history, it would be helpful for the reviewer to have a complete picture of the patient's deficits secondary to the CVA. For example, how severe are the flexor and extensor synergies in terms of affecting function and safety following the recent fracture? Also, since the age of the patient is unknown, will the patient be returning to work or school? Did the patient receive supportive services at home?

3. Is there evidence of the need for skilled intervention?

Yes, evidence is clear given the diagnosis of a recent femur fracture, recent history of a right CVA, and left hip fracture. Functional deficits in transfers, bed mobility, and ambulation are also described.

4. Are there adequate baseline data to develop future comparisons?

Although more data would be beneficial in describing the patient, there was adequate data present to justify future comparisons and the need for skilled physical therapy services. This is especially true for range of motion, strength, bed mobility, transfers, and ambulation.

5. Are the objective data related to functional deficits?

This is the one area that is lacking throughout the case. The relationship regarding data recorded and the patient's function is lacking for range of motion, strength, balance, and pain.

6. Are comparative statements and data clearly outlined?

In general, data are present, although they are not related to function. Data are lacking in the areas of vision/hearing, vital signs, edema, posture, and coordination.

7. (A) Are the three components for goals present (measurable, functional, time frames)?

All goals are functional and measurable, except for the short-term and long-term goal relating to caregiver training. Those goals are not measurable. All goals lack a time frame.

(B) Are the goals realistic for the individual case?

Yes, the goals appear realistic, except for the inability to measure caregiver knowledge and the long-term goal for ambulation. Given the description of the patient's major deficits, such as with standing and the synergistic patterning of the left extremities, a reviewer may question whether 130 feet for ambulation is realistic or necessary for the patient to function in the home environment.

8. Do you feel that the proposed treatment is reasonable and necessary?

Yes, given the functional regression in ambulation and transfers and the patient's challenging medical history, the evaluation and recommended treatment appear appropriate.

Case 17: Subacute, Progress Report

Attendance: 56 visits from SOC.

Current Baseline Data

Bed mobility: Sit to and from supine independent on mat; min/mod A right LE and cues on bed. On bed sit to and from supine min A for BLE's and VC's.

Balance (sit and stand): Pt. performs dynamic standing activity with RUE. Previously required RUE support in standing with walker.

Transfers: W/C to stand CGA; SPT mod A.

Ambulation (level and elevated surfaces): Pregait—Stood with walker min A for wt. shifting on LLE. Pt. demonstrated minimal weight shifting on LLE. Pt. performed unilateral stance on LLE to increase wt. bearing.

Orthotic/prosthetic devices: This month ABC Labs has been involved in reconstruction of LLE shoe for appropriate height and AFO modifications.

Treatment Diagnosis: Left femur fracture, CVA with left hemiplegia.

Assessment

Reason for skilled care: This pt. has made significant progress in transfers sit to and from stand, momentary dynamic balance without UE support, assessment for appropriate AFO and shoe lift and w/c independence with modifications of a left brake extender for safety. Leg length discrep. appears to have been corrected although from hx of compensations, pt. has had more difficulty at times with sit to stand secondary to increase in hip flexion on left, increased torque with old THR. Will cont. to work within pt.'s tolerance. AFO has improved knee stability. Doctor XYZ will be assessing pt.'s LLE stability in two weeks. Progress is expected to cont. to achieve the stated goals. D/C plans to return home with family at level of SBA for transfers, independent bed mobility.

Plan of Care

Specific treatment strategies: Physical therapy for ther. ex. (strengthening and ROM), functional training (bed mobility, balance and transfer training), aquatic therapy, safety awareness training, caregiver instruction.

Frequency: 6x/wk, 7 as tolerated.

Short-term goals and achievement dates:

1. Pt. will be independent in bed mobility.
2. Pt. will perform pivot transfers with min. A/CGA of 1.
3. Pt. will stand up with CGA of 1 consistently.

Long-term goals and achievement dates:

1. Pt. will pivot transfer bed, w/c, chair and toilet with SBA.
2. Pt. will amb. 130ft with hemiwalker and CGA.
3. Pt. will be discharged to live at home.

Case 17: Subacute, Progress Report Worksheet

1. Are the "essential elements" (defined in Chapter 1) for documentation present?

Essential Element	Y, N, or N/A	Comment(s)
Attendance	Y	The therapist indicates "56 visits from SOC." It is recommended that the number of visits scheduled and any reasons for absence be identified.
Current Baseline Data		
Cognition	N/A	Not applicable at this time. Cognition was addressed in the evaluation and no deficits were reported. As this is a progress report, the data need to focus primarily on the areas of functional deficit. However, it would be important to include any changes in cognition that may affect the patient's rehabilitation potential.
Vision/hearing	N	This area was not addressed in the evaluation or progress report. Any deficits in vision/hearing would be important for a reviewer to know when determining the need for skilled care.

Essential Element	Y, N, or N/A	Comment(s)
Vital signs	N	Vital signs are not addressed in the evaluation or progress report. If cardiopulmonary challenges exist, data such as respirations, pulse rate, and blood pressure would provide another reason for skilled intervention.
Vascular signs	N	Not addressed. Vascular changes should be described (if they exist) from the left femur fracture, history of left hip fracture, and left hemiplegia.
Sensation/proprioception	N/A	Not applicable at this time. Sensation/proprioception were described in the evaluation. It would only be necessary to document changes that may affect functional progress, as this area is not the primary focus of treatment.
Edema	N	Edema is not addressed in the evaluation or progress report. If edema is present, it would be important to describe its effect on function, such as the ability to use the left ankle foot orthosis.
Posture	N	Posture is not addressed in the evaluation or progress report. Given the reported leg length discrepancy, the patient may demonstrate postural deficits that are related to function.
AROM/PROM	N	As range of motion is addressed in the plan of care and measurements were provided in the evaluation, a reviewer can reasonably expect comparative data. A description of the strategy used to increase range of motion and the resulting functional improvement is needed. Further, "increased torque with old THR" is at best vague and may not be understood by a reviewer.
Strength	N	It is important to provide comparative data regarding strength. Strength grades were provided in the evaluation, and the plan of care included strengthening as a treatment strategy. A description of the individualized program and any functional improvement is needed.
Pain	N	Pain often produces challenges in functional activities. In the evaluation, the patient did report some pain. A reviewer would want to see a comparison of pain improvement/control, or if pain has not improved, how it is slowing progress.
Coordination	N	Coordination is not addressed in the evaluation or progress report. A description of how left extremity synergies affect functional activities, especially ambulation, would provide the reviewer with further justification for skilled care.
Bed mobility	Y	Bed mobility is described; however, comparative statements are lacking. It would be helpful to provide data regarding the amount of verbal cuing required for future progress comparisons.
Balance (sit and stand)	Y	Comparative data are provided for standing balance. However, a functional description of the deficits is lacking. As examples, does the patient lean posteriorly and to the right or stand longer than ten seconds? The type of walker used needs to be described.
Transfers	Y	The type of transfer and level of assistance are described. A reviewer would find it helpful if comparative data and information regarding how the patient is transferring on the nursing unit were documented. It is also recommended that the abbreviation "SPT" be written out, as a reviewer may not know it means standing pivot transfer.
Ambulation (level and elevated surfaces)	Y	Pregait skills are described. However, comparative data are needed to demonstrate functional improvement.

(continued)

Essential Element	Y, N, or N/A	Comment(s)
Orthotic/prosthetic devices	Y	The therapist appropriately documents that an orthotist is involved in modifying the patient's shoe and ankle foot orthosis. Further descriptions of the therapist's role in this process and how the modifications will affect functional progress are needed. For example, *Leg length discrepancy identified and modifications to the shoe and ankle foot orthosis were completed by ABC Labs on (date) to improve ankle stability during gait training.*
Wheelchair use	N/A	Not applicable at this time. The evaluation indicated that the patient was independent in propulsion skills; therefore, only a change in function would need to be documented.
DME (using or required)	N	This is an oversight, as the patient uses a wheelchair.
Activity tolerance	N	Activity tolerance is not addressed in the evaluation or progress report. A reviewer would find it helpful to know how the patient tolerates rehabilitation. For example, does the patient require frequent rests, or have cardiopulmonary challenges such as shortness of breath that require instruction in energy conservation techniques?
Wound description, including incision status	N/A	Not applicable at this time, as therapy was initiated four months post-op. However, documentation pertaining to soft tissue restrictions should be described, if applicable.
Special tests	N/A	
Architectural/safety considerations	N	The evaluation data indicated that the patient previously lived at home and the mechanism of injury was a fall from a wheelchair. As return to home is a goal, it is important to consider safety and architectural barriers throughout the course of treatment to help justify skilled care.
Treatment Diagnosis	Y	The treatment diagnosis indicates a "Left femur fracture, CVA with left hemiplegia." The reviewer may not understand this, as the medical history indicates that the CVA occurred months before the femoral fracture. The treatment diagnosis may best be described as a *gait disturbance.*
Assessment		
Reason for skilled care	Y	A lengthy description of the reason for skilled care is provided. Anticipated progress is documented, as well as the patient's discharge plans. However, additional detail regarding ambulation would be helpful at this point in the progression of treatment.
Problems	N	The problems are not described in the evaluation or progress report. It is helpful to determine the problems in order to focus treatment (e.g., decreased bed mobility, decreased transfers, inability to ambulate).
Plan of Care		
Specific treatment strategies	Y	The treatment strategies are described. However, data do not indicate the need for or patient performance of aquatic therapy. If billing occurred for this modality, further documentation is needed. Also, gait training was lacking.
Frequency	Y	The frequency is listed as "6x/wk, 7 as tolerated." A nonvariable frequency is recommended. It would be more appropriate to indicate a treatment frequency of *7x/wk* and describe the reason for any absence in the Attendance section of upcoming reports.
Duration	N	The duration is not indicated. This is an apparent oversight by the therapist. A reviewer will analyze the functional progress and goals in relationship to the anticipated duration to determine if the treatment is reasonable and necessary.

Essential Element	Y, N, or N/A	Comment(s)
Patient instruction/home program	N	Particularly in the arena of managed care, reviewers expect a home program to be initiated from the start of care. A reviewer would expect to find a reference to instruction/initiation of a home program and/or restorative nursing recommendations.
Caregiver training	N	Caregiver training is lacking in the evaluation and progress report. Training of caregivers and evidence of restorative nursing program changes requires the skills of a therapist.
Short-term goals and achievement dates	Y	The short-term goals are functional and measurable; however, they lack time frames. It is also helpful to identify the goal status. For example, were the previous goals met?
Long-term goals and achievement dates	Y	Three long-term goals are listed. All goals are functional and measurable; however, they lack time frames.
Rehabilitation potential	N	It is important to identify the rehabilitation potential of the patient to achieve the stated goals. This helps the reviewer determine if skilled care is reasonable and necessary.

2. Is there evidence of the need for skilled intervention?

Yes, there is evidence of the need for skilled intervention because of the numerous functional deficits described, such as transfers, ambulation, leg length discrepancy, and complicating diagnosis of a CVA.

3. Are there adequate baseline data to develop future comparisons?

Although data are present, particularly regarding transfers and ambulation, additional data are lacking for range of motion, strength, edema, balance, vision/hearing, vital signs, coordination, and restorative recommendations. Normally, with so many data lacking, there would not be enough to substantiate an intensive rehabilitation program, except that the deficits are so major in transfers and ambulation. Ongoing rehabilitation may require additional data in the areas lacking for future progress comparisons.

4. Are the objective data related to functional deficits?

In the area of transfers and ambulation, yes. In all other areas, the relationship to functional deficits is minimally described. The reviewer has very little information on how deficits in range of motion, strength, and balance are affecting the patient's ability to perform functional activities and return home.

5. Are comparative statements and data clearly outlined?

Comparative statements are clearly outlined for transfers and ambulation, but are either absent or unclear for the remaining areas of functional deficit.

6. (A) Are the three components for goals present (measurable, functional, time frames)?

The goals are measurable and functional; however, time frames are absent.

(B) Are the goals realistic for the individual case?

Yes, except Goal 2, which states, "Pt. will ambulate 130 ft. with hemiwalker and CGA." A reviewer may question whether 130 feet is realistic or necessary for the patient to function in her home environment.

7. Do you feel that the treatment was reasonable and necessary?

Yes, the patient presented with multiple disabilities. Documentation did demonstrate improvement in functional levels, such as balance, transfers, and standing ability. Additional support for the necessity of this treatment would be more detail on caregiver/nursing assistant instruction, development of a home exercise program/restorative nursing recommendations, and discussion of architectural/safety barriers, as discharge to home was a goal. For example, indication of plans for a home visit to facilitate discharge planning would have been helpful.

Chapter 5

Strategies for Improving Documentation Quality: A Proactive Approach

Introduction

Documenting physical therapy services provides the link between the clinical aspect of delivering quality service and the financial aspect of securing reimbursement for the skilled service rendered. Documentation allows the therapist to share with the reviewer how the skilled service was delivered and captures the resultant functional benefits.

Developing documentation skills is often an overlooked component in various settings. In certain treatment settings, reimbursement is predetermined and therefore documentation quality is not emphasized. However, in any setting, quality documentation is important to the efficacy of physical therapy service.

Why Improve Therapy Documentation?

Improving documentation skills to paint a clear picture of the patient requires a true commitment to excellence. This commitment will affect many aspects of an organization, including clinical and financial. Quality documentation will help focus and direct treatment. This is a necessity in all settings because of health care trends and the emphasis on managed care and prospective payment systems.

Improvements in documentation and documentation systems, although beginning with the therapist, will affect the duration of treatment, functional outcomes, marketing, and financial aspects of delivering physical therapy services. As health care reform continues to evolve, organizations committed to excellence will be better poised to enhance their position in the health care arena. However, what is the process to improve documentation?

Because of the multiple players involved, there is no simple solution to improving documentation. Despite the increasing demand for functional documentation, the challenge to be efficient is prevalent. To balance the essential elements needed from a reviewer's perspective can be frustrating. To add every documentation strategy provided in this book could result in lengthy reports and be extremely time consuming. That is not the inten-

tion of the authors. So, where does the process of improving documentation start?

A Commitment to Excellence

Before the process of improving documentation skills and documentation systems begins, all staff must recognize the reasons for change and be committed to excellence. That includes the management team and the therapists providing treatment. This sounds easy. However, it is not! The therapists who may require the most education may not recognize the need to improve their functional writing skills or be accepting of a documentation system change. All staff must understand the impact these skills will have on the organization, patient care, and the profession. Without a true commitment and defined performance expectations, this process will have limited success.

Therefore, begin by developing a team to compile information on the present documentation system or systems. This compilation may be accomplished through team meetings and surveys. It is helpful to involve all staff, including those who document and those who process the documentation, such as support staff and billing personnel.

It is useful to find out as much as possible about present operations to improve efficiency. It will provide insight into areas of difficulty. For instance, the therapists may not realize that they can code more than one diagnosis, or that certain diagnoses or procedures have resulted in denials. They may not realize that the billing personnel or management receives memos or educational materials from payers that could be provide insight into guidelines and coverage issues. It is surprising how many therapists do not even know their billers or whether they have ever received a denial. Therefore, opening the door for communication can be helpful to all players.

It is beneficial to compile therapists' opinions of the present documentation system. This will help determine whether there are any system needs. It is equally important to do random chart reviews to identify the skill level of each therapist's documentation. What essential elements are documented correctly, and which ones poorly? Trends may be identified that can be remedied through education. If areas are lacking and reimbursement issues surface then documentation criteria can be identified.

Establishing Necessary Documentation Criteria

The easiest way to begin identifying documentation criteria is to find out what elements are requirements. What are the national and state professional physical therapy practice guidelines, regulatory and facility guidelines, and third-party payer requirements? For instance, there are often documentation requirements to be a provider of service. Assess whether the present documentation system meets the established criteria and identify any deficiencies.

Next, the team needs to agree on items that should not be sacrificed while improving quality documentation. These items may include prior level of function, comparative data, functional relationships, and the plan of care. Or perhaps short-term goals are the key element the payer requests for authorization. In any case, it is helpful to identify important items. Information from another organization or an expert in the field may provide valuable insight. Other purposes of documentation, such as the legal aspect, must also be considered.

Providing Staff Education

To foster a positive work environment amid what could be multiple changes, it is helpful to provide continuous educational support regarding functional documentation. The problem with documentation skills is that over time, attention to detail is lost and quality diminishes. Therefore, ongoing education is necessary to ensure efficiency and accuracy.

Education can be provided in many ways. Inservicing is one means. Establishing peer review or quality assurance projects to monitor documentation are other strategies to consider. Try to make the process nonthreatening. However, it must be taken seriously. Too often, therapists complete a checklist without reading the report they are critiquing. Others are fearful of offering constructive feedback. Professional growth is ongoing, and this should be stressed. It may be helpful to request an inservice from the payer, to define areas that need improvement to expedite the payment process.

Does a Perfect Documentation Report Exist?

In the experience of the authors, there is no such thing as a perfect report. Therefore, anyone providing constructive feedback

can probably offer suggestions on any report. It is evident in the Chapter 4 case studies that deficiencies in documentation are easily identified.

Future Trends

The future of documentation is clear. Therapists need to provide information more effectively to justify treatment interventions as reasonable and necessary despite the presence or absence of specific guidelines. Every report is an opportunity to reflect the efficacy of our treatment interventions and the consequent improvement of function and healthy lifestyle in each patient who receives that physical therapy intervention.

Precertifications may continue to increase with health care reform. Therapists frequently report a high degree of discomfort and frustration with precertification of therapy treatments. This is not to be minimized, as precertification is relatively new to the profession and often follows no pattern for diagnoses, loss of function, or comorbidities—further frustrating the therapist, who feels pressured to provide inadequate care in unreasonably short visits or under capitated rates.

There is no easy answer to this dilemma. However, the authors firmly believe that the best chance for consideration of services will occur with solid documentation. In addition, therapists need to be more assertive, encourage their patients to demonstrate more self-management as well as to contact appropriate responsible parties, and diplomatically educate physicians and third-party payers as to the efficiency of treatment intervention.

The future requires therapist involvement. Therapists and rehabilitation providers need to be involved at the policy level. It is the policy level that is going to influence clinical practice. Justifying the need for physical therapy service through documented functional outcomes and research will be the key to the future. The need for research can not be overstressed.

Documenting physical therapy from a reviewer's perspective can help in securing reimbursement and supporting research. As managed care becomes more prominent, physical therapists increasingly need to serve as advocates for the profession, the patient, and the efficacy of treatment interventions.

Review Questions

1. Why should therapists demonstrate a commitment to improving physical therapy documentation?
2. Who should be involved in improving documentation, and why?
3. Describe the process recommended by the authors for improving documentation.

Review Question Answer Sheet

1. Therapists should demonstrate a commitment to improving physical therapy documentation because improvements will affect the duration of treatment, functional outcomes, and the marketing and financial aspects of service delivery.

2. The process of improving documentation starts with a commitment to excellence by all staff, including billing personnel. All staff must be involved in analyzing present operations and must recognize the reasons for change. Without all staff involved, the success of the process will be limited. Communication is important.

3. First, involve all staff.

   Second, develop a team to compile opinions regarding the present system through meetings and/or surveys.

   Third, establish necessary documentation criteria, including national and state professional practice guidelines, regulatory and facility guidelines, and third-party payer requirements.

   Fourth, agree on items that should not be sacrificed, such as legal considerations or payer requirements.

   Fifth, provide staff education.

   Finally, provide ongoing education.

Appendix 1

American Physical Therapy Association Guidelines for Physical Therapy Documentation

Reader note: The APTA amends core documents periodically. Updated documents can be obtained through the APTA (1-800-999-2782).

PREAMBLE

The American Physical Therapy Association (APTA) is committed to meeting the physical therapy needs of society, to meeting the needs and interests of its members, and to developing and improving the art and science of physical therapy, including practice, education, and research. To help meet these responsibilities, the APTA Board of Directors has approved the following guidelines for physical therapy documentation. It is recognized that these guidelines do not reflect all of the unique documentation requirements associated with the many specialty areas within the physical therapy profession. Applicable for both handwritten and electronic documentation systems, these guidelines are intended to be used as a foundation for the development of more specific documentation guidelines in specialty areas, while at the same time providing guidance for the physical therapy profession across all practice settings.

OPERATIONAL DEFINITIONS

Guidelines:

APTA defines "guidelines" as approved, non-binding statements of advice.

Documentation:

Any entry into the client record, such as: consultation report, initial examination report, progress note, flow sheet/checklist that identifies the care/service provided, reexamination, or summation of care.

Authentication:

The process used to verify that an entry is complete, accurate, and final. Indications of authentication can include original written signatures and computer "signatures" on secured electronic record systems only.

I. GENERAL GUIDELINES

A. All documentation must comply with the applicable jurisdictional/regulatory requirements.
1. All handwritten entries shall be made in ink and will include original signatures. Electronic entries should be made with appropriate security and confidentiality provisions.
2. Informed consent: As required by the APTA *Standards of Practice for Physical Therapy and the Accompanying Criteria.*
   2.1 The physical therapist has sole responsibility for providing information to the patient and for obtaining the patient's informed consent in accordance with jurisdictional law before initiating physical therapy.
   2.2 Those deemed competent to give consent are competent adults. When the adult is not competent, and in the case of minors, a parent or legal guardian consents as the surrogate decision maker.
   2.3 The information provided to the patient should include the following: (a) a clear description of the treatment ordered or recommended, (b) material (decisional) risks associated with the proposed treatment, (c) expected benefits of treatment, (d) comparison of the benefits and risks possible with and without treatment, and (e) reasonable alternatives to the recommended treatment. The physical therapist should solicit questions from the patient and provide answers. The patient should be asked to acknowledge understanding and consent before treatment proceeds.

Examples of ways in which to accomplish this documentation:

   Ex 2.3.1 Signature of patient/guardian on long or short consent form.
   Ex 2.3.2 Notation/entry of what was explained by the physical therapist or the physical therapist assistant in the official record.

Ex 2.3.3 Filing of a completed consent checklist signed by the patient.

3. Charting errors should be corrected by drawing a single line through the error and initialing and dating the chart or through the appropriate mechanism for electronic documentation that clearly indicates that a change was made without deletion of the original record.

4. Identification.

4.1 Include patient's full name and identification number, if applicable, on all official documents.

4.2 All entries must be dated and authenticated with the provider's full name and appropriate designation (e.g., PT, PTA).

4.3 Documentation by students (SPT/SPTA) shall be authenticated by a licensed physical therapist.

4.4 Documentation by graduates (GPT/GPTA) or others pending receipt of an unrestricted license shall be authenticated by a licensed physical therapist.

5. Documentation should include the manner in which physical therapy services are initiated.

Examples include:

Ex 5.1 Self-referral/direct access.

Ex 5.2 Attachment of the referral/consultation request by a qualified practitioner.

Ex 5.3 File copy of correspondence to referral source as acknowledgment of the referral.

II. INITIAL EXAMINATION AND EVALUATION/ CONSULTATION

A. Documentation is required at the outset of each episode of physical therapy care.

B. Elements include:

1. Obtaining a history and identifying risk factors:

1.1 History of the presenting problem, current complaints, and precautions (including onset date).

1.2 Pertinent diagnoses and medical history.

1.3 Demographic characteristics, including pertinent psychological, social, and environmental factors.

1.4 Prior or concurrent services related to the current episode of physical therapy care.

1.5 Comorbidities that may affect goals and treatment plan.

1.6 Statement of patient's knowledge of problem.

1.7 Goals of patient (and family members, or significant others, if appropriate).

2. Selecting and administering tests and measures to determine patient status in a number of areas. The following is a partial list of these areas, with illustrative tests and measures:

2.1 Arousal, mentation, and cognition

Examples include objective findings related, but not limited, to the following areas:

Ex 2.1.1 Level of consciousness

Ex 2.1.2 Ability to process commands

Ex 2.1.3 Alertness

Ex 2.1.4 Gross expressive and receptive language deficits

2.2 Neuromotor development and sensory integration

Examples include objective findings related, but not limited, to the following areas:

Ex 2.2.1 Gross and fine motor skills

Ex 2.2.2 Reflex and movement patterns

Ex 2.2.3 Dexterity, agility, and coordination

2.3 Range of motion

Examples include objective findings related, but not limited, to the following areas:

Ex 2.3.1 Extent of joint motion

Ex 2.3.1 Pain and soreness of surrounding soft tissue

Ex 2.3.3 Muscle length and flexibility

2.4 Muscle Performance

Examples include objective findings related, but not limited, to the following areas:

Ex 2.4.1 Strength

Ex 2.4.2 Power

Ex 2.4.3 Endurance

2.5 Ventilation, respiration, and circulation

Examples include objective findings related, but not limited, to the following areas:

Ex 2.5.1 Vital signs

Ex 2.5.2 Breathing patterns

Ex 2.5.3 Heart sounds

2.6 Posture

Examples include objective findings related, but not limited, to the following areas:

Ex 2.6.1 Static posture

Ex 2.6.2 Dynamic posture

2.7 Gait, locomotion, and balance

Examples include objective findings related, but not limited, to the following areas:

Ex 2.7.1 Characteristics of gait

Ex 2.7.2 Functional ambulation

Ex 2.7.3 Characteristics of balance

2.8 Self-care and home management status

Examples include objective findings related, but not limited, to the following areas:

Ex 2.8.1 Activities of daily living

Ex 2.8.2 Functional capacity

Ex 2.8.3 Static and dynamic strength

2.9 Community and work (job/school/play) integration/ reintegration.

Ex 2.9.1 Instrumental activities of daily living

Ex 2.9.2 Functional capacity

Ex 2.9.3 Adaptive skills

3. Evaluation (a dynamic process in which the physical therapist makes clinical judgements based on data gathered during the examination).

4. Diagnosis (a label encompassing a cluster of signs and symptoms, syndromes, or categories that reflects the information obtained from the examination).

5. Goals.

    5.1 Patient (and family members or significant others, if appropriate) is involved in establishing goals.

    5.2 All goals are stated in measurable terms.

    5.3 Goals are linked to problems identified in the examination.

    5.4 Short- and long-term goals are established when applicable (may include potential for achieving goals).

6. Intervention plan or recommendation requirements:

    6.1 Shall be related to realistic goals and expected functional outcomes.

    6.2 Should include frequency and duration to achieve the stated goals.

    6.3 Should include patient and family/caregiver educational goals.

    6.4 Should involve appropriate collaboration and coordination of care with other professionals/services.

7. Authentication and appropriate designation of physical therapist.

III. DOCUMENTATION OF THE CONTINUUM OF CARE

A. Intervention of service provided.

1. Documentation is required for each patient visit/encounter. Authentication is required for every note by the physical therapist or the physical therapist assistant providing the service under the supervision of the physical therapist.

Examples include:

    Ex 1.1 Checklist

    Ex 1.2 Flow sheet

    Ex 1.3 Graph

    Ex 1.4 Narrative

2. Elements may include:

    2.1 Identification of specific interventions provided.

    2.2 Equipment provided.

B. Patient status, progress, or regression.

1. Documentation is required for every visit/encounter. Authentication is required for every note by the physical therapist or physical therapist assistant providing the service under the supervision of the physical therapist.

2. Elements may include:

    2.1 Subjective status of patient.

    2.2 Changes in objective and measurable findings as they relate to existing goals.

    2.3 Adverse reaction to treatment.

    2.4 Progression/regression of existing therapeutic regimen, including patient education and adherence.

    2.5 Communication/consultation with providers/patient/family/significant other.

    2.6 Authentication and appropriate designation of either a physical therapist or a physical therapist assistant.

C. Reexamination and reevaluation

1. Documentation is required monthly for patients seen at intervals of a month or less; if the patient is seen less frequently, documentation is required for every visit or encounter.

2. Elements include:

    2.1 Documentation of elements as identified in III.B.2.1 through III.B.2.5 to update patient's status.

    2.2 Interpretation of findings and, when indicated, revision of goals.

    2.3 When indicated, revision of treatment plan, as directly correlated with documented goals.

    2.4 Authentication and appropriate designation of physical therapist.

IV. SUMMATION OF CARE

A. Documentation is required following conclusion of the current episode in the physical therapy care sequence.

B. Elements include:

1. Reason for discontinuation of service.

Examples include:

    Ex 1.1 Satisfactory goal achievement.

    Ex 1.2 Patient declines to continue care.

    Ex 1.3 Patient is unable to continue to work towards goals due to medical or psychological complications.

2. Current physical/functional status.

3. Degree of goal achievement and reasons for goals not being achieved.

4. Discharge plan that includes written and verbal communication related to the patient's continuing care.

Examples include:

    Ex 4.1 Home program.

    Ex 4.2 Referrals for additional services.

    Ex 4.3 Recommendations for follow-up physical therapy care.

    Ex 4.4 Family and caregiver training.

    Ex 4.5 Equipment provided.

5. Authentication and appropriate designation of physical therapist.

References

1. *Direction, Delegation and Supervision in Physical Therapy Services.* HOD 06-96-30-4

2. *Comprehensive Accreditation Manual for Hospitals.* Oakbrook Terrace, Ill: Joint Commission of Accreditation of Healthcare Organizations; 1996.

3. *Glossary of Terms Related to Information Security.* Schamburg, Ill: Computer-Based Patient Record Institute; 1996.

4. *Guidelines for Establishing Information Security Policies at Organizations Under Computer-Based Patient Records.* Schamburg, Ill: Computer-Based Patient Record Institute; 1995.

Adopted by the Board of Directors
March 1997
Amended March 1993, June 1993, November 1994, March 1995, March 1997

Reprinted from Guide to Physical Therapist Practice; *Phys Ther*; Alexandria, Virginia, APTA; 1997;77(11):1634–1636, with permission of the American Physical Therapy Association.

Appendix 2

American Physical Therapy Association Standards of Practice for Physical Therapy and the Accompanying Criteria

Reader note: The APTA amends core documents periodically. Updated documents can be obtained through the APTA (1-800-999-2782).

The Standards of Practice for Physical Therapy are promulgated by APTA's House of Delegates; the Criteria for the Standards are promulgated by the APTA's Board of Directors. The Criteria are italicized beneath the Standards to which they apply.

PREAMBLE

The physical therapy profession is committed to providing an optimum level of service delivery and to striving for excellence in practice. The House of Delegates of the American Physical Therapy Association, as the formal body that represents the profession, attests to this commitment by adopting and promoting the following *Standards of Practice for Physical Therapy*. These *Standards of Practice for Physical Therapy* are the profession's statement of conditions and performances that are essential for provision of high-quality physical therapy. The *Standards* provide a foundation for assessment of physical therapy practice.

I. LEGAL/ETHICAL CONSIDERATIONS

A. Legal Considerations
The physical therapist complies with all the legal requirements of jurisdictions regulating the practice of physical therapy.

The physical therapist assistant complies with all the legal requirements of jurisdictions regulating the work of the assistant.

B. Ethical Considerations
The physical therapist practices according to the *Code of Ethics* of the American Physical Therapy Association.

The physical therapist assistant complies with the *Standards of Ethical Conduct for the Physical Therapist Assistant* of the American Physical Therapy Association.

II. ADMINISTRATION OF THE PHYSICAL THERAPY SERVICE

A. Statement of Mission, Purposes, and Goals
The physical therapy service has a statement of mission, purposes, and goals that reflects the needs and interests of the individuals served, the physical therapy personnel affiliated with the service, and the community.

Criteria
The statement:
- *Defines the scope and limitations of the service.*
- *Lists the goals and objectives of the service.*
- *Is reviewed annually.*

B. Organizational Plan
The physical therapy service has a written organizational plan.

Criteria
The plan:
- *Describes relationships within the service and, where the physical therapy service is part of a larger organization, between the physical therapy service and other components of the organization.*
- *Ensures that the service is directed by a physical therapist.*
- *Defines supervisory structures within the service.*
- *Reflects current personnel functions.*

C. Policies and Procedures
The physical therapy service has written policies and procedures that reflect the operation of the service and that are consistent with the mission, purposes, and goals of the service.

Criteria
The policies and procedures, which are reviewed regularly and revised as necessary, address pertinent information including (but not limited to) the following:
- *Clinical education.*
- *Clinical research.*
- *Interdisciplinary collaboration.*
- *Criteria for access to, initiation of, continuation of, referral of, and termination of care.*

- *Equipment maintenance.*
- *Environmental safety.*
- *Fiscal management.*
- *Infection control.*
- *Job/position descriptions.*
- *Competency assessment.*
- *Medical emergencies.*
- *Patient/client care policies and protocols.*
- *Patient/client rights.*
- *Personnel-related policies.*
- *Quality/performance improvement.*
- *Documentation.*
- *Staff orientation.*

The policies and procedures meet the requirements of state law and external agencies.

D. Administration

A physical therapist is responsible for the direction of the physical therapy service.

Criteria
The director:
- *Ensures compliance with local, state, and federal requirements.*
- *Ensures compliance with current APTA documents, including Standards of Practice for Physical Therapy, Guide for Professional Conduct, and Guide for Conduct of the Affiliate Member.*
- *Ensures that services provided are consistent with the mission, purposes, and goals of the service.*
- *Ensures that services are provided in accordance with established policies and procedures.*
- *Reviews and updates polices and procedures.*
- *Provides training that assures continued competence of physical therapy support personnel.*
- *Provides for continuous in-service training on safety issues and for periodic safety inspection of equipment by qualified individuals.*

E. Fiscal Management

The director of the physical therapy service, in consultations with staff and appropriate administrative personnel, is responsible for planning for, and allocation of, resources. Fiscal planning and management of the service is based on sound accounting principles.

Criteria
The fiscal management plan includes:
- *Preparation and monitoring of a budget that provides for optimum use of resources.*
- *Accurate recording and reporting of financial information.*
- *Conformance with legal requirements.*
- *Cost-effective utilization of resources.*
- *A fee schedule that is consistent with cost of services and that is within customary norms of fairness and reasonableness.*

F. Quality/Performance Improvement

The physical therapy service has a written plan for continuous improvement of the performance of services provided.

Criteria
The plan:
- *Provides evidence of ongoing review and evaluation of the service.*
- *Provides a mechanism for documentation of performance improvement.*
- *Is consistent with requirements of external agencies, if applicable.*

G. Staffing

The physical therapy personnel affiliated with the physical therapy service have demonstrated competence and are sufficient to achieve the mission, purposes, and goals of the service.

Criteria
The service:
- *Meets all legal requirements regarding licensure and/or certification of appropriate personnel.*
- *Provides staff expertise that is appropriate to the patients/ clients served.*
- *Provides for appropriate staff-to-patient/client ratios.*
- *Provides for appropriate ratios of support staff to professional staff.*

H. Staff Development

The physical therapy service has a written plan that provides for appropriate and ongoing staff development.

Criteria
The plan:
- *Provides for consideration of self-assessments, individual goal setting, and organization needs in directing continuing education and learning activities.*
- *Includes strategies for long-term learning and professional development.*

I. Physical Setting

The physical setting is designed to provide a safe and accessible environment that facilitates fulfillment of the mission and achievement of the purposes and goals of physical therapy service. The equipment is safe and sufficient to achieve the purposes and goals of physical therapy.

Criteria
The physical setting:
- *Meets all applicable legal requirements for health and safety.*
- *Meets space needs appropriate for the number and type of patients/clients served.*
The equipment:
- *Meets all applicable legal requirements for health and safety.*
- *Is inspected routinely.*

J. Interdisciplinary Collaboration

The physical therapy service collaborates with all appropriate disciplines.

Criteria
The collaboration includes:
- *An interdisciplinary team approach to patient/client care.*
- *Interdisciplinary patient/client and family education.*
- *Interdisciplinary staff development and continuing education.*

III. PROVISIONS OF SERVICES

A. Informed Consent

The physical therapist has sole responsibility for providing information to the patient/client and for obtaining the patient's/client's informed consent in accordance with jurisdictional law before initiating physical therapy.

Criteria
The information provided to the patient/client should include the following:
- *A clear description of the proposed intervention/treatment.*
- *A statement of material (decisional) risks associated with the proposed intervention/treatment.*
- *A statement of expected benefits of the proposed intervention/treatment.*
- *A comparison of the benefits and risks possible both with and without intervention/treatment.*
- *An explanation of reasonable alternatives to the recommended intervention/treatment.*

Informed consent requires:
- *Consent by a competent adult.*
- *Consent by a parent/legal guardian as the surrogate decision maker when the adult patient/client is not competent or when the patient/client is a minor.*
- *The patient's/client's acknowledgment of understanding and consent before the intervention/treatment proceeds.*

B. Initial Examination and Evaluation

The physical therapist performs and documents an initial examination and evaluates the results to identify problems and determine the diagnosis prior to intervention/treatment.

Criteria
The examination:
- *Is documented, dated, and signed by the physical therapist who performed the examination.*
- *Identifies the physical therapy needs of the patient/client.*
- *Incorporates appropriate objective tests and measures to facilitate outcome measurement.*
- *Documents sufficient dates to establish a plan of care.*
- *May result in recommendations for additional services to meet the needs of the patient/client.*

C. Plan of Care

The physical therapist establishes and provides a plan of care for the individual based on the results of the examination and evaluation and on patient/client needs.

The physical therapist involves the patient/client and appropriate others in the planning, implementation, and assessment of the intervention/treatment program.

The physical therapist, in consultation with appropriate disciplines, plans for discharge of the patient/client taking into consideration goal achievement, and provides for appropriate follow-up or referral.

Criteria
The plan of care includes:
- *Realistic goals and expected functional outcomes.*
- *Intervention/treatment, including its frequency and duration.*
- *Documentation that is dated and signed by the physical therapist who established the plan of care.*

D. Intervention/Treatment

The physical therapist provides, or delegates and supervises, the physical therapy intervention/treatment consistent with the results of the examination and evaluation and plan of care.

The physical therapist documents, on an ongoing basis, services provided, responses to services, and changes in status relative to the plan of care.

Criteria
The intervention/treatment is:
- *Provided under the ongoing personal care or supervision of the physical therapist.*
- *Provided in such a way that delegated responsibilities are commensurate with the qualifications and legal limitations of the physical therapy personnel involved in the intervention/treatment.*
- *Altered in accordance with changes in individual response or status.*
- *Provided at a level that is consistent with current physical therapy practice.*
- *Interdisciplinary when necessary to meet the needs of the patient/client.*

Documentation of the services provided includes:
- *Date and signature of the physical therapist and/or of the physical therapist assistant when permissible by law.*

E. Reexamination and Reevaluation

The physical therapist reexamines and reevaluates the individual continually and modifies or discontinues the plan of care accordingly.

Criteria
The physical therapist:
- *Periodically documents, dates, and signs the patient/client reexamination and modifications of the plan of care.*

F. Discharge/Discontinuation of Treatment or Intervention

The physical therapist discharges the patient/client from physical therapy intervention/treatment when the goals or projected outcomes for the patient/client have been met.

Physical therapy intervention/treatment shall be discontinued when the goals are achieved, the patient/client declines to continue care, the patient/client is unable to continue, or the physical therapist determines that intervention/treatment is no longer warranted.

Criteria
Discharge documentation shall include:
- *The patient's/client's status at discharge and functional outcomes/goals achieved.*
- *Dating and signing of the discharge summary by the physical therapist.*
- *When a patient/client is discharged prior to goal achievement, the patient's/client's status and the rationale for discontinuation.*

IV. EDUCATION

The physical therapist is responsible for the individual professional development. The physical therapist assistant is responsible for individual career development.

The physical therapist participates in the education of physical therapist students, physical therapist assistant students, and students in other health professions. The physical therapist assistant participates in the education of physical therapist assistant students and other student health professionals.

The physical therapist educates and provides consultation to consumers and the general public regarding the purposes and benefits of physical therapy.

The physical therapist educates and provides consultation to consumers and general public regarding the roles of the physical therapist and the physical therapist assistant.

Criteria
The physical therapist educates and provides consultation to consumers and the general public regarding the roles of the physical therapist, the physical therapist assistant, and other support personnel.

V. RESEARCH

The physical therapist applies research findings to practice and encourages, participates in, and promotes activities that establish the outcomes of physical therapist patient/client management.

The physical therapist supports collaborative and interdisciplinary research.

VI. COMMUNITY RESPONSIBILITY

The physical therapist demonstrates community responsibility by participating in community and community agency activities, educating the public, formulating public policy, or providing pro bono physical therapy services.

Criteria
The physical therapist demonstrates community responsibility by participating in community and community agency activities; educating the public, including prevention and health promotion activities; formulating public policy; or providing pro bono physical therapy services.

Standards:
Adopted by the House of Delegates
June 1980
Amended June 1985, June 1991, June 1996

Criteria:
Adopted by the Board of Directors
March 1993
Amended November 1994, March 1995

Reprinted from Guide to Physical Therapist Practice; *Phys Ther*; Alexandria, Virginia, APTA; 1997;77(11):1625–1628, with permission of the American Physical Therapy Association.

Appendix 3

American Physical Therapy Association Code of Ethics

Reader note: The APTA amends core documents periodically. Updated documents can be obtained through the APTA (1-800-999-2782).

PREAMBLE

This *Code of Ethics* sets forth ethical principles for the physical therapy profession. Members of this profession are responsible for maintaining and promoting ethical practice. This *Code of Ethics*, adopted by the American Physical Therapy Association, shall be binding on physical therapists who are members of the Association.

Principle 1

Physical therapists respect the rights and dignity of all individuals.

Principle 2

Physical therapists comply with the laws and regulations governing the practice of physical therapy.

Principle 3

Physical therapists accept responsibility for the exercise of sound judgment.

Principle 4

Physical therapists maintain and promote high standards for physical therapy practice, education, and research.

Principle 5

Physical therapists seek remuneration for their services that is deserved and reasonable.

Principle 6

Physical therapists provide accurate information to the consumer about the profession and about those services they provide.

Principle 7

Physical therapists accept the responsibility to protect the public and the profession from unethical, incompetent, or illegal acts.

Principle 8

Physical therapists participate in efforts to address the health needs of the public.

Adopted by the House of Delegates
June 1981
Amended June 1987, June 1991

Reprinted from Guide to Physical Therapist Practice; *Phys Ther*; Alexandria, Virginia, APTA; 1997;77(11):1628, with permission of the American Physical Therapy Association.

Appendix 4

American Physical Therapy Association Standards of Ethical Conduct for the Physical Therapist Assistant

Reader note: The APTA amends core documents periodically. Updated documents can be obtained through the APTA (1-800-999-2782).

PREAMBLE

Physical therapist assistants are responsible for maintaining and promoting high standards of conduct. These *Standards of Ethical Conduct for the Physical Therapist Assistant* shall be binding on physical therapist assistants who are affiliate members of the Association.

STANDARD 1

Physical therapist assistants provide services under the supervision of a physical therapist.

STANDARD 2

Physical therapist assistants respect the rights and dignity of all individuals.

STANDARD 3

Physical therapist assistants maintain and promote high standards in the provision of services, giving the welfare of the patients their highest regard.

STANDARD 4

Physical therapist assistants provide services within the limits of the law.

STANDARD 5

Physical therapist assistants make those judgements that are commensurate with their qualifications as physical therapist assistants.

STANDARD 6

Physical therapist assistants accept the responsibility to protect the public and the profession from unethical, incompetent, or illegal acts.

Adopted by House of Delegates
June 1982
Amended June 1991

Reprinted from Guide to Physical Therapist Practice; *Phys Ther*; Alexandria, Virginia, APTA; 1997;77(11):1632, with permission of the American Physical Therapy Association.

Appendix 5

American Physical Therapy Association Guide for Professional Conduct

Reader note: The APTA amends core documents periodically. Updated documents can be obtained through the APTA (1-800-999-2782).

PURPOSE

This *Guide for Professional Conduct (Guide)* is intended to serve physical therapists who are members of the American Physical Therapy Association (Association) in interpreting the *Code of Ethics (Code)* and matters of professional conduct. The Guide provides guidelines by which physical therapists may determine the propriety of their conduct. The *Code* and the *Guide* apply to all physical therapists who are Association members. These guidelines are subject to change as the dynamics of the professional change and as new patterns of health care delivery are developed and accepted by the professional community and the public. This *Guide* is subject to monitoring and timely revision by the Judicial Committee of the Association.

INTERPRETING ETHICAL PRINCIPLES

The interpretations expressed in this *Guide* are not to be considered all inclusive of situations that could evolve under a specific principle of the *Code* but reflect the opinions, decisions, and advice of the Judicial Committee. While the statements of ethical principles apply universally, specific circumstances determine their appropriate application. Input related to current interpretations, or to situations requiring interpretation, is encouraged from Association members.

PRINCIPLE 1

Physical therapists respect the rights and dignity of all individuals.

1.1 Attitudes of Physical Therapists

A. Physical therapists shall recognize that each individual is different from all other individuals and shall respect and be responsive to those differences.

B. Physical therapists are to be guided at all times by concern for the physical, psychological, and socioeconomic welfare of those individuals entrusted to their care.

C. Physical therapists shall not engage in conduct that constitutes harassment or abuse of, or discrimination against, colleagues, associates, or others.

1.2 Confidential Information

A. Information relating to the physical therapist/patient relationship is confidential and may not be communicated to a third party not involved in that patient's care without the prior written consent of the patient, subject to applicable law.

B. Information derived from component-sponsored peer review shall be held confidential by the reviewer unless written permission to release the information is obtained from the physical therapist who was reviewed.

C. Information derived from the working relationships of physical therapists shall be held confidential by all parties.

D. Information may be disclosed to appropriate authorities when it is necessary to protect the welfare of an individual or the community. Such disclosure shall be in accordance with applicable law.

1.3 Patient Relations

Physical therapists shall not engage in any sexual relationship or activity, whether consensual or nonconsensual, with any patient while a physical therapist/patient relationship exists.

1.4 Informed Consent

Physical therapists shall obtain patient informed consent before treatment.

PRINCIPLE 2

Physical therapists comply with the laws and regulations governing the practice of physical therapy.

2.1 Professional Practice

Physical therapists shall provide consultation, evaluation, treatment, and preventive care, in accordance with the laws and regulations of the jurisdiction(s) in which they practice.

PRINCIPLE 3

Physical therapists accept responsibility for the exercise of sound judgment.

3.1 Acceptance of Responsibility

A. Upon accepting an individual for provision of physical therapy services, physical therapists shall assume the responsibility for evaluating that individual; planning, implementing, and supervising the therapeutic program; reevaluating and changing that program; and maintaining adequate records of the case, including progress reports.
B. When the individual's needs are beyond the scope of the physical therapist's expertise, or when additional services are indicated, the individual shall be so informed and assisted in identifying a qualified provider.
C. Regardless of practice setting, physical therapists shall maintain the ability to make independent judgements.
D. The physical therapist shall not provide physical therapy services to a patient while under the influence of a substance that impairs his or her ability to do so safely.

3.2 Delegation of Responsibility

A. Physical therapists shall not delegate to a less qualified person any activity which requires the unique skill, knowledge, and judgment of the physical therapist.
B. The primary responsibility for physical therapy care rendered by supportive personnel rests with the supervising physical therapist. Adequate supervision requires, at a minimum, that a supervising physical therapist perform the following activities:
  1. Designate or establish channels of written and oral communication.
  2. Interpret available information concerning the individual under care.
  3. Provide initial evaluation.
  4. Develop plan of care, including short- and long-term goals.
  5. Select and delegate appropriate tasks of plan of care.
  6. Assess competence of supportive personnel to perform assigned tasks.
  7. Direct and supervise supportive personnel in delegated tasks.
  8. Identify and document precautions, special problems, contraindications, goals, anticipated progress, and plans for reevaluation.
  9. Reevaluate, adjust plan of care when necessary, perform final evaluation, and establish follow-up plan.

3.3 Provision of Services

A. Physical therapists shall recognize the individual's freedom of choice in selection of physical therapy services.
B. Physical therapists' professional practices and their adherence to ethical principles of the Association shall take preference over business practices. Provisions of services for personal financial gain rather than for the need of the individual receiving the services are unethical.
C. When physical therapists judge that an individual will no longer benefit from their services, they shall so inform the individual receiving the services. Physical therapists shall avoid overutilization of their services.
D. In the event of elective termination of a physical therapist/patient relationship by the physical therapist, the therapist should take steps to transfer the care of the patient, as appropriate, to another provider.

3.4 Referral Relationships

In a referral situation where the referring practitioner prescribes a treatment program, alteration of that program or extension of physical therapy services beyond that program should be undertaken in consultation with the referring practitioner.

3.5 Practice Arrangements

A. Participation in a business, partnership, corporation, or other entity does not exempt the physical therapist, whether employer, partner, or stockholder, either individually or collectively, from the obligation of promoting and maintaining the ethical principles of the Association.
B. Physical therapists shall advise their employer(s) of any employer practice which causes a physical therapist to be in conflict with the ethical principles of the Association. Physical therapist employees shall attempt to rectify aspects of their employment which are in conflict with the ethical principles of the Association.

PRINCIPLE 4

Physical therapists maintain and promote high standards for physical therapy practice, education, and research.

4.1 Continued Education

A. Physical therapist shall participate in educational activities which enhance their basic knowledge and provide new knowledge.
B. Whenever physical therapists provide continuing education, they shall ensure that course content, objectives, and responsibilities of the instructional faculty are accurately reflected in the promotion of the course.

4.2 Review and Self Assessment

A. Physical therapists shall provide for utilization review of their services.
B. Physical therapists shall demonstrate their commitment to quality assurance by peer review and self-assessment.

4.3 Research

A. Physical therapists shall support research activities that contribute knowledge for improved patient care.
B. Physical therapists engaged in research shall ensure:
   1. the consent of subjects;
   2. confidentiality of the data on individual subjects and the personal identities of the subjects;
   3. well-being of all subjects in compliance with facility regulations and laws of the jurisdiction in which the research is conducted;
   4. the absence of fraud and plagiarism;
   5. full disclosure of support received;
   6. appropriate acknowledgment of individuals making a contribution to the research;
   7. that animal subjects used in research are treated humanely and in compliance with facility regulations and laws of the jurisdiction in which the research experimentation is conducted.
C. Physical therapists shall report to appropriate authorities any acts in the conduct or presentation of research that appear unethical or illegal.

4.4 Education

A. Physical therapists shall support quality education in academic and clinical settings.
B. Physical therapists functioning in the educational role are responsible to the students, the academic institutions and the clinical settings for promoting ethical conduct in educational activities. Whenever possible, the educator shall ensure;
   1. the rights of students in the academic and clinical setting;
   2. appropriate confidentiality of personal information;
   3. professional conduct toward the student during the academic and clinical educational processes;
   4. assignment to clinical settings prepared to give the student a learning experience.
C. Clinical educators are responsible for reporting to the academic program student conduct which appears to be unethical or illegal.

PRINCIPLE 5

Physical therapists seek remuneration for their services that is deserved and reasonable.

5.1 Fiscally Sound Remuneration

A. Physical therapists shall never place their own financial interest above the welfare of individuals under their care.
B. Fees for physical therapy services should be reasonable for the service performed, considering the setting in which it is provided, practice costs in the geographic area, judgement of other organizations, and other relevant factors.
C. Physical therapists should attempt to ensure that providers, agencies, or other employers adopt physical therapy fee schedules that are reasonable and that encourage access to necessary services.

5.2 Business Practices/Fee Arrangements

A. Physical therapists shall not:
   1. directly or indirectly request, receive, or participate in the dividing, transferring, assigning, rebating of an unearned fee.
   2. profit by means of a credit or other valuable consideration, such as an unearned commission, discount, or gratuity in connection with furnishing of physical therapy services.
B. Unless laws impose restrictions to the contrary, physical therapists who provide physical therapy services in a business entity may pool fees and moneys received. Physical therapists may divide or apportion these fees and moneys in accordance with the business agreement.
C. Physical therapists may enter into agreements with organizations to provide physical therapy services if such agreements do not violate the ethical principles of the Association.

5.3 Endorsement of Equipment or Services

A. Physical therapists shall not use influence upon individuals under their care or their families for utilization of equipment or services based upon the direct or indirect financial interest of the physical therapist in such equipment or services. Realizing that these individuals will normally rely on the physical therapists' advice, their best interest must always be maintained as well as their right of free choice relating to the use of any equipment or service. While it cannot be considered unethical for physical therapists to own or have a financial interest in equipment companies, or services, they must act in accordance with law and make full disclosure of their interest whenever such companies or services become the source of equipment or services for individuals under their care.
B. Physical therapists may be remunerated for endorsement or advertisement of equipment or services to the lay public, physical therapists, or other health professionals provided they disclose any financial interest in the production, sale or distribution of said equipment or services.
C. In endorsing or adverting equipment or services, physical therapists shall use sound profession judgment and shall not give the appearance of Association endorsement.

5.4 Gifts and Other Considerations

A. Physical therapists shall not accept nor offer gifts or other considerations with obligatory conditions attached.
B. Physical therapists shall not accept or offer gifts or other considerations that affect or give an objective appearance of affecting their professional judgment.

PRINCIPLE 6

Physical therapists provide accurate information to the consumer about the profession and about those services they provide.

6.1 Information about the Profession

Physical therapists shall endeavor to educate the public to an awareness of the physical therapy profession through such means as publication of articles and participation in seminars, lectures, and civic programs.

6.2 Information about Services

A. Information given to the public shall emphasize that individual problems cannot be treated without individualized evaluation and plans/programs of care.
B. Physical therapists may advertise their services to the public.
C. Physical therapists shall not use, or participate in the use of, any form of communication containing a false, plagiarized, fraudulent, misleading, deceptive, unfair, or sensational statement or claim.
D. A paid advertisement shall be identified as such unless it is apparent from the context that it is a paid advertisement.

PRINCIPLE 7

Physical therapists accept the responsibility to protect the public and the profession from unethical, incompetent, or illegal acts.

7.1 Consumer Protection

A. Physical therapists shall report any conduct which appears to be unethical, incompetent, or illegal.
B. Physical therapists may not participate in any arrangements in which patients are exploited due to the referring sources enhancing their personal incomes as a result of referring for, prescribing, or recommending physical therapy.
C. Physical therapists shall be obligated to safeguard the public from underutilization or overutilization of physical therapy services.

7.2 Disclosure

The physical therapists shall disclose to the patient if the referring practitioner derives compensation from the provision of physical therapy. The physical therapist shall ensure that the individual has freedom of choice in selecting a provider of physical therapy.

PRINCIPLE 8

Physical therapists participate in efforts to address the health needs of the public.

8.1 Pro Bono Service

Physical therapists should render pro bono publico (reduced or no fee) services to patients lacking the ability to pay for services, as each physical therapist's practice permits.

Issued by Judicial Committee, APTA
October 1981
Last Amended September 1997

Reprinted from Guide to Physical Therapist Practice; *Phys Ther*; Alexandria, Virginia, APTA; 1997;77(11):1629–1631, with permission of the American Physical Therapy Association.

Appendix 6

American Physical Therapy Association Guide for Conduct of the Affiliate Member

Reader note: The APTA amends core documents periodically. Updated documents can be obtained through the APTA (1-800-999-2782).

PURPOSE

This *Guide* is intended to serve physical therapist assistants who are affiliate members of the American Physical Therapy Association in the interpretation of the *Standards of Ethical Conduct for the Physical Therapist Assistant*, providing guidelines by which they may determine the propriety of their conduct. These guidelines are subject to change as new patterns of health care delivery are developed and accepted by the professional community and the public. This *Guide* is subject to monitoring and timely revision by the Judicial Committee of the Association.

INTERPRETING STANDARDS

The interpretations expressed in this *Guide* are not to be considered all inclusive of situations that could evolve under a specific standard of the *Standards of Ethical Conduct for the Physical Therapists Assistant* but reflect the opinions, decisions, and advice of the Judicial Committee. While the statements of ethical standards apply universally, specific circumstances determine their appropriate application. Input related to current interpretations, or to situations requiring interpretation, is encouraged from APTA members.

STANDARD 1

Physical therapist assistants provide services under the supervision of a physical therapist.

1.1 Supervisory Relationships

Physical therapist assistants shall work under the supervision and direction of a physical therapist who is properly creden-tialed in the jurisdiction in which the physical therapist assistant practices.

1.2 Performance of Service

A. Physical therapist assistants may not initiate or alter a treatment program without prior evaluation by and approval of the supervising physical therapist.
B. Physical therapist assistants may modify a specific treatment procedure in accordance with changes in patient status.
C. Physical therapist assistants may not interpret data beyond the scope of their physical therapist assistant education.
D. Physical therapist assistants may respond to inquiries regarding patient status to appropriate parties within the protocol established by a supervising physical therapist.
E. Physical therapist assistants shall refer inquiries regarding patient prognosis to a supervising physical therapist.

STANDARD 2

Physical therapist assistants respect the rights and dignity of all individuals.

2.1 Attitudes of Physical Therapist Assistants

A. Physical therapist assistants shall recognize that each individual is different from all other individuals and respect and be responsive to those differences.
B. Physical therapist assistants shall be guided at all times by concern for the dignity and welfare of those patients entrusted to their care.
C. Physical therapist assistants shall not engage in conduct that constitutes harassment or abuse of, or discrimination against, colleagues, associates, or others.

2.2 Request for Release of Information

Physical therapist assistants shall refer all requests for release of confidential information to the supervising physical therapist.

2.3 Protection of Privacy

Physical therapist assistants must treat as confidential all information relating to the personal conditions and affairs of the persons whom they serve.

2.4 Patient Relations

Physical therapist assistants shall not engage in any sexual relationship or activity, whether consensual or nonconsensual, with any patient while a physical therapist assistant/patient relationship exists.

STANDARD 3

Physical therapist assistants maintain and promote high standards in the provision of services, giving the welfare of patients their highest regard.

3.1 Information About Services

A. Physical therapist assistants may provide consumers with information regarding provision of services within the protocol established by a supervising physical therapist.
B. Physical therapist assistants may not use, or participate in the use of, any form of communication containing a false, fraudulent, misleading, deceptive, unfair, or sensational statement or claim.

3.2 Organizational Employment

Physical therapist assistants shall advise their employer(s) of any employer practice which causes them to be in conflict with the *Standards of Ethical Conduct for the Physical Therapist Assistant.*

3.3 Endorsement of Equipment

Physical therapist assistants may not endorse equipment or exercise influence on patients or families to purchase or lease equipment except as directed by a physical therapist acting in accord with the stipulation in paragraph 5.3.A. of the *Guide for Professional Conduct.*

3.4 Financial Considerations

Physical therapist assistants shall never place their own financial interest above the welfare of their patients.

3.5 Exploitation of Patients

Physical therapist assistants shall not participate in any arrangements in which patients are exploited. Such arrangements include situations where referring sources enhance their personal incomes as a result of referring for, delegating, prescribing, or recommending physical therapy services.

STANDARD 4

Physical therapist assistants provide services within the limits of the law.

4.1 Supervisory Relationships

Physical therapist assistants shall comply with all aspects of law. Regardless of the content of any law, physical therapist assistants shall provide services only under the supervision and direction of a physical therapist who is properly credentialed in the jurisdiction in which the physical therapist assistant practices.

4.2 Representation

Physical therapist assistants shall not hold themselves out as physical therapists.

STANDARD 5

Physical therapist assistants make those judgments that are commensurate with their qualifications as physical therapist assistants.

5.1 Patient Treatment

Physical therapist assistants shall report all untoward patient responses to a supervising physical therapist.

5.2 Patient Safety

A. Physical therapist assistants may refuse to carry out treatment procedures that they believe to be not in the best interest of the patient.
B. The physical therapist assistant shall not provide physical therapy services to a patient while under the influence of a substance that impairs his or her ability to do so safely.

5.3 Qualifications

Physical therapist assistants may not carry out any procedure that they are not qualified to provide.

5.4 Discontinuance of Treatment Program

Physical therapist assistants shall discontinue immediately any treatment procedures which in their judgment appear to be harmful to the patient.

5.5 Continued Education

Physical therapist assistants shall continue participation in various types of educational activities which enhance their skills and knowledge and provide new skills and knowledge.

STANDARD 6

Physical therapist assistants accept the responsibility to protect the public and the profession from unethical, incompetent, or illegal acts.

6.1 Consumer Protection

Physical therapist assistants shall report any conduct which appears to be unethical or illegal.

Issued by Judicial Committee, APTA
October 1981
Last Amended January 1996

Reprinted from Guide to Physical Therapist Practice; *Phys Ther*; Alexandria, Virginia, APTA; 1997;77(11):1632–1633, with permission of the American Physical Therapy Association.

Appendix 7

American Physical Therapy Association Guidelines for Peer Review Training

Reader note: The APTA amends core documents periodically. Updated documents can be obtained through the APTA (1-800-999-2782).

I. Purpose

The *Guidelines for Peer Review Training* provide direction to APTA chapters and sections, to physical therapy services, and to individual physical therapists who want to develop or pursue training in the peer review of the provision of physical therapy. These *Guidelines* are APTA-approved, nonbinding statements of advice intended to promote standardization both in the content of peer review training and in the performance of peer review. They also may be helpful as a tool for self-review. *It is important to note, however, that these* Guidelines *do not provide the training itself.*

Specifically, these *Guidelines*:

- Describe peer review.
- Delineate the underlying principles of peer review.
- Describe the content areas required for peer review training.
- Provide a framework for the training process.
- Provide a list of tools required both for peer review training and for the performance of peer review.

In addition to having the knowledge described in these *Guidelines*, a physical therapist providing external peer review services:

- Should be a licensed physical therapist, with no history of license suspension or revocation.
- Should be a member of APTA.
- Should have current clinical expertise in the area of the review.
- Is recommended to have a minimum of 5 years of clinical experience.

Definitions

Claims review: Review of the billing record that may result in identification of issues that may require medical review.
Guidelines: APTA defines "guidelines" as approved, nonbinding statements of advice (BOD 03-92-12-34).

Medical review: Review of the medical record based on standards of practice in regard to medical necessity and appropriateness of care.
Peer: A person of the same profession who is like-licensed.
Peer review: A system by which peers with similar areas of expertise assess the quality of physical therapy provided, using accepted practice standards and guidelines.
  Internal: The process in which a physical therapist reviews the services provided by peers within a physical therapy service.
  External: The process in which a physical therapist reviews physical therapy provided by a peer outside of the reviewer's physical therapy service at the request of a payer, a medical review organization, a professional organization, or a regulatory agency.
Utilization Review: Utilization review is a system for reviewing the medical necessity, appropriateness, and reasonableness of services proposed or provided to a patient or group of patients. This review is conducted on a prospective, concurrent, and/or retrospective basis to reduce the incidence of unnecessary and/or inappropriate provision of services. Utilization review is a process that has two primary purposes: to improve the quality of service (and patient outcomes) and to ensure the efficient expenditure of money.

II. Description of Peer Review

The purpose of peer review are to educate physical therapists to: (1) uphold professional standards, (2) be accountable to the public, and (3) be consistent in interactions with payers and managed care organizations. Peer review provides a framework to evaluate the quality, the medical necessity, and the appropriateness of the physical therapy provided. It can lead to identification of the need for corrective actions and can provide instructive feedback to practitioners.

Internal peer review and external peer review are based on the same principles and guiding documents (e.g., APTA's *Standards of Practice for Physical Therapy and the Criteria*.) They differ, however, in the source of the request for the review, the party to whom the report is sent, and the final actions. Internal peer review may result in self-correction (by an individual physical therapist or physical therapy service), whereas external peer review may result in a reimbursement, provider status, licensure, accreditation, or credentialing decision. Internal peer review processes may include additional requirements that reflect the type of practice setting or the individual service's policies and procedures.

An *internal peer review process* may assist a physical therapy service with the following:

- Performing quality improvement review.
- Providing for continuing professional competence and growth.
- Assessing medical necessity, effectiveness of intervention, and patient outcomes.
- Identifying problems and possible corrective actions.
- Meeting the requirements of regulatory agencies.
- Preparing for credentialing (e.g., by managed care organizations) of an individual physical therapist or of a physical therapy service.

An *external peer review process* may assist with the following:

- Determining (concurrently or retroactively) medical necessity and appropriateness of care for payers, managed care organizations, provider networks, and governmental agencies (e.g., agencies governing medical assistance and Medicare, state physical therapy licensing boards) that request a review of a physical therapist's performance or a physical therapy service's performance.
- Providing a quality assurance review.
- Determining fair and equitable levels of reimbursement.

III. Training Content

A. Principles of Peer Review

A physical therapist performing peer review must have a working knowledge of the following principles:

- A peer review process performed by a physical therapist assesses the physical therapy provided based on APTA's *Standards of Practice for Physical Therapy and the Criteria*; other core documents; and, when applicable, state laws and chapter documents.

  > It is the position of the American Physical Therapy Association (APTA) that peer review and utilization review of physical therapy services should be provided by physical therapists using criteria based on APTA Standards of Practice for Physical Therapy and other pertinent documents. (*Position on Peer review and Utilization Review of Physical Therapy Services* HOD 06-95-32-19).

- The peer review process is a quality improvement mechanism that applies to all physical therapists and to all patient management provided by physical therapists.
- The peer review process, both internal and external, is appropriate for use in a variety of physical therapy settings.
- APTA core documents, including the *Standards of Practice for Physical Therapy and the Criteria and the Guidelines for Physical Therapy Documentation,* put forth minimal requirements for documentation and practice and apply to all physical therapy settings. The physical therapy service is encouraged to set optimal requirements to promote quality improvement in practice.
- The clinical expertise of the physical therapist providing the peer review should be commensurate with that of the physical therapist(s) whose services are being reviewed.

- A physical therapist should apply the *Guidelines* and standards for peer review of the provision of physical therapy.
- Peer review must be performed with impartiality and objectivity.
- In the performance of peer review, as in other areas of practice, physical therapists are legally and ethically accountable for the services provided.

B. Documentation

A physical therapist performing peer review must have a working knowledge of physical therapy documentation as described by APTA's *Guidelines for Physical Therapy Documentation*. Training should be based on the understanding that documentation is a:

- Chronological record of the physical therapy provided.
- Legal medical document.
- Means of communication with other health care provider.
- Reflection of medical necessity.
- Rationale for care.
- Method to demonstrate outcomes.
- Record of the effectiveness of intervention.
- Means to support reimbursement.

Documentation should reflect the critical thinking and sound professional judgment that are required for patient management. Documentation should show that the physical therapist integrates the five elements of patient care—examination, evaluation, diagnosis, prognosis, and intervention—in a manner designed to maximize a patient's outcome. Training therefore should provide a working knowledge of the following:

- APTA's *Standards of Practice for Physical Therapy and the Criteria, Guidelines for Physical Therapy Documentation, Code of Ethics, Guide for Professional Conduct, Standards of Ethical Conduct for the Physical Therapist Assistant, Guide for Conduct of the Affiliate Member,* and *A Guide to Physical Therapist Practice (Part One: A Description of Patient Management* and *Part Two: Preferred Practice Patterns).*
- Chapter guidelines, when applicable.
- Other regulatory guidelines (e.g., Medicare and Medicaid).
- State practice acts.
- Functional assessment tools and various types of outcomes and their relationship (or lack of relationship) to function.
- Literature-based (including evidence-based) practice and functional outcomes, including preferred practice patterns in *A Guide to Physical Therapist Practice, Part Two: Preferred Practice Patterns.*

C. Billing and Coding

A physical therapist performing peer review must have an understanding of billing and coding, including current or applicable Current Procedural Terminology (CPT) and Relative

Value Resource Based System (RVRBS) guidelines or other accepted codes used for billing. Training should be based on the following principles:

- Documentation must substantiate the number and description of CPT or other accepted codes used for billing.
- Contracts may include specific exclusions or limitation of the services to be provided. Application and interpretation of contracts is the responsibility of the payer. Physical therapist peer review addresses medical necessity and appropriateness of care, not contractual agreements.
- The party requesting peer review may ask the reviewer to comment on the fees associated with the services or codes billed. The peer reviewer may choose to make recommendations concerning appropriate reimbursement based on his or her knowledge of (a) the value of the services and (b) standardized and accepted payment methodologies (e.g., RVRBS). It is not the peer reviewer's role, however, to determine actual payment for services.

D. Record Review

A physical therapist performing peer review must have a working knowledge of record review. Training should address each step of record review. These steps include:

1. Organize and record the documents that are provided.
2. Determine whether the documents are adequate for the purpose of peer review, and request additional information when necessary.
3. Review the claims made.
4. Match the record to the billings.
5. Review the medical record and assess it relative to identified standards, guidelines, state laws, and regulations, including *Standards of Practice for Physical Therapy and the Criteria*. (A checklist may be useful in organizing the review process.)
6. Evaluate findings, answering such key questions as:
   a) Were services provided by appropriate personnel?
   b) Is there evidence of coordination and communication with other health care professionals as appropriate?
   c) Does the record reflect timely patient-related instruction, including a home program and education of patient, family, significant other, and caregiver?
   d) Is there measurable, sustainable, and functional progress toward defined functional outcomes or goals, with reference to ongoing discharge planning?
   e) Does the record reflect appropriate changes in patient management strategy? Is there evidence of critical thinking, professional judgement, and skilled interventions?
   f) Does the documentation link impairment, functional limitation, and disability to predicted functional outcomes and the physical therapy plan of care?
   g) Is the billing supported by the documentation?
7. Develop conclusions and recommendations based on evaluation of the record using the established standards, guidelines, state laws, and regulations.

8. Answer any specific or additional questions that have been posed by the party requesting the review.

E. Report Writing

A physical therapist performing peer review must have a working knowledge of report writing. Training should address each item of a peer review report, including, but not limited to:

- Basic identification information for each file (e.g., patient ID #, claim #).
- The list of records and claims received by the peer reviewer.
- Documents on which the review is based (e.g., *Standards of Practice for Physical Therapy and the Criteria, Guidelines for Physical Therapy Documentation*, state practice act).
- The results of the claims review and the medical review.
- Conclusions.
- Recommendations.
- Answers to specific questions and concerns.
- A disclaimer indicating that the payer is ultimately responsible for the payment or the denial of the claim.
- Invoice, if appropriate.

Training also should encourage the physical therapist reviewer to:

- Substantiate the findings of peer review by quoting from the preamble of APTA's *Standards of Practice for Physical Therapy and the Criteria*: "These *Standards* are the profession's statement of conditions and performance that are essential for provision of high-quality physical therapy. The *Standards* provide a foundation for assessment of physical therapy practice."
- Be as specific as possible, quoting the medical record, APTA's *Standards and the Criteria*, and state statutes to support conclusions.
- Assess overall quality of the physical therapy provided, but be very specific in the report itself regarding whether the physical therapy provided meets APTA's *Standards and the Criteria* and therefore, criteria for medical necessity and appropriateness of care.
- Use language that reflects that recommendations are based only on medical necessity and appropriateness of care. (Recommendations should not indicate whether a claim should be paid.)

F. Claims Appeals

Physical therapists performing peer review must have a working knowledge of the claims appeals process of each payer and should encourage payers to develop an appeals process if one does not exist. Training should emphasize the following:

- When an appeals process is initiated, the peer reviewer may review additional information and write an addendum to the original report.
- The appeals process should include the option for the provider to receive a review by another peer reviewer if the provider and the original reviewer are unable to reach agreement.

G. Communication with Payers

Physical therapists performing peer review should use communication with payers as an opportunity to educate them about the appropriate utilization of physical therapy. Training should emphasize that, at a minimum, communication must convey the following principles:

- Professional guidelines and standards used in peer review can be appropriately applied only by a physical therapist.
- It is critical for the payer requesting the review to supply the entire record, including referral, when applicable; initial evaluation; daily notes; progress reports; billings; and background information from other providers.
- The use of the term "physical therapy" is appropriate only when used in reference to services that are provided by or under the direction of a qualified physical therapist (HOD 06-96-20-32).

Training should also instruct physical therapists in how to do the following as part of the peer review process:

- In all communications regarding the role of the physical therapist and the scope of physical therapist practice, emphasize that physical therapy can be provided or directed only by physical therapists.
- Provide pertinent documents to educate payers about the scope of physical therapy practice and about appropriate utilization of physical therapy (e.g., APTA's *A Guide to Physical Therapist Practice,* and APTA's *Guidelines for Physical Therapy Claims Review*).
- Encourage or support an appropriate appeals process.
- Promote positive communication among payers, reviewers, and providers.
- Encourage payers to inform physical therapy providers of the peer review process.

H. Communication with Providers

Communication with providers should have an educational focus. Training should address the following:

- Different types of review (retrospective, concurrent, prospective) require different means of communication.
- Communication should be based on established guidelines and should direct providers to pertinent resources.
- All conclusions and recommendations should be based on available physical therapy documentation and established standards, guidelines, state laws, and regulations.

I. Marketing the Value of Peer Review

A physical therapist performing peer review must have a working knowledge of how to market the value of peer review to payers and providers. Training should instruct the physical therapist to base marketing efforts on the following:

- The value of peer review, including the value of established guidelines and nationally accepted professional standards as applied by a trained peer reviewer.
- The value of peer review in (a) ensuring adherence to professional standards, (b) promoting appropriate utilization outcomes through the education of physical therapists, and (c) ensuring accountability to the community for the quality of physical therapy provided.

Training also should emphasize:

- The importance of networking to develop relationships, using various marketing vehicles (e.g., telephone, visits, letters, brochures).
- The legal ramifications involved in marketing peer review services.

J. Ethical and Legal Issues

A physical therapist performing peer review must have a working knowledge of ethical and legal issues, including:

- State practice acts both for physical therapists and for non-physical therapists.
- Other state statutes and documents regarding (a) data privacy, (b) patient bill of rights, and (c) confidentiality.
- Facility policies and procedures regarding release of information.
- Reviewer's responsibility for obtaining liability protection coverage for performance of external reviews.
- Confidentiality in all matters related to the review process, with the understanding that the physical therapist reviewer should access information only when there is a need to know.
- Potential conflicts of interest, which might skew the reviewer's judgement.
- APTA's *Code of Ethic, Guide for Professional Conduct, Standards of Ethical Conduct for the Physical Therapist Assistant,* and *Guide for Conduct of the Affiliate Member.*
- Antitrust laws.
- Peer review contract negotiation with insurers, including clarification of (a) whether the reviewer is masked to the provider, (b) insurer expectations, and, (c) reviewer payment guidelines (i.e., paid per review or per hour).

Additional considerations:

- The reviewer should request that the review be referred to another reviewer when that review is beyond his or her own clinical expertise and body of knowledge.
- The reviewer should understand the ethical and legal dimensions of the claims appeals process.

IV. Training Method

Suggested methods of peer review training (which does not have to be limited to a workshop) may include any of the following:

- Lecture and audiovisual presentations.
- Use of a training manual.
- Presentation of case studies during instruction or as part of post-course assessment.
- Use of self-assessment tools.
- Assignment of pre-program readings.
- Testing on course content.
- Small group discussions.
- "Test" reviews conducted with mentors and as a member of a review team.
- Use of interreviewer reliability determination as part of ongoing training.
- When instructors are utilized, the following in suggested:
- The instructor, or at least one instructor of a training team, should be an experienced physical therapist peer reviewer.
- Instructors must ensure confidentiality throughout all sensitive materials, regardless of whether that material is presented verbally or in writing.

The effectiveness of training efforts can be assessed through determination of interreviewer reliability.

V. Recommended Resources

Training should incorporate resources that include, but are not limited to:

- APTA's *A Guide to Physical Therapist Practice (Part One: A Description of Patient Management* and *Part Two: Preferred Practice Patterns).*
- APTA's *Code of Ethics* (HOD 06-91) and *Guide for Professional Conduct* (Judicial Committee 01-96).
- APTA's *Standards of Ethical Conduct for the Physical Therapist Assistant* (HOD 06-91) and *Guide for Conduct of the Affiliate Member* (Judicial Committee 01-66).
- APTA's *Standards of Practice for Physical Therapy and the Criteria* (HOD 06-96-16-31) (BOD 02-97-03-05).
- APTA's *Guidelines for Physical Therapy Documentation* (03-97-23-69).
- APTA's *Resource Guide: Peer Review/Utilization Review* (includes core documents).
- APTA's *Guidelines for Physical Therapy Claims Review.*
- Pertinent state practice acts.
- Pertinent state laws and regulations.
- Other related state statutes (e.g., data privacy; liability protection, if available; patient bill of rights).
- Examples of release forms used and signed by patients.
- Standards of utilization review accrediting bodies (e.g., American Accreditation HealthCare Commission/URAC).
- Confidentiality statements signed by reviewers.

- Bibliography of related topics in *Physical Therapy, PT—Magazine of Physical Therapy,* and other professional publications.
- Common Procedural Terminology (CPT Codes) (year-specific) and CPT definitions.
- Diagnostic classifications systems (e.g., International Classification of Disease-9, Clinical Modification [ICD-9-CM]).
- Disablement classifications and models (e.g., The World Health Organization's International Classification System of Impairment, Disabilities, and Handicaps [ICIDH]; the Nagi model of disablement).[1–4]
- Health Care Financing Administration Common Procedure Coding System (HCPCS).
- Various claim form samples.

Notes

1. Jette AM. Physical disablement concepts for physical therapy research and practice. *Phys Ther.* 1994;74:380–386.
2. *International Classification of Impairments, Disabilities, and Handicaps.* Geneva, Switzerland: World Health Organization; 1980.
3. Nagi SZ. Some conceptual issues in disability and rehabilitation. In: Sussman M, ed. *Sociology and Rehabilitation.* Washington, DC: American Sociological Association; 1965:100–113.
4. Nagi S. Disability concepts revisited: implications for prevention. In: Pope A, Tarlov A, eds. *Disability in America: Toward a National Agenda for Prevention.* Washington, DC: National Academy Press; 1991:309–327.

BOD 06-97-03-06
Adopted by Board of Directors
American Physical Therapy Association
June 1997

American Physical Therapy Association, 1111 N Fairfax St, Alexandria, VA 22314. Order No. P-140.

Guidelines for Peer Review Training reprinted with permission of the American Physical Therapy Association.

Appendix 8
Abbreviations

Note: This list contains common abbreviations found in the text as well as the authors' interpretation of the abbreviations found in the case study examples. Some of the abbreviations are not necessarily common or recommended for use in all settings.

°	Degree
"	Inch
'	Feet
<	Less than
%	Percent
#	Pound
A	Assist
AB	Abduction
ABD	Abduction
ACL	Anterior cruciate ligament
ADD	Adduction
ADL	Activities of daily living
AFO	Ankle foot orthosis
AMB	Ambulation
ANT	Anterior
APTA	American Physical Therapy Association
AROM	Active range of motion
ASHD	Arteriosclerotic heart disease
ASSIST	Assistance
BLE	Bilateral lower extremity
BLT	Bilateral
BU	Bilateral upper
BUE	Bilateral upper extremity
C/O	Complaints of
C	Cervical
CA	Cancer
CABG	Coronary artery bypass graft
CAD	Coronary artery disease
CAT	Computerized axial tomography
CGA	Contact guard assistance
CHF	Congestive heart failure
CM	Centimeter
COPD	Chronic obstructive pulmonary disease
CVA	Cerebrovascular accident
D/C	Discharge
D.O.T.	Department of Transportation
DEC	Decrease
DEC'D	Decreased
DECRD	Decreased
DF	Dorsiflexion
DIST	Distal
DM	Diabetes mellitus
DME	Durable medical equipment
DOL	Department of Labor
DX	Diagnosis
ER	External rotation
EKG	Electocardiogram
EVAL	Evaluation
EX	Exercise
EXT	Extension
F	Fair
F+	Fair plus
F−	Fair minus
FCA	Functional capacity assessment
FIB	Fibrillation
FLEX	Flexion
FLX	Flexion
FT	Feet
FX	Fracture
G	Good
G+	Good plus
G−	Good minus
HEP	Home exercise program
HP	Hot packs
HTN	Hypertension
HVPC	High volt pulsed current
HX	History
I.V.	Intravenous
IDDM	Insulin dependent diabetes mellitus
IEP	Individualized Education Program
INC	Increase
INC'D	Increased
INDEP	Independent
INDEP'LY	Independently
IP	Inpatient
IR	Internal rotation
L	Left
LBS	Pounds
LE	Lower extremity
LLE	Left lower extremity

LTR	Lateral trunk rotation	R	Right
LU	Left upper	REHAB	Rehabilitation
LUE	Left upper extremity	REPS	Repetitions
M.D.	Doctor of Medicine	RLE	Right lower extremity
MAX	Maximal	RN	Registered nurse
MED	Medical	ROM	Range of motion
MID	Middle	RUE	Right upper extremity
MIN	Minimal	S	Same
MIN.	Minute	S/P	Status post
MIN+	More than minimal	SBA	Standby assistance
MM	Millimeter	SEC	Seconds
MMT	Manual muscle test	SH	Shoulder
MOD	Moderate	SHLD	Shoulder
MPH	Miles per hour	SLR	Straight leg raise
MRI	Magnetic resonance imaging	SOAP	Subjective, objective, assessment, plan
MUS	Muscle	SOB	Shortness of breath
N/TESTED	Not tested	SOC	Start of care
N	Normal	SPT	Standing pivot transfer
NA	Not applicable	STIM	Stimulation
NEGLIG	Negligible	SUP	Supination
NMES	Neuromuscular electrical stimulation	T	Trace
		TB	Tuberculosis
NT	Not tested	THER EX	Therapeutic exercise
NWB	Nonweight bearing	THER	Therapeutic
OCC	Occasional	THR	Total hip replacement
ORIF	Open reduction internal fixation	TIA	Transient ischemic attack
ORTHO	Orthopedic	TKE	Terminal knee extension
OT	Occupational therapy	TRAFO	Tone reducing ankle foot orthosis
OZ	Ounce		
P/AAROM	Passive/active assisted range of motion	TRAPS	Trapezius
P	Poor	UBE	Upper body exercise
P.T.	Physical therapy or physical therapist	UE	Upper extremity
		US	Ultrasound
P+	Poor plus	UTI	Urinary tract infection
P–	Poor minus	VC	Verbal cues
PDL	Physical demand level	W/	With
PF	Plantar flexion	W/O	Without
PNF	Proprioceptive neuromuscular facilitation	W/C	Wheelchair
POE	Prone on elbows	WB	Weight bearing
PRO	Pronation	WBAT	Weight bearing as tolerated
PROG	Program	WFL	Within functional limits
PROM	Passive range of motion	WK	Week
PROX	Proximal	WKS	Weeks
PT	Patient	WNL	Within normal limits
PT	Physical therapy or physical therapist	WT	Weight
		X	Times
QUAD	Quadriceps	YR	Year

Glossary

Appeal. The process that allows the patient and/or provider of service to challenge a medical coverage decision.

Appeal letter. A letter that formally requests reconsideration of services.

Comparative data. Data that demonstrate a functional and/or measurable change. Data may be presented in chart or statement form.

Denial. The formal notification that services provided or requested are not covered by the third-party payer.

Descriptive terminology. Documentation that includes specific objective measurements and a functional component. The descriptions help the reviewer determine skilled care.

ERGOS. A functional capacity system manufactured by Work Recovery, Inc., in Tucson Arizona.

Evaluation. Making clinical judgements based on the analysis of data gathered from the examination. (See Examination.)

Examination. The investigation or gathering of data required prior to intervention. It includes three components: the patient history, relevant systems reviews, and tests and measures. It differs from an evaluation. (See Evaluation.)

Expectation statements. Statements that demonstrate to the reviewer of documentation an anticipated functional outcome.

External chart review. Chart review performed by peers outside of the practice setting/facility.

Functional phrase alternatives. Terms or phrases that convey to the reviewer the skilled nature of the service provided.

Internal chart review. Chart review performed by peers within the same practice setting/facility.

Medicaid. A federal and state funded entitlement program.

Medical review. The process of reviewing documentation to ensure that only medically necessary and reasonable physical therapy services are provided within the scope of the insurance plan's coverage criteria.

Medicare. A federally funded health insurance program for individuals 65 years of age or older and for the disabled.

Peer Physical Therapy Review. A system by which physical therapists with similar areas of expertise review documentation to determine the reasonableness of skilled care.

Primary payer. The payer that is billed first for services rendered.

Prior authorization. A procedure that requires the provider to obtain permission from the third-party payer prior to evaluation and/or treatment.

Prospective review. Determination of the medical necessity for treatment prior to the provision of service. It may be based on discounted rates, capitation rates, or specific visits for a certain diagnosis.

Retrospective review. Determination of the medical necessity of treatment after the services have been provided.

Reviewer. An individual who determines whether the services rendered are reasonable and necessary.

Secondary payer. The payer that is billed after the primary payer. (See Primary payer.)

Start of care. First day of the physical therapy evaluation.

Third-party payer. The party responsible for payment of services that are received by a patient. It may include a health maintenance organization or private insurance company.

Index

Date Due

NOV 2 9 2004			